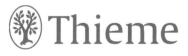

Foundations

An Introduction to the Profession of Physical Therapy

Stephen J. Carp, PT, PhD, GCS
Assistant Professor
Department of Physical Therapy
DeSales University
Center Valley, Pennsylvania, USA

31 illustrations

Thieme
New York • Stuttgart • Delhi • Rio de Janeiro

Executive Editor: Delia DeTurris
Managing Editor: Torsten Scheihagen
Director, Editorial Services: Mary Jo Casey
International Production Director: Andreas Schabert
Editorial Director: Sue Hodgson
International Marketing Director: Fiona Henderson
International Sales Director: Louisa Turrell
Director of Institutional Sales: Adam Bernacki
Senior Vice President and Chief Operating Officer: Sarah Vanderbilt
President: Brian D. Scanlan
Printer: King Printing

Library of Congress Cataloging-in-Publication Data

Names: Carp, Stephen J., author, editor.
Title: Foundations : an introduction to the profession of physical therapy / Stephen J. Carp.
Other titles: Introduction to the profession of physical therapy
Description: New York : Thieme, [2019] | Includes bibliographical references and index. |
Identifiers: LCCN 2018058808 (print) | LCCN 2018059595 (ebook) | ISBN 9781626235403 (electronic) | ISBN 9781626235397 (paperback) | ISBN 9781626235403 (eISBN)
Subjects: | MESH: Physical Therapy Specialty | Physical Therapists | Professional Role
Classification: LCC RM705 (ebook) | LCC RM705 (print) | NLM WB 460 | DDC 615.8/2023–dc23
LC record available at https://lccn.loc.gov/2018058808

Thieme Publishers New York
333 Seventh Avenue, New York, NY 10001 USA
+1 800 782 3488, customerservice@thieme.com

Thieme Publishers Stuttgart
Rüdigerstrasse 14, 70469 Stuttgart, Germany
+49 [0]711 8931 421, customerservice@thieme.de

Thieme Publishers Delhi
A-12, Second Floor, Sector-2, Noida-201301
Uttar Pradesh, India
+91 120 45 566 00, customerservice@thieme.in

Thieme Publishers Rio de Janeiro, Thieme Publicações Ltda.
Edifício Rodolpho de Paoli, 25º andar
Av. Nilo Peçanha, 50 – Sala 2508
Rio de Janeiro 20020-906 Brasil
+55 21 3172-2297 / +55 21 3172-1896

Cover design: Thieme Publishing Group
Typesetting by DiTech Process Solutions

Printed in the United States of America by King Printing Co., Inc.

5 4 3 2 1

ISBN 978-1-62623-539-7

Also available as an e-book:
eISBN 978-1-62623-540-3

Important note: Medicine is an ever-changing science undergoing continual development. Research and clinical experience are continually expanding our knowledge, in particular our knowledge of proper treatment and drug therapy. Insofar as this book mentions any dosage or application, readers may rest assured that the authors, editors, and publishers have made every effort to ensure that such references are in accordance with the **state of knowledge at the time of production of the book.**

Nevertheless, this does not involve, imply, or express any guarantee or responsibility on the part of the publishers in respect to any dosage instructions and forms of applications stated in the book. **Every user is requested to examine carefully** the manufacturers' leaflets accompanying each drug and to check, if necessary in consultation with a physician or specialist, whether the dosage schedules mentioned therein or the contraindications stated by the manufacturers differ from the statements made in the present book. Such examination is particularly important with drugs that are either rarely used or have been newly released on the market. Every dosage schedule or every form of application used is entirely at the user's own risk and responsibility. The authors and publishers request every user to report to the publishers any discrepancies or inaccuracies noticed. If errors in this work are found after publication, errata will be posted at www.thieme.com on the product description page.

Some of the product names, patents, and registered designs referred to in this book are in fact registered trademarks or proprietary names even though specific reference to this fact is not always made in the text. Therefore, the appearance of a name without designation as proprietary is not to be construed as a representation by the publisher that it is in the public domain.

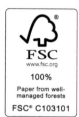

FSC
www.fsc.org
100%
Paper from well-managed forests
FSC® C103101

For my wife and children, whose love, teaching, and generosity can never be repaid. For Kay Shepard and Laurita Hack, for allowing me to stand on your shoulders and for catching me when I fell.

Contents

Foreword

Within the pages of *Foundations: An Introduction to the Profession of Physical Therapy*, the reader is offered an opportunity to explore aspects integral to the physical therapy profession as it exists within the context of the healthcare milieu. The editor, Stephen Carp, has artfully interwoven the full scope of the physical therapy profession beyond that which is readily observed during the traditional pre-physical therapy student experience, thus adding both breadth and depth to the entry level physical therapy student's perspective of a profession they yearn to excel in.

Although traditionally a component of PT curriculum nationally, securing student buy-in to the value of this course material as more than memorizable data is widely accepted as challenging. Acutely aware of this dilemma, Dr. Carp has added features to the beginning of each chapter that provide both intrigue and an opportunity for reflection for the reader. This journey of discovery begins with detailed outlines that preface each chapter and sets the stage for further interest in the scope of the topic, introducing a knowledge gap that is filled, showing the relationship to the healthcare environment, and recommendations for implications to practice for each focused chapter. This explicated lens of both benefits and barriers enables the reader to continue to reflect on the impact of physical therapy and the PT's responsibility within the topic at hand. Finally, Dr. Carp has masterfully captured the reader's interest through the inclusion of a first-person narrative. This short narrative, written by a first-person observer, reveals the personal relevance of the topic and provides an enticement to the reader to continue on their own quest for further information. The use of narratives to introduce each chapter as described here is innovative and thought-provoking and successfully provides the food for thought to encourage personal exploration of the topic.

As a colleague, I can tell you first hand that the Dr. Carp has many gifts. Personally, the gift I value most is his natural ability to connect with people within personal engagements. Those who know Steve share my enjoyment of sharing a cup of tea while candidly exploring relevant issues with him. When you get this opportunity to spend that gift of time with Steve, you always walk away with much more than you came in with. This is what you should expect when reading this book, as each chapter represents the bulk of what would be an intimate conversation with a very well-experienced, revered, and thoughtful colleague about an important and relevant topic. Every chapter delivers on content in ways that make you want to wonder. In today's fast-paced, internet-connected world there is little opportunity to wonder, but it is this gift that Steve has recreated within this collection of papers that have come together so nicely.

The wisdom within this book, crafted chapter by chapter from experts with rich experience in the field, is the raw material from which the physical therapy profession is built upon. From its past evolution through to the future, chapters describe the interplay of physical therapy with relevant systems including legal issues, reimbursement, and the healthcare team. Additionally, expanding on the role of the PT as a clinician, the role and responsibilities of the physical therapist as educator, researcher, and community service provider has particular value to the future of our profession. Issues specific to the physical therapy student are also explored, especially in relation to their own learning environment: clinical education. These topics, as well as other chapter subject areas, permeate our present day and will guide us, if we choose to apply them, into the future. By being inclusive of the many integral aspects of physical therapy as a profession, Dr. Carp creates the mosaic by which physical therapy students can build the knowledge, skill, and behaviors of a consummate professional and thus be equipped to develop into excellent physical therapists who will serve their clients well.

The physical therapy academic community has long since expressed the need for such a valuable text and will revel in its impact on the teaching and learning of this content. Our profession continues to benefit from the ongoing exploration and sharing of the full canvas that is physical therapy today and which is captured so aptly in this text. What better place to start introducing both the content and the responsibility to utilize this knowledge than with our physical therapy students. I congratulate Stephen Carp and his esteemed contributors on creating a compendium that provides the future of physical therapy with a broad and inviting view of their chosen profession in a format that engages their interest and commitment.

—*Anita M. Santasier, PT, PhD, OCS*
Chair and Associate Professor
School of Physical Therapy and Rehabiliation Science
University of Montana

Preface

If you are reading this preface you are most likely a first-year doctor of physical therapy (DPT) student. As a first-year DPT student you are also most likely currently experiencing wide swings in your emotional barometer.

Within the past year you had one of the best days of your life. Years of hard work in your undergraduate program: nights studying past midnight, avoiding social media, forgoing "road trips" with your friends because you had a paper due, studying for the Graduate Record Examination, nervously completing the graduate school applications, interviewing, and waiting, waiting, waiting for an admission's decision—and you were finally rewarded with a DPT acceptance letter. How your heart must have leapt when you read these words: "We at (write the name of your program here) are pleased to inform you that your application for a seat in the Doctor of Physical Therapy Program has been accepted!" That kind of emotional high is seldom felt in life and all of you deserved that moment of absolute, unrestricted glee.

After placing the letter of acceptance on your desk at home, if you are like most students, the thought that "I made it and can now relax a bit" must have entered your mind. And, if you are like most students, that thought quickly exited your mind when you received or reviewed online your doctoral curriculum. The list of courses was spellbinding: anatomy, anatomy laboratory, physiology, physiology laboratory, neuroscience, clinical medicine, geriatrics, pediatrics, clinical decision making, orthopedics, biomechanics, psychology of illness, cardio-pulmonary, neurology, and business management. "Where is the badminton course? Where is archery? Where is the Movies of Martin Scorsese?"

Any first-year DPT student, when asked why he or she decided to train to become a physical therapist, will answer something to the effect that "I wish to serve others." That comment—true but mildly naïve—is only part of the reason why you entered the profession. "Serving others" as a standalone statement indicates an open-looped system—the benefits channel one way from the therapist to the client. Any experienced doctor of physical therapy practitioner, when asked why he or she practices physical therapy, will answer something to the effect that "I wish to serve others because the gifts I receive back from my patient completes me as a person." In a humanistic world, we serve others in order to meet a basic psychic need. A bumper sticker I recently read proclaimed: "We can only find ourselves when we lose ourselves in service to others." Or, as my friend, Vincentian Dan Johnson, often says: "We serve others because that is the way it is supposed to be."

Therefore, do not look at that imposing curriculum as an insurmountable chore. Look at it cheerfully and optimistically as to what it truly represents—a list of preparatory tasks needed to accomplish and master to enable you the amazing opportunity of serving the poor, sick, and impaired for the next forty years! As a physical therapist you will never become wealthy. You will never become famous. You will never fly first class. You will never comfortably eat at the finest restaurants. You will never dress yourself in the most expensive designer clothes. You will not drive a Ferrari. You will, however, live life as a completed person because of the unique opportunity to serve others as a physical therapist.

Foundations: An Introduction to the Profession of Physical Therapy contains the background content every practitioner must incorporate into practice in order to effectively serve clients. Chapter 1, The Evolution of Physical Therapy, describes the development of the profession from its nascent beginnings in early Greece to the high-impact, large-scope, international profession of today. Chapter 2 provides a strong summary of reimbursement—touching broadly on healthcare reimbursement as a whole and focusing strongly on physical therapy reimbursement in particular. Because reimbursement policies and methodology vary from service arena to arena and inpatient to outpatient care, this chapter will match reimbursement method to arena and inpatient/outpatient designation. Chapter 3, The Healthcare Team, provides content related to the physical therapist as a healthcare team member. With the complexity of clinical practice and oversight regulation in 21st century healthcare, no clinician can practice in a silo. Regardless of practice location, the physical therapist is an integral member of the healthcare team. Being an effective healthcare team member requires specific clinical and professional behavior knowledge competence. Documentation schema including regulatory and provider oversight is discussed in Chapter 4. Physical therapists, as are all healthcare practitioners, are required a litany of notes: initial evaluations, assessments, progress notes, discharge summaries, and letters of medical necessity. This chapter includes the requirements for each type of documentation performed by therapists. Chapter 5, Physical Therapy and Community Services, presents the role of the physical therapist as a servant-leader toward the sick, poor, and impaired. This chapter expands upon the anonymous quote: "All teams have a leader by name; the true leader is the member with the servant-heart." Rachel Naomi Remen, MD, who has developed retreats for people with cancer, described the servant heart well: "Helping, fixing, and serving represent three different ways of seeing life. When you help, you see life as weak. When you fix, you see life as broken. When you serve, you see life as whole. Fixing and helping may be the work of the ego, and service the work of the soul."[1] The Code of Ethics for the Physical Therapist[2] specifically calls for physical therapists to provide pro bono services to underserved and underinsured populations.

Chapter 6, The Physical Therapist as a Researcher, discusses the role of the physical therapist as a clinical researcher and as a consumer of clinical research. Dr. Carroll is a classically trained anatomist and researcher and directs the anatomy donor laboratories at DeSales University, Center Valley, Pennsylvania. Clinical Education, a topic of great interest to student therapists, is presented in Chapter 7. Chapter 8, A Student's Perspective of Clinical Education, describes the clinical education experience from a student's perspective, providing excellent insights into clinical education based upon the chapter author's recent history as a doctor of physical therapy student.

Chapter 9 presents a strong overview of our professional organization, the American Physical Therapy Association. Chapter 10 provides an overview of the physical therapist as a professional and leader, and discusses the attributes of professionalism and leadership and how they translate to physical therapist practice. Chapter 11 describes the process of the first professional job search. Chapter 12, the companion chapter to Chapter 11, provides and details an algorithm that can be used to compare competing job offers. Chapter 13, presents the physical therapist as a teacher. Within the scope of physical therapy, therapists teach patients, patient families, community members, other health care professionals, physical therapy and physical therapy assistant students, and insurance representatives. Physical therapy students and physical therapist assistant students are often unaware of the quantity of teaching they will perform in clinical practice and the effect of the quality of teaching on long and short-term clinical outcomes.

In Chapter 14, the importance of a culture and spirituality to healthcare practitioners and healthcare clients is discussed. Victor Frankl, a psychiatrist who wrote of his experiences in a Nazi concentration camp: "Man is not destroyed by suffering; he is destroyed by suffering without meaning."[3] One of the challenges physical therapists face is to help clients find meaning and acceptance in the midst of suffering and chronic illness. Medical ethicists have reminded us that religion and spirituality form the basis of meaning and purpose for many people.[4] Chapter 15 presents an overview of the legal aspects of our profession: the civil, criminal, and administrative laws that all physical therapists must be aware of and incorporate into our practices. Chapter 16 attempts to predict future trends in our profession. The book ends with a comprehensive glossary of common physical therapy terms.

Each chapter is prefaced by a list of keywords and a first-person experience. At the conclusion of each chapter is a list of questions for review. Each chapter is meticulously referenced.

Foundations is not a science book. The reader will not find facts about physiology or anatomy. There is no information related to pharmacology, neurology, or orthopedics. There is no chapter on diagnostic testing. Rather, the aim of *Foundations* is to provide the reader with a comprehensive overview of what many practitioners call the "background music of our profession"—those Foundational items we all, as physical therapists and physical therapist assistants, need to know in order to provide quality clinical care.

I hope you enjoy it!

—*Stephen J. Carp, PT, PhD, GCS*

1. Remen RN. Kitchen Table Wisdom: Stories That Heal. New York: Riverhead Books; 1997.
2. APTA.org (accessed January 10, 2018)
3. Frankl VE. Man's Search for Meaning. New York: Simon and Schuster; 1984.
4. Foglio JP, Brody H. Religion, faith, and family medicine. J Fam Pract. 1988;27:473–474.

Contributors

Stephen J. Carp, PT, PhD, GCS
Assistant Professor
Department of Physical Therapy
DeSales University
Center Valley, Pennsylvania, USA

Melissa A. Carroll, PhD, MS
Assistant Professor
Department of Physical Therapy
DeSales University
Center Valley, Pennsylvania, USA

Sean F. Griech, PT, DPT, OCS, COMT
Assistant Professor
Department of Physical Therapy
DeSales University
Center Valley, Pennsylvania, USA

Laurita M. Hack, DPT, PhD, MBA, FAPTA
Professor Emeritus
Department of Physical Therapy
Temple University
Philadelphia, Pennsylvania, USA

Grace C. Karaman, PT, MPT
Manager
Physical Rehabilitation Services
Chestnut Hill Hospital
Philadelphia, Pennsylvania, USA

Peter J. Leonard, OSFS, M.Div, PhD
Pastor
Immaculate Heart of Mary Church
High Point, North Carolina, USA

Sabrina L. Martha, PT, DPT
Chestnut Hill Hospital
Philadelphia, Pennsylvania, USA

Kim Nixon-Cave, PT, PhD, MS, FAPTA
Associate Professor
Department of Physical Therapy
Program Director of Doctor of Physical Therapy and
    Post-Professional Education
Board-Certified Clinical Specialist in
Pediatric Physical Therapy (PCS)
Jefferson University
Jefferson College of Rehabilitation Sciences
Philadelphia, Pennsylvania, USA

Deborah Smith Brown, CPA
Certified Public Accountant
Hatfield, Pennsylvania, USA

Julie M. Skrzat, PT, DPT, PhD, CCS
Assistant Professor
Department of Physical Therapy
DeSales University
Center Valley, Pennsylvania, USA

Susan Wainwright, PT, PhD
Professor and Chairperson
Department of Physical Therapy
Jefferson College of Rehabilitation Sciences
Philadelphia, Pennsylvania, USA

1 The Evolution of Physical Therapy Practice

Stephen J. Carp

Keywords: American Physical Therapy Association, American Physical Therapy Association Code of Ethics, Autonomous Practitioner Model, Commission on Accreditation in Physical Therapy Education, Federation of State Boards of Physical Therapy, Health Maintenance Organization, Medicaid, Medicare, Physical Therapist, Physical Therapist Assistant, Physical Therapy, Reconstruction Aide, Vision 2020

Chapter Outline

"My entry-level physical therapy degree was awarded in 1981. I have been practicing for 36 years. Thirty-six years in health care practice is an eternity. Change is omnipresent in health care. Describing how I practiced in 1981 would prompt quizzical expressions by today's therapists. The differences in physical therapy practice which have occurred over the past thirty-six years are substantial, and almost entirely positive.

"Reflecting on my 1981 professional curriculum, there were a number of courses which are, in today's scope of physical therapy (PT) practice, irrelevant or nearly irrelevant, but they were relevant back then. As an example, we were required to take two 4-credit courses in massage. Massage was a major component of PT practice thirty years ago; I haven't massaged anyone for decades. I also took two 4-credit courses in modalities. Though we as PTs still use therapeutic modalities, the published evidence and current insurance reimbursement schemas have lessened the clinical impact of these tools. A number of modalities—ultraviolent light, short-wave diathermy, microwave diathermy, and hydrotherapy (the use of whirlpools clinically)—have almost become anachronistic. On the positive side, PT students are now taught the components of evidenced-based practice, neuroscience, ethics, and genetics. They are taught the purpose and aim of laboratory values, radiographic and cardiopulmonary testing. They are taught pharmacology. They are taught differential diagnosis. Today's curricula accurately represent today's physical therapist's practice.

"In 1981 my practice uniform was dark blue pants and a white tunic top. We looked like barbers. Today, I wear dress pants, a dress shirt, and a tie. Less comfortable, perhaps, but definitely more professional.

"In 1981, physical therapy was a 9 to 5 profession. Today, the clinic where I practice is open seven days per week from 6:00 a.m. to 10:00 p.m.

"My first salary as a physical therapist was $14,500. New graduates today are typically offered starting salaries of $65,000 or more. I paid $2,200 for my entire last year of my university professional program. I graduated with no tuition debt. Most PT programs now charge the student more than $30,000 per year and physical therapy students often graduate with more than $100,000 in combined undergraduate and graduate tuition debt.

"My entry-level professional degree was a bachelor's degree; I became a PT in four years. Today, the doctor of physical therapy (DPT) is the required entry-level degree and extends most educational curricula to 7 years.

"In 1981 physical therapy was considered a technical profession. We did what we were 'ordered' to do by a physician. Today, we are consultants, adding richness, a unique knowledge base, professionalism, and positive outcomes to the care of the patient. We are partners in the care of the patient. We are no longer subordinate.

"In 1981 we rarely had to worry about uninsured or underinsured patients. Terms such as copay, therapy cap, deductible, and coinsurance hadn't yet entered the insurance lexicon. Today, along with or evaluative, assessment, and interventional knowledge, we must possess the knowledge to consider and counsel the patient about the financial burden of health care services.

"To whom do we owe this broad evolution of practice? We owe thanks to the historic leaders of our profession who had the foresight, grit, and imagination to lead our profession to where it is now. We owe thanks to the American Physical Therapy Association, our organization which represents and supports physical therapists in all aspects of professional life. And we owe thanks to the physical therapists and physical therapist assistants who labor daily because they believe in the effectiveness of their hard work, using their gifts to better their fellow man.

"I can't wait to see what the next thirty-six years bring!"

—Brian R., Tampa, Florida

1.1 Overview

In just 100 years, the profession of physical therapy has grown from a little-known band of "reconstruction aides" to a large and expanding worldwide group of dedicated professionals at the cutting edge of health care diagnostics, interventions, research, ethics, and altruistic community service. Today's physical therapists (PTs) are highly motivated, respected, service-oriented, well-educated, licensed health care professionals who assist patients to restore mobility though improving strength, balance, and range of motion; improving safety; reducing pain and risk factors; and, the prevention of disease and disease complications —in many instances without expensive surgery and without the requirement for the long-term use of prescription medications.

PTs examine each individual, develop a problem list related to mobility and function with the patient, develop short and long-term goals for treatment, and institute an intervention plan. In addition, PTs work with clients to prevent the loss of mobility and to ameliorate risk factors such as obesity and sedentary lifestyle, by developing prescriptive fitness and wellness-oriented programs for healthier and more active lifestyles.

Physical therapists provide care for clients in a variety of settings, including hospitals, private practices, outpatient clinics, home health agencies, hospices, schools, sports and fitness facilities, work settings, and nursing homes. Physical therapists perform research, teach at colleges and universities, and perform regulatory and utilization work for insurance companies. State licensure is required in each state in which a physical therapist practices. Physical therapists work in many arenas of care. ▶ Table 1.1 is a partial list of employment opportunities delineated by arena and inpatient/outpatient focus.

Physical therapy consistently ranks near the top of desirable professions[1,2] and near the bottom in professional recidivism rates—the percentage of persons who leave the profession for another.[3] Since the early 2000s, there has been a high demand for physical therapists in the workforce. According to the Bureau of Labor Statistics,[4] employment of physical therapists is expected to grow by 36% from 2012 to 2022, a much faster rate than the average for all occupations. Data from the American Physical Therapy Association (APTA, the professional organization of physical therapists and physical therapist assistants) shows that while an increase in graduates from physical therapist (PT) education programs could help to slightly lower projected workforce shortages in the future, the trend toward increased health insurance coverage nationwide through the Affordable Care Act indicates that the demand for PTs will continue to climb between now and 2022.[1] Additional causes of the anticipated need for physical therapists are the expanding scope of physical therapy practice into areas such as wound care, women's health, and diseases of the vestibular system; technological advancements such as robotic orthotics and prosthetics and exoskeletons; and, emerging evidenced-based treatments for specific chronic diseases that heretofore had few intervention indications.

In just 50 years, the entry level degree for the profession has evolved from "certificate" to bachelor's degree to master's degree to doctoral degree. As of January 1, 2016, the Doctor of Physical Therapy entry-level degree (DPT) is the required degree for all entry-level physical therapist education programs. In 2016, there are 233 accredited programs and 22 developing programs.[5]

Table 1.1 Arenas of practice for physical therapists

Pediatric	Inpatient	Acute care hospital
		Acute medical rehabilitation hospital
		Long-term acute care hospital
		Psychiatric/behavioral hospital
		Burn hospital
	Outpatient	Independent outpatient clinic
		Hospital-owned outpatient clinic
		School district
		Home care
Adult	Inpatient	Acute care hospital
		Acute medical rehabilitation hospital
		Long-term acute care hospital
		Psychiatric/behavioral hospital
		Skilled nursing facility
		Transitional unit
		Burn hospital
		Nursing home
		Life-care community
	Outpatient	Independent outpatient clinic
		Hospital-owned outpatient clinic
		Adult day care
		Home care
		Sports medicine: high school, college, university, professional sports team
Industry	Outpatient	Employee health clinics
		Ergonomic assessment
		Insurance reviewer
Research/ Teaching		University faculty
		Industry researcher
		University researcher
Administration		Hospital administrator
		Outpatient clinic administrator
		Home care administrator

1.2 History of the Profession

1.2.1 Origins of the Medical Professions

The merger of history, legislation, wars, epidemics, paradigm shifts, and evidenced-based knowledge has led to the development of the science of physical therapy, the profession of physical therapy, and the recognition of physical therapy as a leading and well-respected provider in the healing arts. The development and use of the physical interventions commonly applied by physical therapists today, including exercise, mobilization, manipulation, massage, heat, cold, water, and later, electricity, dates back at minimum to Greek culture[6] and Hippocrates' influence on clinical practice as the father of Western medicine. Galen (born 129 CE), a prominent Greek physician, surgeon, and philosopher of the Roman Empire, wrote extensively about his belief in physical medicine as a curative modality.[7] Galen was also the first to write about the confluence of medicine and philosophy: about the need to practice healing in a formal, objective, and evidence-based manner with the requirement for the practitioner to consider not only the corporal variables but also the "philosophy" of the patient (today known as mind–body influences).[6,7] Galen was the first to write extensively about the musculoskeletal system including muscle attachments, the importance of sensory and motor innervation, and muscle tone.[6]

1.2.2 The Dark Ages

Sadly, the Dark Ages (also known as the Middle Ages) from the fall of Rome to the initiation of the Renaissance, ushered in a period of medicine characterized by stagnation of medical advancements, the discontinuation of experimentation as an aid to evidence and practice, and the incorporation of astrology, religious, sorcery, witchcraft, and other fringe practices into medical care.[8] Few advancements in medical care were developed during this era.

1.2.3 The Renaissance

As with the arts, philosophy, bench, and qualitative research, medicine experienced a rebirth during the Renaissance. The Renaissance was a study in progressive change from the stagnation and unscientific practices of the Dark Ages-practiced medicine to the adaptation of the scientific method to medicine in the 18th century. During the Renaissance, medical practice was a complex web that incorporated both elite university medicine and a wide-ranging array of historical and unproven healing traditions, all of which competed with and influenced each other. By the early 16th century, broader trends in Renaissance culture, particularly humanism, had begun to affect university-based medical learning. The humanist scrutiny of classical medical texts helped lead to a number of changes including attempts to amend the knowledge of the ancients and a gradual increase in the perceived value of empirical and scientific investigations. Throughout the period, however, university-trained physicians represented only a small proportion of healers. Far more populous were surgeons, barbers, apothecaries, midwives, and a wide variety of unlicensed healers. Although physicians increasingly attempted to bring the licensing of other practitioners under control, the broader healing landscape remained essentially unchanged from the Dark Ages for most citizens. Patients had a wide variety of healers to choose from, and healers had diverse approaches. Religious and magical forms of healing remained inexorably intertwined with naturalistic remedies, and this balance remained until the late 1700s. At the same time, the rapid urbanization that took place in the Renaissance led to an increased need for public health measures as well as poor relief. Individuals and towns struggled with recurrent bouts of epidemic disease. This combination of dynamic change and traditional healing structures makes the Renaissance and Reformation a complex and fascinating epoch in the history of medicine and led to the bridge to today, what we call "modern medicine."[9]

1.2.4 The Origins of Physical Therapy

The 1800s

Physical therapy, known as physiotherapy outside the United States, developed internationally prior to expanding to the United States. Until recently, it was thought that the origins of physical therapy extended to 1894, when a professional group of nurses in England formed the Chartered Society of Physiotherapy.[10] However, recent research conducted throughout several countries in northern Europe identified an established profession of physiotherapy dating back to the early 19th century, which also had a surprisingly scientific-themed basis. In Sweden, the Royal Central Institute of Gymnastics (RCIG) was founded in 1813, which was later referred to as "Medical Gymnastics" in 1865.[11] Patient records from that era detailed documentation of diagnoses and manipulative therapy techniques combined with exercise to help patients overcome their physical problems and injuries. Surprisingly these patient records depict illustrations of some of the same manual and manipulations we use currently (i.e., "pubic symphysis manipulation"). Jonas Kellgren, a graduate of the Medical Gymnastics in 1865 was part of this group; he was the grandfather of James Cyriax, MD, known as the "grandfather of orthopedics."[12] This was the first appearance of the Cyriax family tree in historical physical therapy literature.[12] The Cyriax family promoted the growth of physical therapy in England up to present times. Sadly, the prevailing medical establishment forced the Medical Gymnastics to cede rehabilitation to the physicians and soon the Medical Gymnastics faded into obscurity and is now nearly forgotten. Physical therapy, the original sole providers of physical rehabilitation utilizing exercise and manual therapy techniques, was lost until the 1894 Chartered Society of Physiotherapy in England. The next country to start formal training programs was the School of Physiotherapy at the University of Otago in New Zealand in 1913.[13]

The 1900s

The period from 1916 to 1918 brought two events that forever changed the profession of physical therapy in the United States and worldwide. The first was the severity of the worldwide polio epidemic in 1916 and similar epidemics almost yearly until the development of a preventive vaccine in the 1950s. Polio is a contagious viral disease of the motor neurons often resulting in flaccid paralysis of all or parts of the body. This disease, which most persons tended to survive although in a weakened condition, led to the need for ongoing manual muscle testing, exercise, bracing, and other modalities for which no particular profession, at that time, appeared academically prepared to handle. Secondly, 1917 brought about the involvement of the United States in World War I where battlefield medicine had progressed sufficiently to permit wide-range survival of war-induced injuries and the return of these impaired men, who required significant rehabilitation, back to the United States.

Again, no profession was equipped to meet this medical need. The U.S. Army recognized the need to rehabilitate soldiers and the absence of professionals to direct rehabilitation activity. As a result, a special unit of the Army Medical Department, the Division of Special Hospitals and Physical Reconstruction, developed "reconstruction aide" training programs, which eventually led to the development of two professions: physical therapy and occupational therapy.[14]

In 1917, to respond to the need for medical workers with expertise in rehabilitation, the profession of physical therapy, as it was later termed, had begun with educational programs at Reed College and Walter Reed Hospital. In 1921, a small group of reconstruction aides, formed a professional organization for physical therapists, the American Women's Physical Therapeutic Association.[14] Led by President Mary McMillan, an executive committee of elected officers governed the association, which included 274 charter members. In 1922, the association changed its name to the American Physiotherapy Association (APA) and men were admitted. In the 1930s,[14] the APA introduced its first "Code of Ethics" and membership grew to just under 1,000. Soon the professional organization received its current name, the American Physical Therapy Association (APTA).

During the 1920s, as the growth of the reputation of physical therapists as rehabilitation experts permitted the partnership with the medical and surgical communities, the profession of physical therapy gained public recognition and validation. Into the 1930s and 1940s, the profession continued to grow primarily due to the continued polio epidemics and the United States' involvement in World War II. With improved battlefield medicine and the advent of early antibiotic therapy, World War II resulted in tens of thousands of injured soldiers returning home needing rehabilitation. Physical therapists became the rehabilitation provider of choice for such war-induced diagnoses as spinal cord injury, thermal injury, fracture, wounds, amputation, and traumatic brain injury.

In November 1945, President Harry S Truman delivered a special message to Congress in which he outlined a five-part program for improving the health and health care of Americans.[15] As a result of that call, in 1946, Congress passed the Hill–Burton Act, formally known as the Hospital Survey and Construction Act. Sponsored by Senators Harold Burton of Ohio and Lister Hill of Alabama, the Hill–Burton Act provided inpatient facilities: hospitals, nursing homes and other health facilities, grants, and loans earmarked for construction and modernization and to meet the goal of increasing the nation's hospital beds to 4.5 per 1,000 people. In return, the facilities agreed to provide a reasonable volume of services, including physical therapy services, to persons unable to pay and to make their services available to all persons residing in the facility's area. The program stopped providing funds in 1997, but about 150 health care facilities nationwide are still obligated to provide free or reduced-cost care.

The 1950s was a critical time for the profession in terms of gaining independence, autonomy, and the development of a professional vision. From the early "reconstruction aide" era to the late 1950s, physical therapy was seen as a technical position rather than as a profession. During this period, physical therapy was accredited by the American Medical Association (AMA), and physical therapists by and large performed the technical interventions ordered by physicians. Physical therapists did not

diagnose. They did not make prognoses. They did not perform clinical decision making. Two events in the 1950s contributed to the progression of the physical therapist from technician to professional practitioner. The first was expansion of physical therapist practitioners into the private sector. Prior to the 1950s, physical therapists worked almost exclusively in inpatient settings or inpatient settings with outpatient departments. As more physical therapists moved into independently owned practices, the Self-Employed Section formed as a component of APTA in 1955.[16] This action brought a voice to the needs of the private practitioner and also further popularized the profession as physical therapist-owned independent practices opened in towns across America. Secondly, for a profession to be recognized the profession must perform and publish research. The Physical Therapy Fund was created in 1957 to foster science through research and education within the profession.[14]

Since its inception, physical therapy licensure and accreditation was directed by the AMA. Seeking autonomy, APTA sought to replace the system of registration that had been created through the AMA, which required questionable assessment of professional competence in physical therapy. APTA urged its state chapters to seek licensure through the states, and by 1950, Connecticut, Maryland, and Washington had adopted physical therapy practice acts, joining New York and Pennsylvania, whose initial licensing efforts dated back to 1926 and 1913, respectively. By the end of the decade state licensure existed in 45 states.[17]

Though state regulation and licensure was a positive step toward professional autonomy, the issue of competency assessment continued to challenge the profession. How does one measure competency in those persons applying for licensure? In 1954, to address the issue of professional competency APTA created the first national examination. The exam was a partnership between APTA and the Professional Examination Service of the American Public Health Association.[17]

State practice acts, licensure, professional reputation, and the licensure exam assisted the lobbying efforts of APTA for inclusion in the Medicare and Medicaid Acts of 1965. The Medicare and Medicaid Acts provided insurance coverage to millions of elderly and poor Americans who heretofore lacked insurance and, therefore, often lacked medical care. Overnight, millions of Americans became insured, permitting them to utilize physical therapy services.

The 1950s and 1960s again, sadly, brought new challenges to the profession by the Korean and Vietnam wars. The advent of mobile army surgical hospitals, which permitted battlefield surgery, the increased use of helicopter evacuation of wounded, and the rapid transport of injured soldiers to tertiary care hospitals, saved countless lives and provided a large cohort of severely injured men and women in need of rehabilitation services.

For a number of reasons, including the addition of Medicare and Medicaid money to health care facilities permitting discretionary funding for research and newer and better technology, the 1960s and 1970s brought forth much advancement in all the fields of medicine including physical therapy services. Physical therapist practice in the neuromuscular area developed significantly during this era strongly influenced by the research, writings, and clinical practices of Margaret Rood, Margaret Knott, Dorothy Voss, Signe Brunnström, and the Bobaths,[18] who developed new and innovative intervention techniques for adults and children with stroke, cerebral palsy, and other disorders of the central nervous system. The cardiovascular/pulmonary area of practice also developed during this time, as advancements in medicine and surgery such as open-heart procedures, the heart–lung machine, cardiac stenting, and newer medications became more commonly utilized. These intensive procedures often required long periods of acute hospital stay with resultant functional deficits requiring physical therapy intervention. In the orthopedic practice arena, total joint arthroplasties, experimental in the 1960s but now routine, created an additional need for postoperative physical therapy. Published works by Cyriax, McKenzie, Paris, Grimsby, and Mennell[19] added greatly to the effectiveness of physical therapy interventions for musculoskeletal pathology. The innovation of outcome measures to measure the impact of our interventions proved the effectiveness of our interventions to referrers, insurance companies, and the general public.

The Health Maintenance Organization Act of 1973[20] sponsored by Edward Kennedy and signed by President Nixon and known informally as the Federal HMO Act, provided for a trial federal program to promote and encourage the development of health maintenance organizations. The Federal HMO Act amended the Public Health Service Act which was passed by Congress in 1944. The Federal HMO Act required employers to offer at least one federally approved HMO insurance to its employees. HMOs provided a radical departure from previous standard practices of referral and payment to physical therapists.[20] HMOs reimbursed physical therapists a per member per month (PMPM) fee for outpatient care rather than the typical fee for service charge. The PMPM reimbursement mechanism was the first attempt by a major insurer class to reimburse therapists based on keeping patients healthy rather than reimbursing for treating pathology. An even more impactful change in reimbursement occurred with the passage of the Balanced Budget Act of 1997[21] and its co-legislation, the Medicare Prospective Payment System (PPS), which included the Medicare cap on physical therapy services. The "cap" challenged the profession of physical therapy by limiting episode of care Medicare reimbursement to physical therapists, occupational therapists, and speech and language pathologists. PPS also changed the inpatient reimbursement model of patients with Medicare insurance from an essential fee for service model to a fixed payment per diagnosis. Prior to PPS, the longer the patient stayed in the hospital and the more services delivered to the patient, the greater the hospital was reimbursed by Medicare. Reimbursing based on diagnosis rather than length of stay and services provided forced hospitals to utilize evidence-based data to determine the effectiveness of services and interventions (and avoid those that did not provide benefit to the patient) and also work toward shorter lengths of stay. Although the impact of PPS markedly shortened length of stay for inpatient services thus impacting physical therapy in a negative way, the publication of evidence which detailed the positive impact of physical therapy services in facilitating discharge planning countered the loss of services.

The Education for All Handicapped Children Act[22] was enacted in 1975. This Act required all public schools accepting federal funds to provide equal access to educational opportunities and at minimum and if needed, one free meal per day for students with physical and mental disabilities. Public schools were required to evaluate children with disabilities and create an educational plan with parental input that would parallel as closely as possible the educational experience of nondisabled students. The Act also contains a provision that disabled students should be placed in the least restrictive environment— one that allows the maximum possible opportunity to interact with nonimpaired students. This provision is commonly referred to as "mainstreaming." Separate schooling may only occur when the nature or severity of the disability is such that instructional goals cannot be achieved in the regular classroom. Finally, the law contains a due process clause that guarantees an impartial hearing to resolve conflicts between the parents of disabled children to the school system. One of the important downstream impacts of the Act was that public schools began to provide physical therapy services on the site for children with disabilities to avoid transportation to the outpatient physical therapy arenas, which allowed for a more consistent integration into the classroom.

In the early 1980s, APTA began researching methods to eventually develop physical therapy practice into the ultimate of the independent practitioner schema. This was known popularly as treatment without referral. In the early 1980s APTA adopted a policy indicating that "physical therapy practice independent of practitioner referral was ethical as long as it was legal in the state."[17] Having taken small steps over the previous 50 years to become more independent of the physician, this courageous step punctuated the professionalization of the physical therapist and resulted in states changing their practice acts to provide for the ability to practice without referral. As a part of APTA's vision statement,[23] by the year 2020, physical therapists "will hold all privileges of autonomous practice." This vision statement and the ideals held within it are requisites to the continued growth of physical therapy as a profession.

Also significant during this time was the formation of the Federation of State Boards of Physical Therapy (FSBPT) in 1986. The FSBPT became the organization through which member licensing authorities could coordinate to promote and protect the health, welfare, and safety of the American public through competency assessment. The FSBPT, as a stand-alone agency, is effectively separated from the operational activities of APTA.[17]

The 2000s

The emergence of new diseases and the changes in incidence and prevalence of existing diseases impacted physical therapy practice in the late years of the 20th century and the early years of the 21st century. Human immunodeficiency virus/acquired immunodeficiency syndrome (HIV/AIDs) continues to be a major health problem in the United States and throughout the world. Complications of HIV/AIDs—especially those related to loss of function, muscle wasting and weakness, neuropathy, and cognitive impairment—can benefit from physical therapy intervention. Diabetes mellitus, an illness known for centuries, has, over the past decades, markedly increased in incidence and prevalence especially in the United States. By 2014, an estimated 29.1 million Americans had been diagnosed with diabetes and an additional 8.1 million have diabetes but have yet to be diagnosed.[24] Complications of diabetes—coronary artery disease, cerebrovascular disease, peripheral vascular disease, neuropathy, renal disease, wounds, amputation, and retinopathy—often require intervention by physical therapists.

The 2010s and Beyond

These and related health care system changes identified a need to formally define the role of the physical therapist and to describe the practice of physical therapy, which in part motivated the creation and ongoing development of the *Guide to Physical Therapist Practice* originally published in 1995 and now on its third edition.[25] This document clearly describes in an evidence-based manner, the role and process of the examination, evaluation, diagnosis, prognosis, intervention, reexamination, and assessment of outcomes in the physical therapy management of patients and clients.

Lastly, recent regulations such as The Joint Commission's National Patient Safety Goal Initiative[26] has increased the utilization of physical therapy services. The Fall Risk National Patient Safety Goal requires that all persons admitted to Joint Commission accredited institutions (which are most hospitals and rehabilitation centers) are required to be screened for fall risk. Who better than the experts in mobility to screen for and ameliorate fall risk?

By understanding the past, studying the present, and reflection on the future, one cannot help but be optimistic about the future of the profession of physical therapy. Physical therapists are uniquely positioned to become the "go to" persons for mobility, activity, and functional issues related to disease and impairment, for prevention, and for risk factor modification associated with mobility, obesity, and sedentary lifestyle issues.

1.3 Vision 2020

APTA's current vision statement—"Transforming society by optimizing movement to improve the human experience"—enacted in 2013,[27] and the old vision statement enacted in 2000, is that "by 2020, physical therapy will be provided by physical therapists who are doctors of physical therapy, recognized by consumers and other health care professionals as practitioners of choice whom consumer have direct access for the diagnosis of, interventions for, and prevention of impairments, functional limitations, and disabilities related to movement, function, and health." These statements provide a vision of physical therapy with the following key elements:

- Physical therapists will be the practitioner of choice for movement impairments.
- Physical therapists will practice autonomously.
- All entry-level educational programs will be at the doctoral level.
- Physical therapists will utilize evidence in clinical decision making.
- Physical therapists will practice under strict professional and ethical guidelines.

A concrete understanding of each element is necessary to understanding physical therapist practice in today and in the near future.

1.4 Practitioner of Choice for Movement Impairments

Consumers identify health care practitioners globally individually by an understanding of the scope of care provided by that profession. For instance, consumers with issues related to prescriptive drug interactions may consider asking a pharmacist for assistance. Acute fracture of bones are within the scope of the practice of orthopedic surgeons. Acute coronary syndromes are referred to cardiologists. Physical therapists have become the practitioner of choice for movement disorders—impairments related to pain, joint dysfunction, neurodegenerative disease, acute illness, and such. When movement impairments impact function, the consumer should immediately consider physical therapy.

1.5 Autonomous Practice

Autonomous practice means practice without constraints from others. The others may be considered other health care practitioners or third-party payers. From a legal perspective, autonomous practice means that the physical therapist is solely responsible for the patient's physical therapy diagnosis, evaluation, treatment, and outcome from treatment. This does not indicate silo practice. As an autonomous practitioner, physical therapists will work closely with the health care team to collaboratively develop plans of care, remediate risk factors, and coordinate care. Physical therapists will be responsible for the physical therapy services provided to the patient.

1.6 Doctor of Physical Therapy

By the year 2020, physical therapists entering the profession must have successfully completed a doctor of physical therapy (DPT) degree. Entry-level curricula has expanded from the education of primarily a technician: modalities, exercise, massage, core sciences to an ever-expanding comprehensive education involving robotics, diagnostics, systems review, research methods, assistive technology, pharmacology, and adaptive equipment—all permitting physical therapists to treat impairments and limitations not even dreamed of by the early physical therapists; urinary incontinence, pelvic floor dysfunction, wounds, vestibular pathology, women's health issues, and preventive medicine. Physical therapists, once primarily employed in the inpatient hospital settings, have now expanded their arenas of service to home care, outpatient, schools, industry, research facilities, utilization review, health care administration, and boutique practices.

1.7 Evidence-Based Practice in Clinical Decision Making

Physical therapists make thousands of clinical decisions per day. How these decisions are made often defines the effectiveness of their evaluation and treatment. The best method of clinical decision making is evidenced-based practice. The most commonly utilized definition of evidenced-based practice is by David Sacket and written in 1996:[28] "the conscientious, explicit and judicious use of current best evidence in making decisions about the care of the individual patient. It means integrating individual clinical expertise with the best available external clinical evidence from systematic research." Practically, evidence-based medicine is that the evaluation, intervention, and outcome measures selected by the physical therapist are the most cost-effective, appropriate, and beneficial modality. Physical therapists must constantly and continuously educate themselves and review research for evidence that the modality—evaluation, intervention, and outcome measure—are actually beneficial and appropriate. No longer is what content physical therapists learn in school not sufficient to be an expert clinician; physical therapists need to evolve from a spoon-fed (entry-level curriculum) learner to a lifelong, self-directed learner.

1.8 Physical Therapists Will Practice Under Strict Professional and Ethical Guidelines

A commonly utilized definition of professionalism in physical therapy is "acting with professional character, spirit, and methods." APTA has identified seven Core Values of Professionalism.[29]

1.8.1 The Mission, Vision, and Scope of Accreditation Activities for the Commission on Accreditation in Physical Therapy Education (CAPTE)[30]

CAPTE serves the public by assuring the quality, consistency, and ongoing advancement of physical therapy educational programs.

Mission

The mission of the Commission on Accreditation in Physical Therapy Education (CAPTE) is to serve the public by assuring quality and continuous improvement in physical therapy education.

Vision

CAPTE is an autonomous, self-governing agency that functions globally to model best practices in specialized accreditation.

Scope of Accreditation Activities

CAPTE accredits physical therapist professional education programs offered at the master's and clinical doctoral degree levels by higher education institutions in the United States and internationally. CAPTE also accredits paraprofessional physical therapist assistant technical education programs offered at the associate degree level by higher education institutions in the United States only.

- CAPTE is an accrediting agency that is nationally recognized by the United States Department of Education (USDE) and the Council for Higher Education Accreditation (CHEA). CAPTE grants specialized accreditation status to qualified entry-level education programs for physical therapists and physical therapist assistants. This is the only accreditation agency recognized by the USDE and the CHEA to accredit entry-level physical therapist and physical therapist assistant education programs.

- Has been recognized as an independent agency since 1977 and has been the only recognized agency to accredit physical therapy programs since 1983.
- Currently accredits over 200 physical therapist education programs and over 250 physical therapist assistant education programs in the United States and three physical therapist education programs in other countries (Canada and Scotland).
- Has 29 members from a variety of constituencies: physical therapist and physical therapist assistant clinicians, physical therapist and physical therapist assistant educators, basic scientists, higher education administrators and the public.
- Maintains a cadre of more than 250 volunteers who are trained to conduct on-site reviews of physical therapy programs.
- Conducts on-site visits to approximately 70 programs annually.
- Reviews information from approximately one-third of all accredited programs at each meeting.
- Is an active member of the Association of Specialized and Programmatic Accreditors (ASPA) and subscribes to the ASPA Code of Good Practice.

APTA also defines each value and provides sample indicators for better understanding and implementation. Physical therapists are often quite capable of modeling professional behavior but often lack the eloquence to adequately define these behaviors. Professional behavior is not only a "clinic" behavior. As a member of a profession, physical therapists should practice professional behavior at all times. APTA has also developed a Code of Ethics for Physical Therapists[31] based on the values defined as the Core Values of Professionalism.

1.8.2 APTA Seven Core Values of Professionalism[32]

Members of the physical therapy profession take seriously professional attributes and incorporate them into all aspects of professional life.
1. Accountability.
2. Altruism.
3. Compassion/Caring.
4. Excellence.
5. Integrity.
6. Professional duty.
7. Social responsibility.

The Code of Ethics for the Physical Therapist delineates the ethical obligations of all physical therapists as determined by the House of Delegates of APTA (see ▶ Table 1.2). The Code of Ethics for the Physical Therapist provides the fundamental platform on which all actions of the physical therapist are measured. Much like the Constitution of the United States guiding the legislative process of the United States, the Code of Ethics for Physical Therapists provides the platform on which all actions of the physical therapist are measured.

Table 1.2 American Physical Therapy Association Code of Ethics (APTA)

Principle	Core value	Narrative
Principle 1: physical therapists shall respect the inherent dignity and rights of all individuals	Compassion, integrity	1A. Physical therapists shall act in a respectful manner toward each person regardless of age, gender, race, nationality, religion, ethnicity, social or economic status, sexual orientation, health condition, or disability
		1B. Physical therapists shall recognize their personal biases and shall not discriminate against others in physical therapist practice, consultation, education, research, and administration
Principle 2: physical therapists shall be trustworthy and compassionate in addressing the rights and needs of patients/clients	Altruism, compassion, professional duty	2A. Physical therapists shall adhere to the core values of the profession and shall act in the best interests of patients/clients over the interests of the physical therapist
		2B. Physical therapists shall provide physical therapy services with compassionate and caring behaviors that incorporate the individual and cultural differences of patients/clients
		2C. Physical therapists shall provide the information necessary to allow patients or their surrogates to make informed decisions about physical therapy care or participation in clinical research
		2D. Physical therapists shall collaborate with patients/clients to empower them in decisions about their health care
		2E. Physical therapists shall protect confidential patient/client information and may disclose confidential information to appropriate authorities only when allowed or as required by law
Principle 3: physical therapists shall be accountable for making sound professional judgments	Excellence, integrity	3A. Physical therapists shall demonstrate independent and objective professional judgment in the patient's/client's best interest in all practice settings
		3B. Physical therapists shall demonstrate professional judgment informed by professional standards, evidence (including current literature and established best practice), practitioner experience, and patient/client values
		3C. Physical therapists shall make judgments within their scope of practice and level of expertise and shall communicate with, collaborate with, or refer to peers or other health care professionals when necessary
		3D. Physical therapists shall not engage in conflicts of interest that interfere with professional judgment
		3E. Physical therapists shall provide appropriate direction of and communication with physical therapist assistants and support personnel
Principle 4: physical therapists shall demonstrate integrity in their relationships with patients/clients, families, colleagues, students, research participants, other health care providers, employers, payers, and the public	Integrity	4A. Physical therapists shall provide truthful, accurate, and relevant information and shall not make misleading representations 4B. Physical therapists shall not exploit persons over whom they have supervisory, evaluative or other authority (e.g., patients/clients, students, supervisees, research participants, or employees)
		4C. Physical therapists shall discourage misconduct by health care professionals and report illegal or unethical acts to the relevant authority, when appropriate
		4D. Physical therapists shall report suspected cases of abuse involving children or vulnerable adults to the appropriate authority, subject to law
		4E. Physical therapists shall not engage in any sexual relationship with any of their patients/clients, supervisees, or students
		4F. Physical therapists shall not harass anyone verbally, physically, emotionally, or sexually
Principle 5: physical therapists shall fulfill their legal and professional obligations	Professional duty, accountability	5A. Physical therapists shall comply with applicable local, state, and federal laws and regulations
		5B. Physical therapists shall have primary responsibility for supervision of physical therapist assistants and support personnel

(Continued)

Table 1.2 continued

Principle	Core value	Narrative
		5C. Physical therapists involved in research shall abide by accepted standards governing protection of research participants
		5D. Physical therapists shall encourage colleagues with physical, psychological, or substance-related impairments that may adversely impact their professional responsibilities to seek assistance or counsel
		5E. Physical therapists who have knowledge that a colleague is unable to perform their professional responsibilities with reasonable skill and safety shall report this information to the appropriate authority
		5F. Physical therapists shall provide notice and information about alternatives for obtaining care in the event the physical therapist terminates the provider relationship while the patient/client continues to need physical therapy services
Principle 6: physical therapists shall enhance their expertise through the lifelong acquisition and refinement of knowledge, skills, abilities, and professional behaviors	Excellence	6A. Physical therapists shall achieve and maintain professional competence
		6B. Physical therapists shall take responsibility for their professional development based on critical self-assessment and reflection on changes in physical therapist practice, education, health care delivery, and technology
		6C. Physical therapists shall evaluate the strength of evidence and applicability of content presented during professional development activities before integrating the content or techniques into practice
		6D. Physical therapists shall cultivate practice environments that support professional development, lifelong learning, and excellence
Principle 7: physical therapists shall promote organizational behaviors and business practices that benefit patients/clients and society	Integrity, accountability	7A. Physical therapists shall promote practice environments that support autonomous and accountable professional judgments
		7B. Physical therapists shall seek remuneration as is deserved and reasonable for physical therapist services
		7C. Physical therapists shall not accept gifts or other considerations that influence or give an appearance of influencing their professional judgment
		7D. Physical therapists shall fully disclose any financial interest they have in products or services that they recommend to patients/clients
		7E. Physical therapists shall be aware of charges and shall ensure that documentation and coding for physical therapy services accurately reflect the nature and extent of the services provided
		7F. Physical therapists shall refrain from employment arrangements, or other arrangements, that prevent physical therapists from fulfilling professional obligations to patients/clients
Principle 8: physical therapists shall participate in efforts to meet the health needs of people locally, nationally, or globally	Social responsibility	8A. Physical therapists shall provide pro bono physical therapy services or support organizations that meet the health needs of people who are economically disadvantaged, uninsured, and underinsured
		8B. Physical therapists shall advocate to reduce health disparities and health care inequities, improve access to health care services, and address the health, wellness, and preventive health care needs of people
		8C. Physical therapists shall be responsible stewards of health care resources and shall avoid overutilization or underutilization of physical therapy services
		8D. Physical therapists shall educate members of the public about the benefits of physical therapy and the unique role of the physical therapist

Source: http://www.apta.org/uploadedFiles/APTAorg/About_Us/Policies/Ethics/CodeofEthics.pdf.

1.8.3 American Physical Therapy Association

APTA[33] is an individual membership professional organization representing more than 93,000 member physical therapists, physical therapist assistants (PTAs), students of physical therapy (SPT), foreign trained PTs living in the United States, physical therapist post-professional students, and retired or life members. APTA seeks to improve the health and quality of life of individuals in society by advancing physical therapist practice, education, and research, and by increasing the awareness and understanding of physical therapy's role in the nation's health care system.

APTA is headquartered in Alexandria, Virginia, and has an operating budget of $43.5 million.[33] With over 180 paid employees and countless more volunteers, APTA, led by a senior staff, is tasked to serve the needs of the profession of physical therapy. APTA is organized into sections and chapters. Each state has an individual chapter with a leadership team and operational groups consisting of committees, districts, and special interest groups. The state chapters are tasked with representing and empowering members in the individual states and working to meet the goals of Vision 2020. Like APTA, the chapters advocate for physical therapy, conduct continuing education programs, sponsor conferences, and promote research. In addition, state chapters advocate for the profession with insurance companies that are licensed in the particular state. APTA sections provide practicing therapists with resources needed to stay current in specific areas of expertise and to facilitate forums to connect professionals with like interests.

Physical Therapy Sections[34]

APTA's special-interest sections for physical therapists, physical therapist assistants and students—resources which facilitate currency in specific areas of specialty and also assist with connecting with others sharing common interests.
- Acute care.
- Aquatic physical therapy.
- Cardiovascular and pulmonary.
- Clinical electrophysiology and wound management.
- Education.
- Federal physical therapy.
- Geriatrics.
- Hand rehabilitation.
- Home health.
- Neurology.
- Oncology.
- Pediatrics.
- Private practice.
- Research.
- Sports physical therapy.
- Women's health.

APTA provides valuable information to consumers. This information includes data related to finding a physical therapist, applying to physical therapist and physical therapist assistant educational programs, disease-specific information, prevention tips, and links to beneficial websites. APTA also facilitates research through the Foundation for Physical Therapy.

1.8.4 Commission on Accreditation in Physical Therapy Education

CAPTE[35] is an accrediting agency that is nationally recognized by the USDE and the CHEA. CAPTE grants specialized accreditation status to qualified entry-level education programs for physical therapists and physical therapist assistants.

Role of the Commission on Accreditation of Physical Therapy Education[36]

CAPTE performs a number of roles related to the accreditation of physical therapy educational programs, as cited in section 1.8.1.

Accreditation is a process used in the United States to assure the quality of the professional education received by students. Accreditation is a voluntary, nongovernmental, peer-reviewed process that occurs on a regular basis. Failure to meet strict accreditation standards may result in program closure. CAPTE accredits programs and not institutions.

CAPTE comprises a broad representation from the educational community, the physical therapy profession, and the public. Members include physical therapy educators who are basic scientists, curriculum specialists, and academic administrators; physical therapy clinicians and clinical educators; administrators and leaders from institutions of higher education; and public representatives. The wide-ranging experience, content knowledge, and expertise of this group in education in general and physical therapy education in particular provide ongoing assurance that the accreditation process of physical therapy education programs is fair, reliable, and effective.

CAPTE employs approximately 250 PTs, PTAs, basic scientists, and higher education leaders and administrators to conduct the distance and on-site program evaluation.[35] Accreditors measure program compliance against published elements. Elements are periodically updated based on evidence, input from content experts, and contemporary practice guidelines.

1.8.5 Federation of State Boards of Physical Therapy

The FSBPT is tasked to protect the public by structuring and enforcing laws, regulations, and tools to assess entry-level professional competence (▶ Table 1.3).[17] The mission of FSBPT is "To protect the public by providing service and leadership that promote safe and competent physical therapy practice" and the vision is "To achieve a high level of public protection through a strong foundation of laws and regulatory standards in physical therapy, effective tools and systems to assess entry-level and continuing competence, and public and professional awareness of resources for public protection."[17]

Table 1.3 The six areas of focus for the Federation of State Boards of Physical Therapy

Focus	Narrative
Examinations	To ensure the ongoing excellence, reliability, defensibility, security and validity of the NPTE and related examinations
Membership	To enhance the Federation's value to its membership by developing and maintaining programs and services responsive to membership needs
States' rights, States' responsibilities, and professional standards	To identify and promote effective regulation in physical therapy that ensures the delivery of safe and competent physical therapy care, while respecting states' rights and responsibilities
Education	To provide and promote educational programs and products for board members, administrators, the public and other stakeholders
Leadership	To broaden the Federation's leadership role and recognition within the regulatory, professional and related communities
Organizational and financial stability	To ensure the long-term organizational and financial stability and viability of the Federation

Abbreviation: FSBPT, Federation of State Boards of Physical Therapy
Source: http://fsb.org.money.usnews.com/careers/best-jobs/rankings/the-100-best

1.9 Contemporary Physical Therapy Practice

Contemporary physical therapy practice crosses the entire human lifespan from neonate to frail elderly, directly addressing many of the systems of the human body, including musculoskeletal, neuromuscular, integumentary, genitourinary, cardiovascular, and pulmonary. Physical therapists practice in a number of arenas including hospitals, outpatient practices, schools, universities, research facilities, home care, and rehabilitation centers. Due to the expanse of knowledge and skills involved for such diverse populations and settings, and the challenge of constantly learning and translating to clinical practice new evidence, most physical therapists have a focus or area of practice that allows them to concentrate their expertise. Entry-level physical therapy students are well-versed in the need, on graduation, to evolve from a "spoon-fed" (faculty and curriculum-based) learning model to becoming a self-regulated, self-determined, lifelong learner. Medical evidence changes rapidly and those practitioners who do not practice lifelong learning skills quickly become anachronistic in practice. Being a lifelong learner requires reflection in practice and reflection on practice. Identified weak clinical or knowledge areas need to be remediated; new knowledge must be identified, digested, and translated into practice.

Licensed therapists can update their knowledge in a variety of venues. Most states require physical therapists to amass a specified number of continuing education units (CEUs) on a yearly basis. These courses are often offered on weekends or online and aid to facilitate emerging knowledge and clinical practices. Attendance at national or state conferences often offer CEUs based on attendance. Most states also require mandatory CEUs in specified areas such as ethics or child abuse.

Formal programs such as clinical residencies, clinical fellowships, and certified clinical specializations permit PTs to expand their expertise within defined areas of practice, or "specialties"—much like the medical model of specialization and board certification. A clinical residency program, which terminates with the successful passing of a specialization board examination, is the process by which a physical therapist builds on a broad base of professional education and practice to develop a greater depth of knowledge and skills related to a particular area of practice. There are currently 221 accredited physical therapy residency programs in the United States and are typically 1-year educational and clinical programs with demanding curricula including mentored clinical practice, educational classes, presentations, research, and teaching modules.[37] The specialist certification program was established to provide formal recognition for physical therapists with advanced clinical knowledge, experience, and skills in a special area of practice and to assist consumers and the health care community in identifying physical therapists whose skills and content knowledge meet their impairment need. Licensed physical therapists can sit for the specialization board examination with or without completing the residency. Currently, The American Board of Physical Therapy Specialties (ABPTS) coordinates and oversees the specialist certification process, is the governing body for certification and recertification of clinical specialists, and offers nine areas of clinical residencies and specialization:

- Cardiovascular and pulmonary.
- Clinical electrophysiology.
- Geriatrics.
- Neurology.
- Oncology.
- Orthopedics.
- Pediatrics.
- Sports.
- Women's health.

A clinical fellowship program is designed to provide PTs greater depth in a specialty or subspecialty area than that covered in a residency program. Fellowship programs are post-professional programs intended to train physical therapists in a subspecialty area (beyond specialty training). The fellowship experience combines opportunities for ongoing mentoring and formal and informal feedback to the physical therapist fellow-in-training, including required written and live patient practical examinations, with a foundation in scientific inquiry, evidence-based practice, and course work designed to provide a theoretical basis for advanced practice. Each program is based on a well-defined, systematic process for establishing content validity of the curriculum that describes practice in a defined area. Fellowships should have a curriculum based in one or more subspecialty areas. In subspecialty areas where validated competencies have been identified, the curriculum should be based on those competencies.[38]

1.10 Review Questions

1. The use of physical agents to improve function and decrease pain dates back to which era?
   a) Ancient Greece.
   b) Dark Ages.
   c) The United States Revolutionary War.
   d) World War I.
2. Emerging research indicate that the modern practice of physical therapy began in which country?
   a) England.
   b) Scotland.
   c) The United States.
   d) Sweden.
3. The development of the profession of physical therapy was greatly hastened during the period from 1916 to 1930 by which events?
   a) The use of molded plastics in prosthetic manufacturing and the Spanish flu.
   b) The availability of federally funded school loans in the United States.
   c) World War I and the polio epidemics.
   d) The availability of health insurance and the development of advanced surgical techniques.
4. During Harry Truman's presidency a law was passed by Congress providing inpatient facilities: hospitals, nursing homes, and other health facilities, grants, and loans earmarked for construction and modernization and to meet the goal of increasing the nation's hospital beds to 4.5 per 1,000 people. This Act is formally known as which of the following?
   a) The Medicare and Medicaid Act.
   b) No Child Left Behind Act.
   c) The Hill–Burton Act.
   d) The Affordable Care Act.
5. During the 1950s physical therapy educational programs received accreditation through which agency/association?
   a) The American Medical Association.
   b) The American Physical Therapy Association.
   c) The American Dental Association.
   d) The Joint Commission.
6. Which law, passed in 1965, provided medical insurance to Americans over age 65 and those who were poor and were disabled?
   a) The Medicare and Medicaid Act.
   b) No Child Left Behind Act.
   c) The Hill–Burton Act.
   d) The Affordable Care Act.
7. The Medicare Cap limits Medicare spending by the federal government by which of the following mechanisms?
   a) Prohibiting persons over age 80 from receiving outpatient physical therapy services.
   b) Limiting reimbursement for physical therapists providing wound care services.
   c) Requiring a referral from the primary care practitioner for physical therapy services.
   d) Limiting episode of care Medicare reimbursement to physical therapists, occupational therapists, and speech and language.

8. "Autonomous practice" means which of the following?
   a) Practicing without constraints from others.
   b) Receiving appropriate reimbursement for services provided.
   c) Owning one's own physical therapy practice.
   d) The mandatory inclusion of reimbursement by the employer for continuing education activities.
9. By the year 2020 all physical therapists entering the profession in the United States must have which degree?
   a) Associate's.
   b) Bachelor's.
   c) Master's.
   d) Doctorate.
10. The American Physical Therapy Association is headquartered in which U.S. city?
    a) Memphis.
    b) Philadelphia.
    c) Alexandria.
    d) Washington.

1.11 Review Answers

1. The use of physical agents to improve function and decrease pain dates back to which era?
   a. Ancient Greece.
2. Emerging research indicate that the modern practice of physical therapy began in which country?
   d. Sweden.
3. The development of the profession of physical therapy was greatly hastened during the period from 1916 to 1930 by which events?
   c. World War I and the polio epidemics.
4. During Harry Truman's presidency a law was passed by Congress providing inpatient facilities: hospitals, nursing homes, and other health facilities, grants and loans earmarked for construction and modernization and to meet the goal of increasing the nation's hospital beds to 4.5 per 1,000 people. This Act is formally known as which of the following?
   c. The Hill–Burton Act.
5. During the 1950s physical therapy educational programs received accreditation through which agency/association?
   a. The American Medical Association.
6. Which law, passed in 1965, provided medical insurance to Americans over age 65 and those who were poor and were disabled?
   a. The Medicare and Medicaid Act.
7. The Medicare Cap limits Medicare spending by the federal government by which of the following mechanisms?
   d. Limiting episode of care Medicare reimbursement to physical therapists, occupational therapists, and speech and language.
8. "Autonomous practice" means which of the following?
   a. Practicing without constraints from others.
9. By the year 2020 all physical therapists entering the profession in the United States must have which degree?
   d. Doctorate.
10. The American Physical Therapy Association is headquartered in which U.S. city?
    c. Alexandria.

References

[1] U.S. News. Available at: http://money.usnews.com/careers/best-jobs/rankings/the-100-best-jobs. Accessed October 21, 2016

[2] PT in Motion. Available at: http://www.apta.org/PTinMotion/News/2014/12/02/ForbesTop10Jobs/ Accessed October 30, 2016

[3] Forbes. Available at: http://www.forbes.com/forbes/welcome/?toURL=http://www.forbes.com/2011/04/18/jobs-people-stay-at-leave.html. Accessed October 21, 2016

[4] Bureau of Labor Statistics. Available at: http://bls.gov. Accessed November 2, 2016

[5] CAPTE. Available at: http://capteonline/programs/. Accessed November 1, 2016

[6] Nutton V. The chronology of Galen's early career. Class Q. 1973; 23(1):158–171

[7] De Lacy P. Galen's Platonism. Am J Philol. 1972: 27–39

[8] Proceedings of the Conference 1001 Inventions: Muslim Heritage in Our World Organized by FSTC, London, 25–26 May 2010

[9] Cook HJ. Medicine in the Cambridge History of Science. Vol. 3. Early Modern Science. Park K, Daston L, eds. New York, NY: Cambridge University Press, 2006:407–434

[10] Chartered Society of Physiotherapy. Available at: http://csp.org.UK/. Accessed October 10, 2016

[11] Ottosson A. The first historical movements of kinesiology: scientification in the borderline between physical culture and medicine around 1850. Int J Hist Sport. 2010; 27(11):1892–1919

[12] Holt PJ. Jonas Henrik Kellgren 1911–2002. Rheumatology. 2003; 42(5):708–709

[13] University OTAGO. Available at: http://www.otago.ac.nz/physio/index.html. Accessed November 1, 2016

[14] Moffat M. Three quarters of a century of healing the generations. Phys Ther. 1996; 76(11):1242–1252

[15] Dowell MA. Hill–Burton: the unfulfilled promise. J Health Polit Policy Law. 1987; 12(1):153–175

[16] MacDonald C. Recognizing 200 Years of International OMT Practice. Proceedings from the 2013 AAOMPT Annual Conference

[17] Financial Stability Board. Available at: http://fsb.org. Accessed October 15, 2016

[18] Academy of Neurologic Physical Therapy. Available at: http://neuropt.org/about-us/our-history. Accessed October 15, 2016

[19] Pettman E. A history of manipulative therapy. J Manual Manip Ther. 2007; 15(3):165–174

[20] Rosoff AJ. The Federal HMO Assistance Act: helping hand or hurdle? Am Bus Law J. 1975; 13(2):137

[21] Battaglini M. On the case for a balanced budget amendment to the U.S. Constitution. 2009 Meeting Papers 131, Society for Economic Dynamics

[22] Coates KM. The Education for All Handicapped Children Act. Marquette Law Rev. 1985; 69:122–124

[23] American Physical Therapy Association. Available at: http://www.apta.org/Vision2020/. Accessed November 1, 2016

[24] American Diabetes Association. Available at: http://diabetes.org. Accessed November 1, 2013

[25] Guide to Physical Therapist Practice. Available at: http://guidetoptpractice.apta.org. Accessed October 15, 2016

[26] The Joint Commission. Available at: http://thejointcommission.org. Accessed October 15, 2016

[27] American Physical Therapy Association. Available at: www.apta.org/Vision. Accessed October 15, 2016

[28] Sackett DL, Rosenberg WM, Gray JA, Haynes RB, Richardson WS. Evidence based medicine: what it is and what it isn't. BMJ. 1996; 312(7023):71–72

[29] American Physical Therapy Association. Available at: http://www.apta.org/Professionalism/. Accessed October 15, 2013

[30] CAPTE. Available at: http://capteonline.org. Accessed November 1, 2016

[31] American Physical Therapy Association. Available at: https://www.apta.org/uploadedFiles/APTAorg/About_Us/Policies/Ethics/CodeofEthics.pdf. Accessed November 1, 2016

[32] American Physical Therapy Association. Available at: https://www.apta.org/uploadedFiles/APTAorg/About_Us/Policies/BOD/Judicial/ProfessionalisminPT.pdf. Accessed November 1, 2016

[33] American Physical Therapy Association. Available at: http://apta.org. Accessed November 1, 2016

[34] American Physical Therapy Association. Available at: http://www.apta.org/Sections/. Accessed November 1, 2016

[35] CAPTE. Available at: http://www.capteonline.org/WhoWeAre/. Accessed October 2, 2016

[36] The Federation of State Boards of Physical Therapy. Available at: https://www.fsbpt.org/AboutUs/AreasofFocus.aspx. Accessed October 2, 2016

[37] American Board of Physical Therapy Residency and Fellowship Education. Available at: http://www.abptrfe.org/home.aspx. Accessed October 2, 2016

[38] American Board of Physical Therapy Residency and Fellowship Education. Available at: http://www.abptrfe.org/FellowshipPrograms/Overview/. Accessed October 2, 2016

2 Insurance and Reimbursement

Grace C. Karaman and Stephen J. Carp

Keywords: Advance Beneficiary Notice, Affordable Care Act, bundled payments, capitation, coding, current procedural terminology, Eight-minute rule, health insurance, health maintenance organization, HMO Act, International Classification of Diseases, managed care, Medicaid, Medicare, Medicare Fee Schedule, modifiers, national health insurance, one on one versus group therapy, per member per month fee, private insurance, single payer system, Therapy Cap, World Health Organization

Chapter Outline

1. Overview: The Pursuit of Health Insurance: A Brief History
   a) Attempts to Enact Health Insurance
   b) Rising Medical Costs for Doctors: Medical Licensure and Manpower Issues
   c) The Blues
   d) Continued Growth in Health Insurance
   e) The National Health Insurance Dream
   f) Truman's Support: Another Failed Attempt
   g) President Johnson and the Medicare/Medicaid Compromise
   h) Rising Costs and Managed Competition
   i) Affordable Care Act
   j) Where We Are Now
2. Physical Therapy Reimbursement
   a) Overview
   b) International Classification of Diseases
   c) Current Procedural Terminology
   d) CPT Structure
   e) CPT Development Process
   f) CPT Category III Process
      1. One-on-One Services Versus Group Services
      2. Advance Beneficiary Notice
      3. Modifiers
   g) Reimbursement by Arena
      1. Inpatient Arenas
      2. Outpatient Reimbursement

"I am the Director of Physical Therapy Services at a very large health care organization in Chicago. Our therapists work at many levels of the continuum of care within our organization: acute care, skilled nursing care, acute medical rehabilitation, outpatient care, and home care. Physical therapists are naturally driven to update and maintain their clinical knowledge. Professional programs do an excellent job at teaching new graduates the transition from being spoon fed to lifelong learners. Therapists always have their noses in textbooks and journal articles; they perform literature searches to answer pending clinical questions; they attend continuing educational courses; and, they perform scholarly work such as research and textbook writing. However, a challenge for me as director is to convince my therapists to maintain state-of-the-art knowledge of reimbursement guidelines and procedures. Reimbursement is simply not as sexy as clinical care. If physical therapists loved reimbursement more than clinical care they would work in accounting instead of patient care.

"The challenge in maintaining knowledge of reimbursement is the sheer scope of the content. The first challenge is that most private insurances and Medicaid insurances are regulated by each individual state. Rules and benefits from one state differ from a neighboring state. The second challenge is the number of insurers licensed in a particular state. Some states, like mine—Illinois—have dozens of licensed health insurance carriers, with each carrier having different leadership, policies, procedures, and benefits. Adding to the confusion, many of the carriers offer a number of plans, each with unique benefits. In addition, each health care organization must have a contract with each insurance carrier. I have found it the norm rather than the exception that patients arrive at our organization for care and have no idea of what their physical therapy benefits entail. Along with providing clinical care, staff of the physical therapy department must also verify that the insurance is active and verbally and in writing provide counsel the patient as to his or her benefits.

"Even Medicare is confusing. One would think that Medicare, a federal insurance program, would offer consistent benefits to all subscribers across the country. This is not true. Medicare is governed by 'local entities'—companies contracted by Medicare to run the Medicare program. Each health care organization is assigned a local entity. Therefore, it is entirely possible that the entity governing the Medicare rules at a local hospital may deny coverage for a procedure but a different entity governing the Medicare rules at another local hospital may approve coverage of the same procedure.

"Consider also that tens of millions of Americans are either uninsured or underinsured. Lastly, consider that the reimbursement rules for all insurances vary not only based on insurance carrier and state but also vary by level of care. The rules vary for inpatient acute care, skilled nursing care, acute medical rehabilitation care, home care, and outpatient care—each has a unique set of reimbursement guidelines.

"Reimbursement is an extremely complex subject whose rules change almost daily. Most therapists would agree that maintaining up-to-date knowledge of reimbursement is onerous and challenging. However, we all believe that to provide the best care for our patients we must be aware of the rules of insurance."

—Abby J., Chicago, Illinois

2.1 Overview: The Pursuit of Health Insurance: A Brief History

The history of health insurance—insurance coverage that pays for all or part of the medical and surgical expenses of the covered individual which is incurred due to illness or injury—may date back centuries, possibly to the Norman Conquest. King Henry I introduced sweeping health care reforms to the newly combined kingdoms of England and Normandy. Soon thereafter, at least one "physician," John of Essex, was receiving an honorarium of one penny per day for his efforts. The reimbursement of medical services coming from the Crown appears to be the first evidence of medical insurance at the national level. John of Essex's reimbursement of a penny per day was essentially equal to that of a day's wages for Crown foot soldier or local a shopkeeper.[1]

There is much clearer historical evidence to suggest that American doctors were receiving capitation-like payments—now linked as a reimbursement method of managed care insurers and "boutique" insurance plans. Mark Twain, in a 1959 biography, indicated that during his boyhood in Hannibal, Missouri, his parents paid the local doctor $25 per year for taking care of the entire family regardless of their state of health.[2]

From the inception of the United States as a country until the late 1800s those who became sick or injured typically stayed at home for treatment. Even President Garfield convalesced at the White House and then at the New Jersey shore from the time of his attempted assassination on July 2, 1881 until his death due to septicemia on September 19, 1881.[3] Hospitals, then located primarily in a separate wing of an almshouse, jail, or inn, served primarily the poor and destitute who could not afford care at home. As late as 1873, there were only 178 hospitals with 35,064 beds in the entire United States. Only 36 years later, in 1909, the number had grown to 4,359 hospitals with 421,065 beds, and by 1929 to 6,665 hospitals with 907,133 beds.[4]

Prior to 1920, due to the low salaries of health care providers, including physicians, nurses, dentists, and pharmacists, and the lack of expensive technology, interventions, and medications, the cost to provide medical services per episode of care in the United States was very low. The primary expense of any illness was not the actual health care costs but the lost wages associated with work time loss due to illness. According to a study conducted by the state of Illinois in 1919, lost wages from illness were four times larger than the expenses associated with treating the illness. Most families purchased "sickness" insurance (akin to current disability insurance) which did not provide reimbursement for medical interventions but rather for missed work.[5] Medical services were either directly reimbursed to the practitioner (a fee-for-service model) or not reimbursed at all and provided as charity care.

2.1.1 Attempts to Enact Health Insurance

In the early part of the 20th century, several states and the federal government routinely proposed to enact compulsory health insurance, but all proposals failed. Popular support was low. Physicians, surgeons, and pharmacists opposed the insurance because they feared that it would limit their fees. Commercial insurance companies opposed it because in most cases the proposed compulsory insurance legislation included provisions for "burial insurance." Burial insurance was a significant part of the business portfolios of life insurance companies at the time.

However, in the 1920s to 1930s, the U.S. population was shifting from rural to urban. Families from rural America, who frequently lived in larger homes that could house two or three generations with plenty of human resources to permit direct care for the ill, were moving to the cities, where they lived in smaller homes or apartments. Many of these homes did not have room to care for the sick. Moreover, as the scientific era began, hopes and expectations were raised for better health and recovery from illness. For the first time in history "science" provided hope that illness was not simply a part of life but rather an unfortunate episode which might be overcome by improving medical care.

Along with the population shift from rural to urban environments in the 1920s and early 1930s, significant advancements in the areas of pharmaceuticals, surgery technique, diagnostics, the use of evidence as a method of making clinical decisions, and the understanding of incorporations of practices to improve cleanliness and sterility as a method to prevent disease facilitated the development of hospitals as treatment centers. By the late 1920s a paradigm shift occurred where prospective patients were influenced by the opportunity for healing and by the image of "hospital"—the brick and mortar, technology, science, and professionalism of the caregivers—as the future of wellness. This scientific aura began to develop in part as licensure and standards of care among practitioners increased, which led to a rising cost of providing medical care.[6,7,8]

2.1.2 Rising Medical Costs for Doctors: Medical Licensure and Manpower Issues

The American Medical Association (AMA) brought about several changes in the 1910s that led to an increase in the quality of physicians. In 1904, the Council on Medical Education was formed to standardize the requirements for medical licensure.[8] The Council invited Abraham Flexner of the Carnegie Foundation for the Advancement of Teaching to evaluate the status of medical education. Flexner's highly critical report on medical education was published in 1910. According to Flexner, the methods of medical education had "resulted in enormous overproduction of physicians at a low level, and that, whatever the justification in the past, the present situation … can be more effectively met by a reduced output of well-trained men than by further inflation with an inferior product."[9] Flexner argued for stricter medical school entrance requirements, better training facilities, higher tuition, and tougher academic standards and outcome measures. Following the publication of the Flexner Report, the number of U.S. medical schools dropped from 131 in 1910 to 95 in 1915. By 1922, the number of medical schools in the United States had fallen even further to 81.[4] The improved requirements resulted in two important changes[1]: an improvement in the quality of physician education and practice standards and expectations resulting in improved outcomes and thus a perceived and actual increase in value for physician services by the public; and[2] restriction of physician supply increasing demand and putting an upward arc on physician salaries.

2.1.3 The Blues

Improved technology, increased costs associated with building hospitals, the movement from home care to hospital based medical care, and a rise in physician salaries resulted in a slow and gradual push for health insurance. Another factor, the Great

Depression, also facilitated the development of health insurance. In the early 1930s, at the height of the Great Depression, the biggest health concern of America was how to pay for medical needs of the population.[10] The national income was less than half of what it had been in 1929, and in several states as many as 40% of the people were unemployed and receiving government-sponsored relief. Many Americans could not pay their medical bills or the visits to physicians and hospitals. Before the Depression, physicians charged patients via a fee-for-service reimbursement model. During the Depression this evolved to a sliding scale model (pay what you can afford) and physicians collected their bills as best they could. They also saw patients on a charity basis and passed the expenses along to those who could pay. Loss of medical services and reduced ability to pay meant lower incomes for physicians, too. While physicians as a group fared better than many other professions during the Depression, many saw their income levels cut in half. Hospitals were in similar trouble. Beds went empty as patients could no longer afford a 2-week hospitalization stay, which was the average in 1933. Bills were unpaid, and charitable contributions to hospital fund-raising efforts fell.[10]

Blue Cross and Blue Shield developed separately, with Blue Cross plans providing coverage for hospital services and Blue Shield covering physicians' services.[9] Blue Cross is a name currently used by an association of health insurance plans throughout the United States. Originally developed by Justin Ford Kimball, vice president of Baylor University Hospital in Dallas, Texas in 1929, the plan was an effort to ease the health care cost burden of Dallas teachers. His plan guaranteed teachers 21 days of fully reimbursed hospital care for $6 per year.[10] Eventually, the plan was extended to other employees working in Dallas and then eventually nationwide. The American Hospital Association adopted the Blue Cross symbol in 1939 as the emblem for medical insurance plans meeting predetermined standards of quality and services covered.[10]

While Blue Cross covered hospital costs, Blue Shield was developed by employers in lumber and mining camps of the Pacific Northwest to provide outpatient medical care to employees. The original plan was financed by the employers who paid monthly fees to a local medical service bureau composed of health care practitioners. The bureau provided the medical care to the employees in return for the monthly stipends.[10] In 1939, the first official Blue Shield plan was founded in California. In 1948, the symbol was informally adopted by nine plans called the Associated Medical Care Plan and was later renamed the National Association of Blue Shield Plans.

2.1.4 Continued Growth in Health Insurance

In the 1940s to 1960s, there was a slow, steady, but apparently reluctant growth in health insurance coverage. Insurance companies realized the profitability in providing health insurance products to workers. By providing insurance products to persons capable of working full time, insurance companies avoided "adverse selection"—an industry term indicating the provision of coverage to nonworking and perhaps older persons who may naturally have more costly health care needs than those employed. Those who were healthy enough to work were going to

be healthier by natural selection. By the 1940s, the provision of most commercial health care insurances became part of the standard benefits package for working Americans. Along with salary, vacation days, and sick days, employers began providing medical insurance coverage to their employees. The terminology evolved from medical "insurance" to medical "benefits." Medical insurance became a low-cost draw to pull skilled workers into the booming postwar U.S. industry. Governmental policies also encouraged the provision of health benefits to employees. Employers did not have to pay taxes on money contributed to health insurance plans, and employees did not have to pay income tax on the benefit (an IRS administrative ruling in 1943).[11]

2.1.5 The National Health Insurance Dream

As the 20th century dawned, the United States benefitted from the industrial revolution, inexpensive energy, ample environmental and human resources to become a world power. As salaries and opportunities rose, most Americans changed their life aims from simply survival to the quality of life lived. Subsistence living was replaced for many (but certainly not all!) by accumulation of wealth and improved quality of life. Americans began to believe the "American Dream"—the promise that if one works hard enough, success will follow. And, along with monetary success, Americans, for the first time, began to consider adding health care to the list of "unalienable rights" discussed by Thomas Jefferson in the Declaration of Independence. Americans began to believe that health was part of Jefferson's "life, liberty, and the pursuit of happiness." This movement prompted Theodore Roosevelt, first as president and later as a candidate for reelection of the newly formed Progressive Party, to consider "national health insurance" as provided by the states, as a right for all Americans.[12] In addition, improved international communication permitted many Americans to learn that many European countries have been providing health insurance to its citizens for decades.[13] However, opposition from doctors, labor, insurance companies, and business contributed to the failure of Roosevelt and the Progressives to achieve compulsory national health insurance.[14]

The second major attempt to develop a national insurance benefit was by the Committee on the Cost of Medical Care (CCMC).[14] Altruistic concerns over the cost and distribution of medical care led to the formation of this self-created, privately funded group. The committee was funded by eight philanthropic organizations including the Rockefeller, Millbank, and Rosenwald Foundations. Representatives first met in 1926 and ceased meeting in 1932. The CCMC was composed of fifty economists, physicians, public health specialists, and major interest groups. Their research determined that there was a need for more medical care for everyone, and they published these findings in 26 research volumes and 15 smaller reports over a 5-year period.[14] The CCMC recommended that more national resources go to medical care and saw voluntary, not compulsory, health insurance as a means to covering these costs. Most CCMC members opposed compulsory health insurance, but there was no consensus on this point within the committee. The AMA treated its report as a radical document advocating socialized medicine, and the acerbic, conservative, protectionist, and hyperbolic editor of the *Journal of the American Medical Association* called it "an incitement to revolution."[15]

Franklin D. Roosevelt, whose presidential tenure (1933–1945) can be characterized through seismic events such as World War II, the Great Depression, and the New Deal (including the Social Security Bill) advocated for consideration of compulsory health insurance benefits. As with his distant cousin Theodore's attempts two decades earlier to enact compulsory health insurance, Franklin Roosevelt's attempt also failed primarily due to prioritization of government-sponsored benefits for the unemployed and the elderly—primarily food and job creation—rather than insurance. Roosevelt's Committee on Economic Security feared that inclusion of health insurance in its bill, which was opposed by the AMA, would threaten the passage of the entire Social Security legislation. Therefore, compulsory health insurance was excluded from the bill.[16]

During Roosevelt's presidency, Congress attempted to enact The Wagner National Health Act of 1939. Never receiving Roosevelt's full support, the proposal grew out of his Tactical Committee on Medical Care, established in 1937. The essential elements of the technical committee's reports were incorporated into Senator Wagner's bill, the National Health Act of 1939, which gave general support for a national health program to be funded by federal grants to states and administered by states and localities. However, the 1938 election brought a conservative resurgence and any further innovations in social policy proved untenable.[16]

The Wagner Bill evolved and shifted from a proposal for federal grants-in-aid to a proposal for national health insurance. Reintroduced in 1943, it became the Wagner–Murray–Dingell Bill. The Bill called for compulsory national health insurance financed through a special payroll tax. In 1944, the Committee for the Nation's Health (which grew out of the earlier Social Security Charter Committee), a group of representatives from labor, agriculture, and liberal physicians who were the foremost lobbying group for the Wagner–Murray–Dingell Bill. Prominent members of the committee included Senators Murray and Dingell, the head of the Physician's Forum, and Henry Sigerist, a prominent Johns Hopkins University public health scholar. Opposition to this bill was enormous and the antagonists launched a scathing red baiting/anticommunist attack on the Committee stating that one of its key policy analysts, I.S. Falk, was a conduit between the International Labor Organization (ILO) in Switzerland and the U.S. government. Those against the bill vigorously proclaimed that the ILO was redbaited as "an awesome political machine bent on world domination." Although the Wagner–Murray–Dingell Bill generated extensive national debates, the bill was never approved by Congress despite its reintroduction every session for the next 14 years. Had the Wagner–Murray–Dingell Act been enacted, it would have established compulsory national health insurance for all Americans funded by payroll taxes.[17]

2.1.6 Truman's Support: Another Failed Attempt

After Roosevelt's death, Harry Truman became president (1945–1953) and compulsory national health received his unreserved support. "Socialized medicine" became a code word for compulsory health insurance and thus became entangled in Cold War politics of the day. Opponents were able to equate "socialized medicine" with communism—a symbolic issue in the growing crusade against communist influence in America and the world.[18] During this time period the fear of communists was omnipresent in American society. Exacerbated by the witch hunts associated with the activities of Senator Joseph McCarthy and others and the House Un-American Activities Committee, anything associated with communism was particularly avoided for risk of being tainted with the communist stigma.

Truman's plan for national health insurance in 1945 differed from Roosevelt's 1938 plan because Truman was strongly committed to a single universal comprehensive health insurance plan. Whereas Roosevelt's 1938 program had a separate proposal for medical care of the needy, it was Truman who proposed a single payer system that included all classes of society, not just the working and disadvantaged classes. He emphasized that this was not "socialized medicine." He also dropped the funeral benefit that contributed to the defeat of national insurance in the Progressive Era. Congress had mixed reactions to Truman's proposal. The chairman of the House Committee was an antiunion conservative and refused to hold hearings. Senior Republican Senator Taft declared, "I consider it socialism. It is to my mind the most socialistic measure this Congress has ever had before it."[17] Taft suggested that compulsory health insurance, like the Full Unemployment Act, came right out of the Soviet constitution and walked out of the hearings.[17] The AMA, the American Bar Association, and the conservative press had no mixed feelings; they hated the plan. The AMA claimed it would make doctors "slaves"—a statement of particular jarring injustice to those Americans who fewer than 80 years previously were in fact slaves.[18] The Republican successes in the 1946 congressional elections delayed further action by Truman until his surprise 1948 reelection. With renewed vigor, Truman again introduced a national health care insurance bill to Congress. The AMA responded angrily by assessing their members an extra $25 each to resist Truman's plan and during the years 1945 to 1948 spent what was up to then the most expensive lobbying effort in American history.[18] The AMA distributed one pamphlet that read, "Would socialized medicine lead to socialization of other phases of life? Lenin thought so. He declared socialized medicine is the keystone to the arch of the socialist state."[17] The link to communist rhetoric sealed the victory for the AMA and Truman's plan died in a congressional committee.

Discouraged by yet another defeat, the advocates of universal health insurance now turned toward a more modest proposal: hospital insurance for the aged and poor and, thus, the beginnings of the Medicare and Medicaid debates. The hopes of a universal health insurance with a one-payer system for all Americans, financed by the federal or state governments had ended. Today almost seven decades have passed since President Truman's quixotic attempts at health care legislation failed and hopes of a national health insurance in the United States appear more unlikely than ever. The reasons for failure are many and include many actors, philosophies, tenets, and beliefs: interest group influence (code words for upper class), ideological differences, anti-communism, anti-socialism, fragmentation of public policy, the entrepreneurial character of American medicine, the fear of greater governmental influence in yet another aspect of our lives, a tradition of American voluntarism and self-reliance, removing the middle class from the coalition of advocates for change through the alternative of Blue Cross private insurance plans, and the association (and perceived successes) of current and past public and nongovernmental programs providing health care to the poor and uninsured.

2.1.7 President Johnson and the Medicare/Medicaid Compromise

By 1958, 75% of Americans had some form of private insurance. The number of working Americans with employer-financed health care insurance gradually increased over this period owing primarily due to worker expectation of health insurance coverage and from union pressure. However, the figurative doughnut hole of the time was coverage for the poor, disabled, and elderly. Employer-financed coverage ended at employment termination: voluntary or involuntary separation retirement, illness, or disability. Unfortunately, the elderly, sick, and recently disabled Americans were often unable to be the sole financer of their health insurance premiums. By advocates of compulsory health insurance concentrating on the vulnerable uninsured and underinsured cohorts, public opinion began to change in favor of a minimum compulsory program providing assistance to these particular groups. Rhode Island congressman Aime Forand introduced a new proposal in 1958 to cover hospital costs for the aged on social security.[19] Predictably, the AMA undertook a massive campaign to portray a government insurance plan as a threat to the patient–doctor relationship. Counter to the AMA proposal was major grassroots support from seniors and advocacy groups which assumed the proportions of a crusade. In the entire history of the national health insurance campaign, this was the first time that a ground swell of grassroots support forced an issue onto the national agenda. The AMA countered by introducing the "Eldercare Plan," which was voluntary insurance with broader benefits and coverage for physician services.[20] In response, the government expanded its proposed legislation to cover physician services. The necessary political compromises and private concessions to the doctors (reimbursements of their customary, reasonable, and prevailing fees), to the hospitals (cost plus reimbursement), and to the Republicans (quid pro quo arrangements) permitted the Democratic administration to create a three-part compulsory health care plan for seniors, the poor, and the disabled. The plan called for comprehensive inpatient health insurance ("Part A"), the revised Republican Eldercare Plan for outpatient coverage ("Part B"), and, inpatient and outpatient coverage for the poor, Medicaid. In 1965, President Johnson signed the legislation into law, The Medicare Act, as part of his Great Society initiative. The largest and most comprehensive fundamental health care reimbursement initiative, initially proposed more than 50 years earlier from President Theodore Roosevelt—though certainly not compulsory for all Americans—came to pass. Overnight millions of Americans (older adults, the old, the poor, the disabled) were provided with unprecedented health insurance benefits by the federal and state governments.

Thus began the golden age of U.S. health care, an era in which the vulnerable, the aged, the disabled, and most working Americans were provided health care insurance, either from their employer or from the government. The increasing number of Americans insured provided reimbursement money to hospitals and physicians facilitating the building of new and more modern hospital facilities. Money became available for health care diagnostic and intervention technology purchases by hospitals and physicians funneling money back to the manufacturers for further research and development. MRIs, CTs, laparoscopic surgeries, interventional radiology, new medications, electrophysiological testing, lithotripsy, and arthroscopy—all had their origins during this golden age of U.S. health care inspiration.

Medicaid and Medicare met all expectations of service to the poor, disabled, and elderly, plus one. The big "one" was the cost. No one fully anticipated the cost directly and indirectly to the federal and state governments, local governments, and employers. Yearly health care cost of living indices greatly exceeded those of the consumer price index. From 1965 through today, insurance companies, including Medicare and Medicaid, have attempted to reduce this Sisyphean burden by attempting to rein in costs through internal and external policy and legislation.

2.1.8 Rising Costs and Managed Competition

Health maintenance organization (HMO) is a term first conceived of by Dr. Paul Ellwood Jr who today is often referred to—initially respectfully but now perhaps dubiously—as the "Father of the HMO." Dr. Ellwood coined the term "health maintenance organization," or HMO, in a 1970 Fortune magazine article and became a strong and vocal advocate for this novel type of health care delivery/reimbursement schema.[21] The concept for the HMO Act began with discussions Ellwood and his Interstudy group members had with President Richard Nixon's administration advisors who were looking for methods to curb medical inflation. Medical inflation, since the enactment of the Medicare Act of 1965, was consistently outpacing the consumer price index and thus, with Medicare and Medicaid program reimbursement being the responsibility of state and federal governments, taking a larger and larger percentage of government spending. Ellwood's work led to the eventual HMO Act of 1973.[22]

The HMO Act provided grants and loans to develop or expand HMOs across the United States, removed certain state restrictions for federally qualified HMOs, and required employers with 25 or more employees to offer federally certified HMO options to employees. The HMO Act did not require employers to offer health insurance. The HMO Act solidified the HMO as a permanent option for health insurance and gave HMOs greater access to the employer-based health care market.[22]

With the passage of the HMO Act of 1973,[22] many naysayer traditionalists, especially those aligned with traditional commercial health insurance plans, thought that the world of health care would come to an end. Advocates for the HMO Act felt the HMO revolution would provide health care value and improved outcomes to all citizens and care and coverage for those previously underserved. Neither outcome came to fruition.

Briefly, managed care is a synonym for HMO and is so named because the design was for the primary care physician (PCP)—previously known as the "general practitioner: and later as the "family doctor"—to be the "manager" or gatekeeper of health care services for the patient. All requests for services, save for some types of emergent care, were required to be performed by the PCP or approved for provision by others by the PCP via referral. Unnecessary or nonevidence-based requests for care by the patient or consultant would be theoretically denied by the PCP thus saving the insurer from paying for unnecessary or ineffective care. PCPs were financially incentivized (rewarded) by limiting referrals. Regular visits to the PCP (preventive medicine) were encouraged and facilitated by very low copays for PCP visits. "Networks" of practitioners were formed by the managed care insurer limiting the pool of possible referrals. "Out of network referral" cost was shifted to either the PCP or patient. The system was formulated to contain costs while simultaneously increasing the quality of care. Previous traditional fee-for-service medicine (paying by product or service) had led to health care inflation because it encouraged caregivers to maximize the number of procedures they performed while not prioritizing preventive services. Medicare, Medicaid, and traditional commercial insurances did not reimburse doctors and hospitals to keep patients well; they were paid to treat them when they were sick. HMOs were designed to significantly change that paradigm.

In reality, HMO plans had a short-range focus to save money. HMOs did not provide greater fiscal value or improved health metrics. Published outcome measures of patients cared for in the HMO model did not validate the expected quality of life and clinical improvements expected and, in some instances, studies indicate poorer outcome measures in patients insured through HMOs as compared with those insured by traditional fee-for-service reimbursement insurers.[23,24] HMOs, critics complained, remained solvent by what was alleged to be appropriate care denied and lives ruined.[24] Patients jumped from managed care company to managed care company looking for bargains, improved customer service, and ease of navigation of the referral process. Those HMOs that did have preventive care programs found them ineffective because patients in large numbers did not stay with one plan for a sufficient duration to show, for example, lower long-term health care costs for better managing the acute complications of diabetes. By the end of the 1990s, the public and the providers had complained and rebelled enough that plans had to start loosening their hold on the insurance marketplace.[23,25]

2.1.9 Affordable Care Act

The Patient Protection and Affordable Care Act (PPACA or simply ACA), commonly called the Affordable Care Act (ACA) or Obamacare, is a U.S. federal law proposed by and enacted by President Barack Obama. The legislation became law on March 23, 2010. Together with its sister legislation, the Health Care and Educational Reconciliation Act, the ACA represented the most significant regulatory overhaul of the U.S. health care system since the 1965 Medicare Act. Under the ACA, hospitals and primary physicians transformed their practices financially, technologically, and clinically to drive better health outcomes, lower costs, and improve their methods of distribution and accessibility.[26]

The ACA was also intended to improve health insurance quality and affordability for all Americans and lower the uninsured rate by expanding insurance coverage and reducing health care costs. The ACA introduced innovative mechanisms and practices including health care mandates, reimbursement subsidies, and insurance exchanges to the lexicon of all Americans. The ACA, among its

many provisions, requires insurers to accept all applicants, cover a specific list of conditions, charge the same rates regardless of pre-existing conditions, and permit young adults up to age 26 to remain on their parents' insurance (see ▶ Table 2.1).[27]

The ACA has resulted in a significant reduction in the number and percentage of people without health insurance. The Centers for Disease Control (CDC) reported that the percentage of people without health insurance fell from 16.0% in 2010 to 8.9% during the January to June 2016 period.[28] The Congressional Budget Office reported in March 2016 that there were approximately 23 million people with insurance due to the law, with 12 million people covered by the exchanges (10 million of whom received subsidies to help pay for insurance) and 11 million made eligible for Medicaid.[29] By 2017, nearly 70% of those on the exchanges could purchase insurance for less than $75 per month after subsidies, which rose to offset significant pre-subsidy price increases in the exchange markets.

Efforts to invalidate, repeal, or limit the ACA have moved forward in courts, Congress, and state legislatures. Politicians and lawyers opposing the ACA have delineated a set of presumptive problems with it. For instance, many believed Congress lacked authority to provide for the ACA's central provisions (e.g., the so-called "individual mandate"), that implementing the ACA

Table 2.1 The Affordable Care Act

Coverage	Ends preexisting condition exclusions for children	Health plans can no longer limit or deny benefits to children under 19 due to a preexisting condition
	Keeps young adults covered	If you are under 26, you may be eligible to be covered under your parent's health plan
	Ends arbitrary withdrawals of insurance coverage	Insurers can no longer end coverage just because you made an honest mistake
	Guarantees your right to appeal	You now have the right to ask that your plan reconsider its denial of payment
Costs	Ends lifetime limits on coverage	Lifetime limits on most benefits are banned for all new health care insurance plans
	Reviews premium increases	Insurance companies must now publicly justify any unreasonable rate hikes
	Helps you get the most from your premium dollars	Your premium dollars must be spent primarily on health care—not administrative costs
Care	Covers preventive care at no cost to you	You may be eligible for recommended preventive health services. No copayment
	Protects your choice of doctors	Choose the primary care doctor you want from your plan's network
	Removes insurance company barriers to emergency services	You can seek emergency care at a hospital outside of your health plan's network

Source: http://www.hhs.gov/healthcare/about-the-law/index.html. Accessed December 1, 2016 will increase the nation's deficit, and that the Act fundamentally limits freedom and choice. To date, all attempts at repeal or limiting the Act in court have been unsuccessful.[28] At the writing of this chapter, President Donald Trump has vowed to repeal the ACA and replace it with a "terrific" alternative.[30]

2.1.10 Where We Are Now

The brief review of U.S. health care reimbursement provided in the previous pages may appear to be a history of multiple attempts offered by multiple constituencies resulting in multiple successes and multiple failures to develop and implement a consensus plan for health care reform. The results we see today are a hodgepodge of public, private, governmental, patient, and "lack of" financed health care insurance with a varied menu of benefits which confuse and bewilder the provider and customer of health care services. Wide health disparities exist in the United States based on income, race, ethnicity, age, and location. Payment rules and policies vary yearly and new products continuously emerge. The only true consistency in the U.S. health care system is that Americans pay more for health care than any other nation and our outcomes continue to drift downward in comparison with other countries' outcomes.[31] Inaction, too much action, poor decisions, wasted money, political partisanship, and self-serving interests have negatively affected our health care system.

With the U.S.'s amalgam of private, not-for-profit, and public insurances, the expansion of the insurance industry has not been based on a demand for quality by the public or employers but on the insurers' ability to make a profit or to sustain a business model. This practice continues and deepens as more and more hospitals, physician practices, and physical therapy practices are "owned" by corporations many of which are for-profit and/or publicly traded companies. We remain the only "industrialized" country with no compulsory health care system for all citizens. Many Americans see a national health insurance with equal benefits for all—with either a single or multiple payer system—as the ultimate goal.

Physicians opposed health care insurance from the onset of discussions, opposed Medicare, opposed managed care, and generally opposed the ACA. Maggie Mahar, noted insurance blogger, has pointed out how the medical industrial complex—pharmaceutical and device companies—has caused an explosion of costs and cost increases.[32] The politicians, the presidents, and the Democrats and the Republicans, all failed to enact health care legislation and reform that they all agree at the outset and most continue to believe so currently, is a national moral imperative.

At this writing, as Washington readies itself for President Trump and Republican-led houses of Congress, one can only guess the course of our health care system over the next four years. President Trump has stated his intention to do away with the Affordable Care Act but has not yet proposed replacement legislation. As Washington fiddles, health disparities in this country grow and the quality chasm deepens.

2.2 Physical Therapy Reimbursement

2.2.1 Overview

The key concept in understanding reimbursement for physical therapy services is that each arena in which physical therapy services are provided: acute care inpatient, skilled nursing facility (SNF) inpatient, acute medical rehabilitation inpatient, long-term acute care inpatient, specialty hospital inpatient, home care, emergency department, preoperative examination, outpatient clinic, prosthetic clinic, lymphedema therapy, and so forth, has its unique reimbursement policies, patterns, and processes. What may be a covered service in the outpatient arena may be considered an uncovered service in the acute care hospital inpatient arena. Billing procedures mandated in one arena are prohibited in another. In most inpatient arenas, there is no direct reimbursement for physical therapy services provided. Newer bundled payment practices combine specific inpatient and outpatient intervention reimbursement for the same episode of care. The best way to learn reimbursement is by arena. However, prior to discuss billing related to arena, the physical therapist needs to have a strong understanding of the terms of billing and of how billing is performed (see ► Table 2.2). Reimbursement remains one of the more confusing aspects of health care services. With a unique lexicon, providers and those receiving services must fully understand the language in order to make cogent health care decisions.

2.2.2 International Classification of Diseases

In any arena where physical therapy services are provided, insurers require a diagnosis—or more specifically, a diagnosis code. The International Statistical Classification of Diseases and Related Health Problems, usually referred to by the short-form name International Classification of Diseases or the abbreviation ICD, is the international "standard diagnostic tool for epidemiology, health management, and clinical purposes."[33] The ICD is maintained by the World Health Organization (WHO). The ICD is designed as a health care diagnostic classification system providing a system of diagnostic codes for classification of disease including a nuanced classification of a wide spectrum of signs, symptoms, abnormal testing results, complaints, downstream social and psychological impacts of diseases, and etiology of injury and disease. This system is designed to map health conditions to corresponding generic categories together with specific variations assigning for these a designated code up to six characters long. Major categories are designed to include a set of similar diseases.[34]

The ICD is published by the WHO and used worldwide for a basis for common terminology used in global health, public health, and medical record systems and research, morbidity and mortality statistics, billing and reimbursement systems, and automated decision support in health care. This system is designed to promote international comparability in the collection, processing, classification, and presentation of these statistics. ICD's analog in behavioral disorders is the Diagnostic and Statistical Manual of Mental Disorders.[35,36]

The ICD is revised periodically and is currently in its tenth revision.[34] The ICD-10, as it is known—the "10" indicating the revision number—has been used since 1992 to track health statistics. The United States adopted the ICD-10 in 2015.[36] ICD-11 was planned for 2017[34] but has been delayed to 2018. Annual minor updates and triennial major updates are published by the WHO. The ICD is part of a "family" of guides that can be

Table 2.2 Glossary of physical therapy reimbursement terms

Acute medical rehabilitation	A hospital, or part of a hospital, that provides an intensive rehabilitation program to inpatients
Advanced beneficiary notice	In Original Medicare, a notice that a doctor, supplier, or provider gives a person with Medicare before furnishing an item or service if the doctor, supplier, or provider believes that Medicare may deny payment
Benefits	The health care items or services covered under a health insurance plan. Covered benefits and excluded services are defined in the health insurance plan's coverage documents
Claim	A request for payment that the patient submits to Medicare or other health insurance when the patient receives items and services that the patient believes are covered
Coinsurance	An amount you may be required to pay as your share of the cost for services after you pay any deductibles. Coinsurance is usually a percentage (e.g., 20%)
Copayment	An amount the patient may be required to pay as share of the cost for a medical service or supply, like a doctor's visit, hospital outpatient visit, or prescription drug. A copayment is usually a set amount, rather than a percentage. For example, the patient may pay $10 or $20 for a doctor's visit or prescription drug
Custodial care	Non-skilled personal care, like help with activities of daily living like bathing, dressing, eating, getting in or out of a bed or chair, moving around, and using the bathroom. It may also include the kind of health-related care that most people do themselves, like using eye drops. In most cases, Medicare doesn't pay for custodial care
Deductible	The amount the patient must pay for health care or prescriptions before Original Medicare, the prescription drug plan, or your other insurance begins to pay
Department of Health and Human Services	The federal agency that oversees CMS, which administers programs for protecting the health of all Americans, including Medicare, the Marketplace, Medicaid, and the CHIP
Durable medical equipment	Certain medical equipment, like a walker, wheelchair, or hospital bed, that's ordered by the doctor for use in the home
Health care provider	A person or organization that's licensed to give health care. Doctors, nurses, and hospitals are examples of health care providers
Health insurance marketplace	A service that helps people shop for and enroll in affordable health insurance. The federal government operates the Marketplace, available at HealthCare.gov, for most states. Some states run their own Marketplaces The Health Insurance Marketplace (also known as the "Marketplace" or "exchange") provides health plan shopping and enrollment services through websites, call centers, and in-person help
Health Insurance Portability and Accountability Act (HIPAA)	The "Standard for Privacy of Individually Identifiable Health Information" (also called the "Privacy Rule") of HIPPA assures health information is properly protected while allowing the flow of health information needed to provide and promote high quality health care and to protect the public's health and well-being
Home health care	Health care services and supplies a doctor decides are necessary to receive in the home under a plan of care established by the doctor. Medicare only covers home health care on a limited basis as ordered by the doctor
Homebound	To be homebound means • Difficulty leaving your home without assistance because of an illness or injury, or • Leaving your home isn't recommended because of a medical condition • The patient may leave home for medical treatment or short, infrequent absences for nonmedical reasons, like attending religious services. • The patient can receive home health care if you attend adult day care
Hospice	A special way of caring for people who are terminally ill. Hospice care involves a team-oriented approach that addresses the medical, physical, social, emotional, and spiritual needs of the patient. Hospice also provides support to the patient's family or caregiver
Inpatient prospective payment system	Hospitals that have contracted with Medicare to provide acute inpatient care and accept a predetermined rate as payment in full
Long term care	Services that include medical and nonmedical care provided to people who are unable to perform basic activities of daily living, like dressing or bathing. Long-term supports and services can be provided at home, in the community, in assisted living, or in nursing homes. Individuals may need long-term supports and services at any age. Medicare and most health insurance plans don't pay for long-term care
Medicaid	A joint federal and state program that helps with medical costs for some people with limited income and resources. Medicaid programs vary from state to state
Medically necessary care	Health care services or supplies needed to diagnose or treat an illness, injury, condition, disease, or its symptoms and that meet accepted standards of medicine
Medicare advantage plan (Part C)	A type of Medicare health plan offered by a private company that contracts with Medicare to provide all Part A and Part B benefits. Medicare Advantage Plans include health maintenance organizations, preferred provider

(Continued)

	organizations, private fee-for-service plans, special needs plans, and Medicare medical savings account plans. If enrolled in a Medicare Advantage Plan, most Medicare services are covered through the plan and aren't paid for under Original Medicare. Most Medicare Advantage Plans offer prescription drug coverage
Medicare Part A	Part A covers inpatient hospital stays, care in a skilled nursing facility, hospice care, and some home health care
Medicare Part B	Part B covers certain doctors' services, outpatient care, medical supplies, and preventive services
Medicare prescription drug plan (Part D)	Part D adds prescription drug coverage to Original Medicare, some Medicare cost plans, some Medicare private-fee-for-service plans, and Medicare Medical savings account plans. These plans are offered by insurance companies and other private companies approved by Medicare. Medicare Advantage Plans may also offer prescription drug coverage that follows the same rules as Medicare prescription drug plans
Medicare summary notice	A notice the patient receives after the doctor, other health care provider, or supplier files a claim for Part A or Part B services in Original Medicare. It explains what the doctor, other health care provider, or supplier billed for, the Medicare-approved amount, how much Medicare paid, and what the patient must pay
Medicare	Medicare is a single-payer, national social insurance program, administered by the US federal government since 1966, currently using about 30–50 private insurance companies across the United States under contract for administration. Medicare is funded by a payroll tax, premiums and surtaxes from beneficiaries, and general revenue. It provides health insurance for Americans aged 65 and older who have worked and paid into the system through the payroll tax. It also provides health insurance to younger people with some disabilities status as determined by the Social Security Administration, as well as younger people with end stage renal disease and amyotrophic lateral sclerosis
Medigap insurance	Medicare Supplement Insurance sold by private insurance companies to fill "gaps" in Original Medicare coverage
National health insurance	NHI—sometimes called SHI—is a legally enforced scheme of health insurance that insures a national population against the costs of health care. It may be administered by the public sector, the private sector, or a combination of both. Funding mechanisms vary with the particular program and country
National health service	The NHS is the name of the public health services in the United Kingdom. Founded after World War II, the NHS was established as a major social reform on the founding principles of being comprehensive, universal and free at the point of delivery
Order (referral)	A physician (and depending on the jurisdiction, a dentist, nurse practitioner, or physician assistant) provides an order for service. The order typically contains a diagnosis and recommendations for intervention. In some jurisdictions, qualified physical therapists do not require an order prior to evaluating and treating specific outpatient conditions
Preventive services	Health care to prevent illness or detect illness at an early stage, when treatment is likely to work best (e.g., preventive services include Pap tests, flu shots, and screening mammograms)
Primary care physician	The doctor seen first for most health problems. He or she ensures the patient receives the needed care. Many insurances require the primary care doctor to approve a referral to a specialist
Referral	A written order from the primary care doctor to see a specialist or get certain medical services. In many HMOs, a referral must be generated prior to receiving medical care from anyone except the primary care doctor
Respite care	Temporary care provided in a nursing home, hospice inpatient facility, or hospital so that a family member or friend who is the patient's caregiver can rest or take some time off. Typically not covered by insurance
Service-based supervised or untimed) CPT codes	Specific codes to permit services such as conducting and evaluation or applying hot/cold packs. Time is not important; only one code can be billed regardless of the time to perform the evaluation or assessment
Skilled nursing facility	A nursing facility with the staff and equipment to give skilled nursing care and, in most cases, skilled rehabilitative services and other related health services
Time-based (constant attendance) CPT codes	Specific codes which allow for variable billing in 15-minute increments when a practitioner provides a patient with one-on-one services such as manual therapy or gait training
Treatment	The intervention; the therapeutic service received by the patient
Worker's compensation health insurance	Workers' compensation is a form of insurance providing wage replacement and medical benefits to employees injured in the course of employment in exchange for mandatory relinquishment of the employee's right to sue his or her employer for the tort of negligence.

Abbreviations: CHIP, children's health insurance program; CPT, current procedural terminology; HMO, health maintenance organization; NHI, national health insurance; NHS, national health service; SHI, statutory health insurance.
Source: https://www.medicare.gov/glossary/a.html. Accessed December 13, 2016.

used to complement each other, including also the International Classification of Functioning, Disability and Health which focuses on the domains of functioning (disability) associated with health conditions, from a medical and social perspective.[37]

From a physical therapy viewpoint, all bills for services must contain the diagnosis and ICD-10 diagnostic code.

2.2.3 Current Procedural Terminology

Physical therapists and all providers of medical and wellness services rely on the Current Procedural Terminology (CPT) to report their services for payment to the Centers for Medicare and Medicaid Services (CMS) and other third-party payers. Historically, CPT codes were used to translate the diagnostic testing and interventions performed by the health care worker or facility to payers to quantify reimbursement. Recently, however, CPT coding has begun to capture quality and outcome measures —a feature that is likely to have increasing importance in the era of Pay for Performance[38] and the Physician Quality Reporting Initiative.[39] In the health care industry, pay for performance (P4P), also known as "value-based purchasing" is a payment model that offers financial incentives to physicians, hospitals, medical groups, and other health care providers and in the future, physical and occupational therapists, for meeting benchmark performance measures. For most medical specialties, clinical outcomes such as longer survival and infant mortality are difficult to measure due to the quantity of confounding variables associated with these outcomes. Therefore, pay for performance systems usually utilize outcome measures such as process timeliness, quality, and efficiency. Examples include measuring blood pressure at each outpatient visit, the administration of prophylactic influenza vaccinations, performance of regular and routine hemoglobin A1C testing in persons with diabetes, and the documentation of smoking cessation counseling. The Physician Quality Reporting System (PQRS) is a quality reporting program that encourages individual eligible professionals (EPs) and group practices to report information on the quality of care to Medicare. PQRS gives participating EPs and group practices the opportunity to assess the quality of care they provide to their patients, helping to ensure that patients receive the right care at the right time. By reporting on PQRS quality measures, individual EPs and group practices can also quantify how often they are meeting a particular quality metric. In 2015, the program began applying a negative payment adjustment to individual EPs and PQRS group practices who did not satisfactorily report data on quality measures for Part B Medicare physician fee schedule (MPFS) for covered professional services in 2013.[39]

Currently, physical therapists are not responsible for PQRS reporting and are not reimbursed under a pay for performance model.

CPT is owned and maintained by the AMA of the United States and maintains copyright protection on CPT. CPT dates back to 1966 with the first edition focusing on codes for surgical procedures. The second edition, published in 1970, expanded CPT's scope to include nonsurgical interventions. The third and fourth editions were released in the 1970s. The fourth edition was a major update, and introduced a system for periodically monitoring and updating CPT. In 1983, the Health Care Financing Administration (HCFA), now CMS, adopted CPT for reporting of physician services for Medicare Part B Benefits. In 1987, HCFA also adopted CPT for reporting outpatient surgical procedures.[40,41]

The Health Insurance Portability and Accountability Act of 1996 (HIPAA) required that the Department of Health & Human Services develop standards for electronic data storage and transmission. Four years later, the department published the *Final Rule*, which selected CPT for reporting physician services (and other medical services) and the ICD-9 for reporting diagnosis codes.

2.2.4 CPT Structure

CPT codes are divided into three categories[40,41]:
- **Category I.** CPT codes are assigned to procedures that are deemed to be within the scope of medical practice across the United States. In general, such codes report services whose effectiveness is well supported in the medical literature and whose constituent parts have received clearance from the U.S. Food and Drug Administration (FDA). The Relative Value Scale (RVS) Update Committee (RUC) process assigns relative value units (RVUs) for all Category I CPT codes.
- **Category II.** CPT codes are tracking codes designed for the measurement of performance improvement. The concept is that the use of these codes should facilitate the administration of quality improvement projects by allowing for standardized reporting that captures the performance (or nonperformance) of services designated as subject to process improvement efforts.
- **Category III.** CPT codes are temporary codes for new or emerging technology or procedures. Such codes are important for data collection and serve to support the inclusion (or exclusion) of new or emergency technology in standard medical practice. Category III CPT codes are not assigned a value through the RUC process.

Therefore, only diagnostic and intervention services performed for which there exists a CPT code are eligible for reimbursement. For all medical services there is a finite list of approved codes. For example, in physical therapy there are codes for evaluation, reevaluation, modalities such as ultrasound and electrical stimulation, and procedures such as gait training and therapeutic activities. Procedures performed for which there are no codes are not reimbursable.

2.2.5 CPT Development Process

The AMA CPT Editorial Panel maintains CPT. The panel consists of 11 physicians nominated by the National Medical Specialty Societies, one physician nominated by the Blue Cross and Blue Shield Association, one physician nominated by America's Health Insurance Plans, one physician nominated by the American Hospital Association, and one physician nominated by CMS. The AMA Board of Directors approves all nominations. The CPT Health Care Professionals Advisory Committee sends two representatives.

The CPT Advisory Committee supports the CPT Editorial Panel, which consists of physicians nominated by national medical societies that are part of the AMA House of Delegates. The CPT Advisory Committee provides important information on specialty-specific issues and suggests CPT revisions. The

Performance Measures Advisory Committee (PMAC), which focuses on performance metrics, also provides input. The AMA's regular staff also provides an important role.[41]

Proposals for a new code pass through the following steps[42]:

- The specialty society develops the initial proposal. A new code may be proposed based on the recent literature, contemporary practice, technological intervention, an emerging need, and changing practice guidelines—often with written input from professional national organizations such as the American Physical Therapy Association.
- The AMA staff reviews the code proposal. This preparatory step confirms that the issue has not been previously addressed and that all of the documentation is in place and organized.
- The CPT Specialty Advisory Panel then reviews the code proposal. All members are given the opportunity to comment, and those comments are then shared with all participants in the process, but not with the general public.
- The CPT Editorial Panel then reviews the code proposal at its regularly scheduled meeting. The group can approve the code, table the proposal, or reject the proposal.
- Approved Category I codes are then submitted to the RUC for valuation.

CPT codes are the common billing language for services provided by all health care practitioners in the United States (see ▶ Table 2.3).

2.2.6 CPT Category III Process

All CPT Category III codes are removed after 5 years from the time of publication. If the original requestors of the code want to continue use of the code, they must submit a proposal for continuing the code as a Category III code or promoting it to Category I status. Due to the difficulty imagining why the fate of an emerging technology would not be clear within 5 years, no Category III code has been renewed for a second 5-year term.

Table 2.3 Examples of common CPT codes utilized by physical therapists[43]

97110	Therapeutic exercises to develop strength and endurance, range of motion, and flexibility (15 minutes)
97140	Manual therapy techniques (e.g., connective tissue massage, joint mobilization and manipulation, and manual traction) (15 minutes)
97010	Hot or cold pack application
97014	Electrical stimulation (unattended)
97112	Neuromuscular reeducation of movement, balance, coordination, kinesthetic sense, posture, and/or proprioception for sitting and/or standing activities (15 minutes)
97001	Physical therapy evaluation
97530	Dynamic activities to improve functional performance, direct (one-on-one) with the patient (15 minutes)
97035	Ultrasound (15 minutes)
97032	Electrical stimulation (manual) (15 minutes)
97116	Gait training (includes stair climbing) (15 minutes)
97012	Mechanical traction
97016	Vasopneumatic devices
97535	Self-care/home management training (e.g., ADL and compensatory training, meal preparation, safety procedures, and instructions in use of assistive technology devices/adaptive equipment), direct one-on-one contact (15 minutes)
97113	Aquatic therapy with therapeutic exercises (15 minutes)
97124	Massage, including effleurage, petrissage, and/or tapotement (stroking, compression, percussion) (15 minutes)
97033	Iontophoresis (15 minutes)
97150	Group therapeutic procedure(s) (two or more individuals)
97026	Infrared
97039	Unlisted modality (specify type and time if constant attendance)
92507	Treatment of speech, language, voice, communication, and/or auditory processing disorder; individual
97250	Myofascial release (no longer a CPT code, but billable under the California workers compensation system in lieu of 97140)
97003	Occupational therapy evaluation
97018	Paraffin bath
97022	Whirlpool
98960	Education and training for patient self-management by a qualified, nonphysician health care professional using a standardized curriculum, face-to-face with the individual patient (could include caregiver/family) (30 minutes)
29530	Knee strapping
98941	CMT of the spine (three to four regions)
29540	Ankle and/or foot strapping
29240	Shoulder strapping (e.g., Velpeau)
97139	Unlisted therapeutic procedure (specify)
97750	Physical performance test or measurement (e.g., musculoskeletal, functional capacity), with written report (15 minutes)
97004	Occupational therapy reevaluation
95831	Extremity (excluding hand) or trunk muscle testing, manual (separate procedure) with report
90901	Biofeedback training by any modality

Abbreviations: ADL, activities of daily living; CMT, chiropractic manipulative treatment; CPT, current procedural terminology.

Category III codes are important for maintaining the integrity of the CPT process, since they permit a means to track the use of new technology before such technology is widely clinically adopted. The use of similar Category I codes for new technology is clearly discouraged by the CPT rules; in fact, the rules, in their strictest sense, actually prohibit this. The other alternative is the use of unlisted procedure Category I code, but when physicians do this, it becomes impossible to measure the actual usage of a specific technology. Thus, the preferred route for coding new technology is the development and application of a Category III code.

One-on-One Services versus Group Services

Physical therapists may provide services in a group environment (one PT and more than one patient) or in a one-on-one environment (one PT and one patient). Specific insurers (notably Medicare and some Medicaid) reimburse differently for group and one-on-one care. An example of a group therapy is a physical therapist leading an aquatics exercise class for five persons who recently underwent hip arthroplasty. An example of one-on-one therapy is one physical therapist providing gait training to a client who has recently received a new prosthesis. To facilitate the performance of group versus one-on-one billing CPT provides a list of "group" and "individual" (one-on-one) codes. The rationale for group versus individual reimbursement is that if the physical therapist is sharing his time equally among five patients, he should only "bill" each patient for a percentage of his time and effort. In addition, by fiscally encouraging physical therapists to preferentially bill individually rather than group (reimbursement dollars are much greater for individual than group) there is a perception that the quality of care performed will improve due to a greater percentage of attention provided to one patient than shared among individual members of the group.

One-on-one services are individual therapy services—ones that involve direct, one-on-one contact with a patient. These codes are cumulative, require constant attendance, and are time-based, which indicates the 8-minute rule (see below) applies. The Center for Medicare and Medicaid Services does permit one-to-one billing in a group situation but only for the exact time spent with each patient. For instance, if a therapist has two patients with Medicare insurance and both arrive in the clinic at 10 a.m. and leave at 11 a.m., the therapist, can count the minutes spent with each patient over the course of that hour, and bill individual codes for the time spent—as long as those intervals are "of a sufficient length of time to provide the appropriate skilled treatment in accordance with each patient's plan of care."[44] For these two patients the total minutes billed for both patients cannot exceed 60. In this instance, the therapist may bill patient A for 45 minutes of therapy and patient B for 15 minutes of therapy.

Group therapy still requires constant attendance, but it does not involve one-on-one contact with the patient. Rather, CMS writes that it "consists of simultaneous treatment to two or more patients who may or may not be doing the same activities."[44] So, if you are providing attention to more than one patient at a time with only "brief, intermittent personal contact," you should bill one unit of group therapy to each patient.

Advance Beneficiary Notice

An advance beneficiary notice (ABN), also known as a waiver of liability, is a notice patients should receive when a provider or supplier offers a service or item they believe Medicare will not cover, or—in the case of ongoing outpatient physical therapy services—will no longer cover.[45] Providers must provide an ABN when the service or item could be covered by Medicare, but the provider expects that Medicare will not find the care to be medically necessary or no longer medically necessary and will, therefore, deny coverage. ABNs only apply to Medicare and not Medicare Advantage programs. The ABN must list the reason why the provider doubts Medicare will cover care. For example, the physical therapist may write on the ABN that, "In my professional opinion, I feel that the patient has plateaued in outpatient physical therapy and no longer requires skilled care." Providers are not required to provide an ABN for services or items that are never covered by Medicare, such as hearing aids.[46]

The ABN serves as warning that Medicare may not pay for the care that a provider has recommended or the patient requests. However, it is still possible that Medicare will approve coverage.

Following the diagnostic testing, intervention, or provision of equipment, if the Medicare Summary Notice (MSN) received by the physical therapist from Medicare indicates that Medicare has denied payment for a service or item, the patient should file an appeal for reimbursement. If the appeal fails, the patient is then responsible for the cost of the services received.

Medicare has rules about when the patient should receive an ABN and how it should be written. If these rules are not followed, the patient may not be responsible for the cost of the care. However, the patient will have to file an appeal to prove this.

The patient may not be responsible for charges if the ABN[45,46,47]
- Is given by the provider (except a lab) to every patient with no reason to believe claims may be denied.
- Is poorly written and lacks sufficient rationale for the presumed denial of services.
- Does not list the actual service provided or is signed after the date the service was provided.
- Is given to the patient during an emergency or is given just prior to receiving a service (i.e., on the way into the MRI machine).

Modifiers

Procedure codes may be modified under certain circumstances to more accurately represent to the insurer the service or item rendered. For this purpose, modifiers are used to add information or change the description of service in order to improve accuracy or specificity. The documentation in the medical record of the service provided must support the use of the modifier. Insurers often request the medical record to ensure linearity of the documentation with the service provided and to document medical necessity. There are two levels of modifiers, one for each level of CPT codes. The CPT and HCPCS (primarily durable medical equipment) Coding Manuals contain a complete list of all available modifiers.[48]

Coding provides a common language throughout health care organizations and health care payers. The use of modifiers is an important part of coding and billing for health care services. Due to changes in rules and regulations with Medicare and various commercial payers modifier usage is increasing yearly.

Correct modifier use is also an important part of avoiding fraud and abuse or noncompliance issues. One of the top billing errors determined by federal, state, and private payers involves the incorrect use of modifiers.[49]

Physical therapists utilize a number of common modifiers, as given below.

Modifier 59

Under certain circumstances, the practitioner may need to indicate that a procedure or service was distinct or independent from other services performed on the same day. Modifier 59 is used to identify procedures and services that are not normally or permitted to be reported together, but are appropriate under the circumstances. Most 59 modifiers are utilized by physicians and surgeons but there are instances when they may be appropriate for use by therapists. As an example, if the therapist is providing two wholly separate and distinct services during the same treatment period, the 59 modifier may be indicated. The National Correct Coding Initiative has identified procedures that therapists commonly perform together and labeled these "edit pairs."[50] Thus, if a therapist bills a CPT code that is linked to one of these pairs, the therapist will receive payment for only one of the codes. Therefore, it is the therapist's responsibility to determine whether the services provided are linked or wholly separate. This, in turn, determines whether modifier 59 is appropriate.[50] An example is as follows: typically, evaluation and reevaluation codes are not permitted to be billed on the same day of service. If a therapist evaluates a patient with a nonhealing wound, which is impacting ambulation at 10 a.m., the therapist appropriately charges an initial evaluation charge. Then, for instance, the patient visits the physician who locally debrides the wound resulting in increased pain which disallows the patient from walking safely. The physician refers the patient back to the therapist at 2 p.m. the same day for gait training to reduce the risk of falls. The therapist may charge the insurance company a reevaluation charge using the 59 modifier.

KX Modifier/Therapy Cap

Introduced as part of the Balanced Budget Act (BBA) of 1997, the therapy cap[50] was intended as a health care cost containment solution to, along with many other measures, control Medicare costs. However, despite a long-standing push to repeal the cap, Congress has continued to renew it each year. For 2016, the cap amount is $1,960 for physical and speech pathology combined and $1,960 for occupational therapy (no suitable explanation has been found to rationalize the cost of physical therapy and speech pathology services being combined and occupational therapy services not being combined). The cap does not reset for each diagnosis; so, even if a patient seeks therapy related to multiple diagnoses over the course of the benefit period, all of those services would count toward that patient's $1,960 limit. Still, to ensure the cap does not prevent Medicare patients from obtaining medically necessary care, Congress also has passed legislation every year that allows exceptions for exceeding the cap. In 2016, there is a two-tiered exceptions process.[51]

Historically, the rules for application of the therapy cap to services furnished in critical access hospitals differed significantly from pre-2014 policy. Beginning in 2014, the therapy cap—along with the rules governing the therapy cap exceptions and manual medical review processes—applies to critical access hospitals in the same manner as all other settings. Therefore, if a patient continues treatment in a critical access hospital, after he or she exceeds the $1,960 cap for therapy services, the critical access hospital would need to follow the rules of the exceptions process for that patient.[52]

The Physical Therapy Cap originated as a method to reduce the federal budget deficit by limiting outpatient physical therapy services to those persons insured by Medicare. Advocates from all areas of society—patients, lobbying groups, therapists, and physicians—have been working for a repeal for many years.

According to CMS, the therapy cap applies to all Part B outpatient therapy services furnished in

- Private practices.
- Physician offices.
- SNFs (Part B).
- Rehabilitation agencies (also known as outpatient rehabilitation facilities, or ORFs).
- Comprehensive outpatient rehabilitation facilities (CORFs).
- Home health agencies (type of bill [TOB] 34X).
- Critical access hospitals.
- Hospital outpatient departments (HOPDs).
- Outpatient hospitals.

G Codes

"G Codes" is the common term for functional limitation reporting (FLR). As health care professional reimbursement begins its eventual shift from payment for specific services performed to a value based/outcome basis, CMS and other insurers will derive the reimbursement value based on the effectiveness of care provided. Philosophically, insurers will pay more for good outcomes and pay less for poorer outcomes. A paradigm shift as large as this one will require not only time but a large amount of data collection by the insurers in order to develop benchmark algorithms. G codes are the first attempt to begin the data collection related to functional outcomes. Currently, functional reporting applies to all claims for therapy services furnished under the Medicare Part B outpatient therapy benefit and to physical therapy (PT), occupational therapy (OT), and speech-language pathology (SLP) services furnished under the Comprehensive Outpatient Rehabilitation Facility (CORF) benefit. Therefore, FLR applies to PTs, OTs, and SLPs who provide outpatient therapy services under Medicare Part B. FLR is mandatory.

CMS requires therapists required to perform and provide FLR to do so on all Medicare Part B patients at the initial examination, at each recertification period and at discharge. Unlike the expansive new ICD-10 code set, the FLR code set is relatively small. In fact, there are only 42 G-codes to choose from when completing FLR.

FLR G-codes are part of a claims-based data collection strategy for outpatient therapy services. The G-codes are quality data codes designed to provide information on patient function during the episode of therapy to provide CMS with a better understanding of beneficiary functional limitations and outcomes. In other words, CMS is utilizing the G codes to determine which therapy interventions are successful at improving patient/client function and the time frames to do.

As current process dictates, the attending therapist identifies the patient/client's primary functional limitation and assigns the appropriate G code. Once the G code is assigned the therapist, at initial evaluation, recertification, and at the termination of care, assigns the appropriate severity modifier. The severity modifier is derived from a combination of the therapist's clinical expertise and the results of valid tests and outcome measures.

Automatic Exceptions to the Therapy Cap

CMS does provide for an exception to the therapy cap. If the therapist believes that continuing therapy with a patient is medically necessary there is a potential that the patient will qualify for additional therapy even if the cap has been met. The KX modifier along with clear and objective documentation may permit continued therapy. The KX modifier and appropriate documentation permit therapy charges to rise to $3,700.00 from the cap limit of $1,960.00. This is known as the automatic exceptions process.[52] Medical record documentation detailing the request for the automatic exception to the cap should include the following:

- Professional rational utilizing objective, measurable, valid, and reliable metrics and outcomes for the automatic exception.
- Documentation that the therapy need is reasonable and necessary.
- Documentation that the intervention requires the skills of a therapist.

Manual Medical Review

The Medicare Access and CHIP Reauthorization Act of 2015 (MACRA)[53] replaced the manual medical review process for claims that exceed the $3,700 threshold with a targeted review process. With this change, MACRA now prohibits the use of recovery auditors to conduct these reviews; instead, CMS has selected Strategic Health Solutions[54] as the supplemental medical review contractor (SMRC) and tasked it with performing the reviews for all payers on a post-payment basis. The SMRC will select claims for review when

- Providers with a high percentage of patients receive therapy beyond the thresholds as compared to other industry professionals.
- Therapy is provided in SNFs, private practices, or outpatient physical therapy, speech–language pathology, or occupational therapy clinics.

Advance Beneficiary Notice Modifiers

There are three common modifiers utilized related to the use or nonuse of an ABN[47,48]:

- GX: indicates the therapist issued a voluntary ABN for a perceived noncovered service.
- GY: indicates that the therapist performed a noncovered service but an ABN is not on file. (In this case the patient is inherently liable for charges because the service performed was noncovered.)
- GZ: indicates the therapist expects the service to be denied by Medicare because it strongly appears to be medically unnecessary but no ABN has been filed. (In this case, the patient will not be responsible for charges.)

Eight-Minute Rule

The 8-minute rule determines how many service units the physical therapist can bill to Medicare for a particular date of service.[55] According to the rule, the therapist must provide treatment for at least 8 minutes in order to receive reimbursement from Medicare for time-based codes. In addition, when two or more codes are billed, the total time must meet specific benchmarks to allow billing.

Physical therapists are reimbursed for time-based charges based on what is commonly known as the "8-minute rule" (see ▶ Table 2.4).

Bundled Payments

Bundled Payments for Care Improvement (BPCI) is a value-based reimbursement model, which is the basis for the recently instituted Comprehensive Care for Joint Replacement (CJR) reimbursement model developed by CMS,[56] which strongly impacts physical therapy reimbursement. The CJR model is a new payment model being tested for episodes of care related to total knee and total hip replacements under Medicare. The model is being tested in 67 metropolitan statistical areas for 5 years beginning April 1, 2016. Programs under the model will be administered by hospitals in the participating areas, and physical therapist practices will be impacted in those areas.

Every Medicare total hip and total knee replacement procedure within the designated areas will be administered through CJR, including rehabilitation components of the episode of care.

An alternative payment model uses a payment structure that is not based on fee for service and generally ties payment to quality measurement and improved outcomes of care. Examples include accountable care organizations, the BPCI initiative, and CJR.[57]

A CJR episode is triggered by an anchor hospitalization in which MS DRG (medical severity diagnostic-related group) 469 or 470 is billed—major joint replacement (or reattachment) of the lower extremity with or without major complication or comorbidity. The episode includes the hospitalization and 90 days of care after discharge (the date of discharge counts as the first day in the 90-day period). The episode includes all related post-acute and outpatient care and includes readmissions if related.

Table 2.4 The 8-minute rule

Units of service	(Medicare 8-minute rule)
8 to 22 minutes total for all time-based modalities	1 unit
23 to 37 minutes total for all time-based modalities	2 units
38 to 52 minutes total for all time-based modalities	3 units
53 to 67 minutes total for all time-based modalities	4 units
68 to 82 minutes total for all time-based modalities	5 units
83 minutes total for all time-based modalities	6 units

Table 3.2 Examples of health care teams by arena

Arena of health care	Physical therapy department team	Organizational team
Acute care inpatient	Performance improvement	Performance Improvement Committee
	Weekly staff meeting	Utilization Review Committee
	Journal Club	Safety Committee
	Evidenced-Based Medicine Committee	Infection Control Committee
		Institutional Research Board
		New Product Safety Evaluation Committee
Acute medical rehabilitation inpatient	Outcomes Development Committee	Initial Patient Care Conference Committee
		Ethics Committee
		Infection Control Committee
Skilled nursing facility inpatient	Long Stay Committee	Ongoing Patient Care Conference Committee
	Competency Development Committee	Marketing Committee
Home care outpatient	Compliance Committee	Multidisciplinary team meeting
General outpatient	Budget Committee	Technology Committee

Additional formal roles within the team are either defined directly by the team leader or by negotiation among the team members.

Ideally, individuals, with the approval of the leader, should be able to negotiate their roles to perform unique and meaningful tasks. However, many health care team members are unable to choose with whom they work and professional specialization and uniqueness of content area limits the transferability of roles. An even more impactful variable for effective health care teams to overcome is the inherent inconsistency between a professional's role and the way others perceive it. This inconsistency between professional role and perception is due to differences in status, skills, historical representation of the profession, learned behavior, perceived value, and the perceived relationship between income and authority. Although health care team role conflict can be exacerbated by these variables, conflict can be avoided when health care professionals work confidently and without pridefulness across disciplinary boundaries in the best interests of the patient. In fact, a symbiotic and effective health care team, which meets its assigned aims, is an effective exercise in breaking barriers between professions, enhancing the knowledge of other professions, and, most importantly, improving clinical outcomes.

3.3.3 Suitable Leadership

The team leader is always important in team dynamics but researchers have found strong and competent leadership even more important as the complexity of the team's aims and objectives increases.[23,24,25] The quality and effectiveness of the leader chosen to lead the health care team should reflect administration's perception of the importance of the team's aims.

Specific behavioral characteristics have been identified with strong health care team leaders. These characteristics include emotional intelligence, ability to delegate effectively, empathy, item-specific and panoramic content knowledge, organization, ability to control, respect of team members, and consistency.[24,25,26,27]

Traditionally, doctors have been accorded leadership of health care teams regardless of their competence.[28] This practice was most likely based on education level, salary, experience, perceived intelligence, and an extension of the historic role of the physician as the "gatekeeper" for the provision of health care to the patient. However, as the educational standards of the entry-level curricula of nonphysician members of the health care team rises new roles for health care leaders are emerging that incorporate sharing of leadership duties. Leaders chosen for content and leadership expertise have shown to be more effective leaders than leaders chosen based on historical status.[29] In today's health care it is not unusual to see a multidisciplinary health care team led by a physical therapist or case manager.

3.3.4 Members Chosen for What They Can Add to the Team

Teams require the correct number of members with the appropriate diversity of content knowledge, experience, team skills, and interpersonal abilities. A balance between homogeneity and heterogeneity of members' skills, interests and backgrounds is preferred. Homogenous teams are composed of individuals with similar experience and skill sets who complete tasks efficiently with minimal conflict. In contrast, heterogeneous teams incorporate membership diversity and therefore, through their diverse views, facilitate innovation, uniqueness of ideas, and problem solving.[30]

3.3.5 Adequate Resources

Organizations need to provide teams with adequate financial resources, administrative and technical support and professional education in order to facilitate the team in meeting its aims.[31] The most efficient and organized method of doing this is for administration to provide the team leader with a budget for available resources. Upfront budget negotiations may lead to avoidance of downstream misunderstandings.

A readily accessible private physical environment with adequate technological resources where team members work in close proximity to each other can promote communication and cohesion. Team members must be provided "work relief" from daily duties in order to exact attention to the requirements of the team. When performing team work, team members should not be concerned about assigned patient care work not being addressed. Beverages and snacks provided by administration for the team is a small cost which can greatly improve morale. Meeting times should be consistent to facilitate scheduling.

3.3.6 Individual Contribution

Potential individual team member contributions are normally considered as antecedent conditions in assisting the leader with staffing of the team. In addition to the obvious content knowledge, leaders typically choose members based on evidence of outstanding team skills such as organization, writing, negotiation, and compromise. At a minimum, individual participation on teams requires content knowledge, trust, commitment and flexibility.

3.3.7 Self-Actualization

Each individual brings to the team a unique professional position, personality, content knowledge, team skills, and historical experience which impacts team processes.[31] Team members need to be independent and self-aware before they can be productive and respectful of others, and, before then can enjoy the satisfaction of the team's success. In health care environments, Horwitz[32] described four images that each individual contributes to a team. These are a personal and professional self-image, professional expectations, an understanding of colleagues' skills and responsibilities, and a perception of colleagues' images of the individual. Of these four images, the professional's self-image was the most influential in team members understanding and interacting with each other (see ▶ Fig. 3.1).

3.3.8 Trust

The ability to trust team members originates from self-knowledge, confidence, experience, and competence. Trust is slowly developed across the team. Most members chosen for the team are disparate, often with little or no social contact with other team members prior to being assigned to the team. Contrary to content knowledge, position, and professional qualifications which are easily identified, behavioral characteristics of team often take time to be understood. This lack of knowledge delays trust. Trusting individuals are willing to share their knowledge and skills without fear of being diminished or exploited. They maintain confidences. Incorporated with trust is respect for another's skills and expertise. To develop respect, health care professionals need to discuss openly any similarities and differences in their professional values and standards. Trust develops as team members recognize and appreciate the unique skills and contributions of each other to coordinated patient care.[33]

3.3.9 Commitment

A clear understanding with buy-in of the team's aims, self-confidence, self-knowledge, and an ability to trust others are the building blocks of commitment. Commitment to a mutually agreed-upon set of team aims and ground rules provides direction and motivation for individual members. Committed individuals are willing to make short term personal sacrifices on behalf of the team, believing that sacrifices will generate a greater good. In addition, high levels of commitment enable team members to thrive among challenges and pressures that may otherwise be perceived as stressful situations.

Health care teams generate commitment through a shared goal, typically discovered during their entry-level professional education and maturing over the work history, of comprehensive, evidence-based, quality patient care—a belief in a patient-centered philosophy of care. This noble and powerful aim, common among health care workers, strongly facilitates health care team activities. In many other industries this lack of noble commitment negatively influences team activities. Committed team individuals are willing to invest personally in the team, contribute to the decision making, and respect the balance of interdependence and collaboration. Trust, especially in the highly technical world of medicine, is facilitated by a perception of competence. Competent and effective performance during meetings is often an antecedent element to building a trusting relationship.

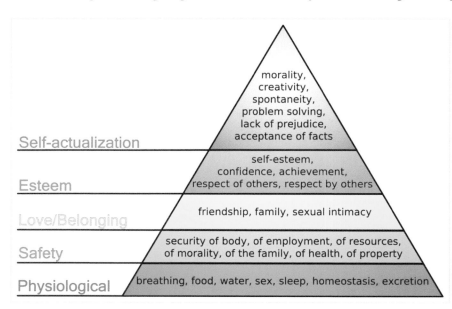

Fig. 3.1 The self-actualization pyramid, one of the seminal works of A.H. Maslow, provides an excellent conceptual framework of the necessary prerequisites for the development of self-actualization. (Adapted from Maslow AH. Critique of self-actualization theory. In: Future Visions: The Unpublished Papers of Abraham Maslow. Hoffman E, ed. Thousand Oaks, CA: Sage; 1996:26–32.)

3.3.10 Flexibility

Flexibility is the ability to temporarily alter or suspend one's process and solution biases, maintain an open attitude, accommodate varied personal, professional, and social values, and be receptive to the ideas of others. Flexibility requires self-assuredness, confidence, honesty, self-knowledge, reflection, and filtering. Flexibility also requires a celebration of diversity, the nonjudgmental openness to new ideas, experiences, processes, and solutions.

3.4 Formal and Informal Team Roles

3.4.1 Formal Roles

In order for a team to work in an organized process toward meeting team aims, several formal roles are often allocated within the group. Allocation may be at the will of the leader or by negotiation by members of the group. Although the leader is the most common role, other positions of specific responsibility provide focus and organization to specific activities and ensure formal tasks are completed.

Leader

The team leader is typically assigned the role by an individual in administration who is organizationally responsible for the aims, scope, and processes of the team. The administrator can cede authority associated with team activities to the team leader but cannot cede responsibility for the team's actions and decisions.

The culture, values, behavior, and methodology employed by the group leader strongly influence the style of how the team will operate. This style should be more participative than directive based on the belief that the leader has been assigned to his or her role for his leadership and process characteristics and not necessarily for his or her content knowledge related to the aims of the team. The key functions of the leader are to assign members to the team, motivate the team into having a strong focus on succeeding in meeting team objectives, and acting as the communication conduit between the team and administration. An effective way to improve success is for the leader to be employed as a functioning team member and not simply as a director "from above." Respect of the leader and an appreciation for his or her process knowledge by the team are important variables in team success.

Facilitator

The facilitator is closely connected with the team, especially with the team leader. The facilitator is an expert in team dynamics and in the improvement process, and thus acts as an advisor and teacher to the team members. The facilitator never owns the problem, but does have a strong interest in the success of the group. The facilitator sets the agenda, directs the meeting, is the timekeeper, and ensures acceptable group dynamics. The facilitator can also, if needed, bring additional members or consultants to the team.

An effective way of allowing the facilitator to lead the team in specific activities—without undermining the leader's role—is for the leader to introduce the facilitator as someone who will help them achieve the team's aims through knowledge of process and group dynamics. The facilitator assumes control by standing in front of the group with the clear mandate of assisting the group while the leader sits with the group.

Recorder

Historically referred to by the nomenclature as "secretary," "scribe," "historian," or "librarian," "recorder" is the currently acceptable term for this role. The recorder is responsible for developing, collating, and storing all written records from the team activities save for the agenda, which is developed by the facilitator. The recorder also disseminates the meeting minutes for review. The information gathered, minutes of meetings, output from tool use, references, artifacts, and communications within and external to the team forms the "group memory" of the team. Without proper development, collating, and storage of written materials the team itself can become disorganized and ineffective. Complete, thorough, well-written, and on-time documentation adds immeasurably to the team's success.

The role of the recorder is thus to record and gather all the data and present it in a format which the team can easily understand and reference. The key skills for the recorder are a clear and concise writing style and an ability to organize information for easy access.

Analyst

Data extracted during the team's work are seldom directly interpretable and must be translated into an understandable format. This is accomplished by appropriate statistical analysis from which decision points may be identified. The analyst's key focus is on the recommendation of the particular statistical analysis tool to employ and the measurement and interpretation of data to enable these decisions to be made.

The exact skills of the analyst will vary with the type of team. Most health care teams, especially for those directly related to a patient care activity, have little need for an ongoing analyst. However, year-end reports and analysis of outcomes and trends do offer the need for the expertise of an analyst who is especially knowledgeable in parametric and nonparametric statistical analysis and the translation of the data into long-term clinical recommendations. Analysts may also be a necessary conduit to the organization's institutional review board if there are questions related to appropriateness and confidentiality of data collection and potential future publication.

Team Member

Team members, often times referred to as "experts," have specialized knowledge which is required by the team for background information, data collection, and decision making. It is important for a health care team to either have appropriate expertise within the team or to have it readily available. Examples include nurse, social worker, case manager, physical therapist, occupational therapist, speech and language pathologist, specialty physician, and insurance specialist (see ▶ Table 3.3).

Table 3.3 Members of the health care team

Case manager

Number practicing	138,500
Entry-level education requirements	There is no unique curriculum for case managers. Most case managers are registered nurses or social workers
Licensing	Case managers are typically not licensed as case managers but they are often licensed based on their educational and clinical specialty such as registered nurse or social worker
Average annual salary for a full-time equivalent	$63,530
Job description	In the health care arena, case managers are the coordinators of discharge planning. Using data pulled from the various clinical members of the health care team, case managers identify the best disposition (discharge) options for the inpatient or outpatient in the health care continuum. The discharge may be as simple as home with no services to home with home health care, to acute medical rehabilitation, to hospice, or to a skilled nursing facility. Case managers are typically the information conduit between the health care team, the family, and the insurance company. Case managers may also be employed in areas such as insurance review and appeal, utilizations review, and quality management

Chaplain

Number practicing	13,080 paid; many others are volunteers
Entry-level education requirements	At least 100 hours of didactic and 300 hours of clinical training in a health care setting. Many health care chaplains have a master's or doctor of divinity degree or equivalent
Licensing	No required state license. Several organizations offer certifications in clinical pastoral services which require a master's degree
Average annual salary for a full-time equivalent	$48,610
Job description	Health care chaplains are responsible for attending to the spiritual needs of patients, patient families, visitors, and employees especially in inpatient facilities and hospices. Approximately 55% of U.S. hospitals employ chaplains on a full or part-time basis. Chaplains may be trained clergy or lay persons of any religious affiliation. Chaplains spend one on one time with patients, work with patients' families, provide spiritual support for the hospital and medical staffs, and may lead regular or as needed services in hospital chapels. In many arenas such as hospices, acute rehab facilities, and long-term care facilities, chaplains may be part of the interdisciplinary health care team. Hospital chaplains are consulted to perform spiritual assessments and make spiritual recommendation for the patient. Chaplains are often called to provide bereavement counseling to families

Counselor

Number practicing	302,540
Entry-level education requirements	Master's degree in counseling, psychology, or social work
Licensing	All states require at last a master's degree and voluntary national certification requires passing the National Board of Certified Counselor's examination
Average annual salary for a full-time equivalent	Varies considerably based on role. Substance abuse and behavioral disorders counselor: $41,090; mental health counselors: $43,700; rehabilitation counselors: $37,660
Job description	*Substance abuse and behavioral disorder counselors:* assist persons with problems with alcohol, drugs, sexual addiction, gambling, and eating disorders. Counseling sessions may be in individual or group settings. May also include crisis counseling *Mental health counselors:* treat mental and emotional health disorders. Are trained in a variety of therapeutic techniques to address issues such as depression, anxiety, stress, grief, and low self-esteem *Rehabilitation counselors:* help people with disability related to congenital causes, illness, or injury. They provide personal and vocational counseling, run support groups, and offer case management support

Dietician

Number practicing	59,530
Entry-level education requirements	Two educational paths are common and each occurs at the undergraduate and graduate level. The first involves entering a coordinated program where didactic science and liberal arts courses are interspersed with clinical experiences. The second is where the didactic portion of the educational program ends prior to the initiation of the clinical internships. All dieticians are required to take a certification examination prior to practicing independently

(Continued)

Licensing	Licensing laws vary by state. Some states require licensing and some do not. The title "registered dietician" denotes graduation from an accredited dietetics program and passage of the national certification examination.
Average annual salary for a full-time equivalent	$56,170
Job description	Dieticians may see clients by referral or via screening. Dieticians take detailed nutritional histories, assess metabolic and functional status, review diagnostic and prognostic tests, and work with other health care professionals to develop a nutritional support plan. This plan may include oral feedings, parenteral feedings, and other nutritional supports. Dieticians are often part of the comprehensive health care team in acute and specialty inpatient hospitals, skilled nursing facilities, acute care hospitals, and extended care facilities

Health care administrator

Number practicing	300,180
Entry-level education requirements	Education level is not mandated and therefore, varies greatly. Fifty-two percent of administrators hold bachelor's degrees, 31% hold master's degrees, and 10% have completed a post-bachelor's certificate program. Master's degrees are typically in health administration (MHA), public health (MPH), business (MBA), or public administration (MPA). Other health care administrators may be promoted licensed health care workers such as physicians or physical therapists with no formal management training
Licensing	Licensing is required for nursing home administrators. Licensing is not required for other areas of health care administration
Average annual salary for a full-time equivalent	Varies widely based on type, scope, and size of facility. Entry levels salaries in small facilities may be as low as $50,000 while CEO's of large academic medical centers earn in the millions of dollars
Job description	Health care administrators plan, direct, control, coordinate, supervise, and staff the health care system. They may direct one department, groups of departments, or entire facilities Often they are employed by the facility but many act in a consultant role

Home health aide/personal health aide

Number practicing	1.9 million
Entry-level education requirements	No specific requirement. Most employers do not require a high school diploma. Aides are often "on the job trained." Are required to meet minimum health, vaccination, and competency education
Licensing	Voluntary certification is available from the National Association for Home Care and Hospice.
Average annual salary for a full-time equivalent	$20,990
Job description	Typically employed by agencies and placed in the home of persons needing assistance with self-care activities such as bathing, grooming, feeding, and toileting. Do not provide skilled medical care. Often assist with light cleaning and other housework. May run errands for the client and accompany client to doctor's appointments

Medical assistant

Number practicing	571,690
Entry-level education requirements	Educational practices vary greatly, from a 1-year certificate/diploma program to a 2-year associate's program. Programs are available in high schools, technical schools, community and junior colleges, and within hospitals and nursing homes
Licensing	There are no state licensing requirements
Average annual salary for a full-time equivalent	$30,780
Job description	Medical assistants fill many roles within the health care system. They assist physicians and other health care workers with office care such as taking blood pressures, weighing patients, preparing areas for treatment, changing dressings, collecting and processing specimens and assisting with registration and billing functions

Medical coder

Number practicing	188,600
Entry-level education requirements	Some receive no formal training and learn on the job while others complete a 6-month or 12-month certification program. Others receive an associate's degree. Training programs are available in high schools, technical and vocational schools, and community and junior colleges
Licensing	Coders are not licensed in any state

(Continued)

Average annual salary for a full-time equivalent	$37,100
Job description	Medical records and health information technicians, commonly referred to as health information technicians, organize and manage health information data. They ensure that the information maintains its quality, accuracy, accessibility, and security in both paper files and electronic systems. They use various classification systems such as the ICD-10 and CPT to code and categorize patient information for insurance reimbursement purposes, for databases and registries, and to maintain patients' medical and treatment histories

Registered nurse

Number practicing	2.7 million
Entry-level education requirements	There are several career paths to become a nurse or to advance within the nursing field: • Associate's degree (ASN): typically, a 2-year program at a community or junior college • Bachelor's degree (BSN): 4-year degree at a college or university • Accelerated bachelor's degree in nursing: 12–18 month accelerated program for students with non-nursing bachelor's degrees. Leads to a BSN. • Diploma: a 3-year program at a hospital based school affiliated with a college or university • Master's entry level (MSN): 3–4-year program for students with a non-nursing bachelor's degree
Licensing	Licensed in all states
Average annual salary for a full-time equivalent	$67,930
Job description	Nurses are the largest group of employees in the health care field. Employed in inpatient, outpatient, office, and community arenas. The job description varies according to the role in which the nurse is employed

Advanced nursing professions: most require a graduate degree such as a masters or doctorate. In the United States there are approximately 200,000 nurses with advanced nursing degrees.

- Nurse practitioners (NP, CNP, and CRNP) perform many of the duties physicians classically perform such as history taking, ordering tests and measures, ordering medications, making a diagnosis and prognosis, and performing limited invasive and noninvasive procedures. In many states they must be supervised or work in a collaborative practice with a licensed physician. Average yearly salary is $95,070.
- Clinical nurse midwives (CNM, CNMW, CM, NM, and CPM) provide obstetrical and gynecological services with an emphasis on pregnancy and childbirth. Requirements and clinical scope vary from state to state. Average salary is $92,230.
- Clinical nurse specialty has similar educational backgrounds as nurse practitioners but with a particular focus such as labor and delivery, oncology, or orthopedics. Clinical nurse participates in teaching, mentoring, research, management, and clinical practice.
- Nurse anesthetists (CRNA and NA) specialize in administering sedation and anesthesia. The scope of practice varies from state to state. In some rural areas, Nurse anesthetists are the sole provider of anesthesia. Average salary is $157,690.
- Doctor of nursing practice typically work in hospital leadership, research, or as an educator in nursing programs.

Licensed practical nurse

Number practicing	705,200
Entry-level education requirements	Licensed practical nurse programs require a high school diploma and typically are 12–18 months in duration. They may be found at technical schools, community and junior colleges, and some vocational schools
Licensing	Licensed in all 50 states

(*Continued*)

Average annual salary for a full-time equivalent	$42,200
Job description	Provide patient care under the direction of a registered nurse or physician. Perform many of the same duties as an registered nurse but are unable to make diagnoses or perform certain procedures. May be found in all arenas of health care but especially in hospitals and physicians' offices

Occupational therapist (OT, OTR, MOT, OTD, MSOT)

Number practicing	108,800
Entry-level education requirements	Entry level degree may be either a master's degree or doctoral degree. Master's programs are typically 2.5 years post bachelor's degree. Doctoral programs are 3 years post bachelor's degree. Both degrees require a moderate amount of clinical fieldwork
Licensing	Licensed in all 50 states
Average annual salary for a full-time equivalent	$76,400
Job description	Occupational therapists assist persons with functional disabilities achieve greater functional independence in their lives by promoting meaningful functional activities and training such as activities of daily living, dressing, cooking, bathing, and specific work-related performances. Occupational therapists work primarily in acute care hospitals, acute medical rehabilitation facilities, skilled nursing facilities, home care, and school districts

Occupational therapist assistants

Number practicing	41,900
Entry-level education requirements	Most programs are at the associate's level requiring two years of college/university
Licensing	Occupational therapist assistants are licensed in all 50 states
Average annual salary for a full-time equivalent	$54,520
Job description	Occupational therapist assistants assist the physical therapist in the provision of care. The scope of services permitted by the occupational therapist assistant varies significantly from state to state. Generally, occupational therapist assistants are permitted to provide an intervention determined by the treating occupational therapist but cannot perform evaluations, interpret data, or advance clinical interventions

Pharmacist (PharmD, RPh, BS Pharmacy)

Number practicing	286,400
Entry-level education requirements	Doctoral programs are typically 3–4 years post bachelor's degree though some provide accelerated alternatives. Postgraduate residency programs such as clinical pharmacy, research, and pain control are not yet mandatory but often required in order to work in specific clinical arenas
Licensing	Licensed in all 50 states
Average annual salary for a full-time equivalent	$116,670
Job description	Pharmacists receive prescriptions and prepare medications for patients. They also provide education to the patient about the medications. Pharmacists work in all areas of the health care continuum including hospitals, acute medical rehabilitation facilities, skilled units, research, and retail. Pharmacists are important members of the health care team by providing input, advice, and counsel to members of the team regarding medications

Physical therapist

Number practicing	204,200
Entry-level education requirements	The clinical doctorate is mandated as the entry level degree in the United States. Most clinical doctorate programs are 3 years post bachelor's degree with an included minimum of 38 weeks of clinical education. Many physical therapists complete a postdoctoral residency in a focus area such as electrophysiology, sports medicine, and geriatrics though residencies are not yet mandatory. Fellowships are also available in specialty areas
Licensing	Licensed in all 50 states
Average annual salary for a full-time equivalent	$79,860

(*Continued*)

Job description	Physical therapists are the movement specialists among the health care team. Any illness or disability related to movement should include the services of a physical therapist. The scope of care is extremely broad from newborn to geriatric, from neurological illness to orthopedic to wound to cardiopulmonary. Physical therapists work in all arenas of health care

Physical therapist assistants

Number practicing	127,000
Entry-level education requirements	Most programs are at the associate's level requiring two years of college/university
Licensing	Physical therapist assistants are licensed in all 50 states
Average annual salary for a full-time equivalent	$42,980
Job description	Physical therapist assistants assist the physical therapist in the provision of care. The scope of services permitted by the physical therapist assistant varies significantly from state to state. Generally, physical therapist assistants are permitted to provide an intervention determined by the treating physical therapist but cannot perform evaluations, interpret data, or advance clinical interventions

Physician/Surgeon (MD, DO)

Number practicing	623,380
Entry-level education requirements	Four-year professional doctoral program post bachelor's degree. The last two years of the professional program are highly clinically based. Typically, the 4-year entry level professional program is followed by a 1–7 year clinical residency for specialization and board certification
Licensing	Physicians and surgeons are licensed in all 50 states
Average annual salary for a full-time equivalent	Salary varies widely based on arena of specialization. Primary care average salary is $149,050. Subspecialty average salary is $235,815. Surgical specialty average salary is $260,830
Job description	Physicians diagnose and treat injuries and illnesses. They examine patients, obtain histories, order, perform, and interpret diagnostic tests, prescribe medications, provide education and follow-up care, and perform surgeries. Many physicians are employed in nonclinical practices such as administration, insurance and reimbursement, and research

Physician assistant

Number practicing	94,400
Entry-level education requirements	Most programs are at the master's level requiring 2–3 years post-bachelors education
Licensing	Physician assistants are licensed in all 50 states
Average annual salary for a full-time equivalent	$98,100
Job description	Physician assistants perform many of the duties physicians classically perform such as history taking, ordering tests and measures, ordering medications, making a diagnosis and prognosis, and performing limited invasive and noninvasive procedures. In many states they must be supervised or in a collaborative practice with a licensed physician. Average yearly salary is $95,070

Social worker (SW, MSW)

Number practicing	649,300
Entry-level education requirements	Programs may be at the bachelor's or master's level. Many arenas in which social workers practice require the master's degree
Licensing	Social workers are licensed in all 50 states
Average annual salary for a full-time equivalent	$45,900
Job description	There are two main types of social workers: direct-service social workers, who help clients (such as patients in a hospital, pregnant women at risk due to illness or poverty) solve and cope with problems in their everyday lives, and clinical social workers, who diagnose and treat mental, behavioral, and emotional issues. A social worker can work in a variety of settings, including mental health clinics, schools, hospitals, and private practices

Source: bls.gov. Accessed December 24, 2016.

Consultant

Consultants are not full-time team members. Consultants are brought into the team by the leader or facilitator to provide a short-term unique perspective or needed data. Once the consultant's duty is completed, he or she is dismissed from the team. Consultants have little need to understand the aims of the team, the roles of the members, or the reporting structure. Consultants are called to provide short-term expertise.

3.4.2 Informal Roles

There are a number of interpersonal behavior roles that members of a team tend to naturally assume. The migration to these roles may be due to learned experience, a perception of expertise in a specific role, or that the role is empty and requires filling. To ensure team success individual team members and the roles they fill must work well together. Lack of partnership may result in overt or subliminal conflict. Subliminal conflicts are particularly problematic because often neither party recognizes or admits to conflict.

In practice, informal roles may vary along a spectrum between extremes. Team members may act at different positions along the spectra depending on a particular situation. Nevertheless, individuals do tend toward particular groups of behaviors and if these are recognized, a cohesive and effective mix may be found in the group to enable its members to work well together. This statement is often true on long-standing teams where informal roles have been established and are tacitly agreed upon by all participants. The sample application vignette describing the development of a hospital safety committee details the important formal and informal roles of team members (see ▶ Table 3.4).

3.5 Social Style: Self Versus Group Think

Social style can be divided into two types: self and group think. It is natural to consider one's own opinions and feelings important and many people are largely self-based in their thinking. This is especially true in solitary work or solitary social experiences. However, in team settings, members are required to consider other members' opinions and feelings in addition to their own. Group think is important in that it facilitates compromise and majority opinion and also lends harmony to the group.

Table 3.4 Application vignette illustrating formal and informal team roles in a hospital team environment

Team name	Hospital Safety Committee		
Team mission statement	"It is our belief that an effective Hospital Safety Committee engaged in a process of continuous quality improvement in safety staffed by a multidisciplinary group responsible for analyzing and resolving environment of care issues in the hospital will better ensure safety for patients, visitors and staff."		
Operational responsibilities	1. Develop hospital-wide and department specific PI plans to provide the Committee with reliable and validated data related to safety and safety policies 2. Review PI data using a validated methodological approach to systematically and ongoing review policies related to safety; develop and implement new policies as indicated 3. Develop and provide ongoing safety education to staff		
Meeting dates	First Monday of every month		
Permanent members	Representative from	Formal role (assigned)	Informal role (evolves)
	Administration	Leader	Board liaison
	Surgery	Facilitator	Expert on safety related to the operating room processes
	Medicine	Staff member	Expert on office practice, acts as team facilitator when Surgery unavailable
	Risk management	Secretary	Expert on safety regulations and reporting; acts as Leader when Administration not available
	Nursing	Staff member	Liaison with the nursing department
	Pharmacist	Staff member	Expert on medication and medication regulations
	Board member	Staff member	Board liaison
	Physical therapy	Staff member	Expert on fall risk and fall prevention
	Engineering	Staff member	Expert on environment of care and environment of care regulations
	Community member	Staff member	Community liaison

Abbreviation: PI, process improvement.

Members with strong self-image may tend toward a leadership role, but unless they also consider the people in the team and the group as a whole, there is a danger of becoming dictatorial and turning the focus away from the problem and onto personalities. Members with weak self-image tend to migrate toward a subservient, withdrawn "rubber stamp" role. Without understanding and appreciating one's role within the team the weak self-image member will add little to the team's outcome.

In effective groups, team members are made to feel comfortable verbalizing their individual ideas but also take seriously the opinion of others and work toward an agreeable solution. It is an important role of the leader to bring about this state of constructive cohesion.

3.6 Work Style: Project Man Versus Dreamer

Some people have a practical work style where joy is derived from organization, setting priorities, collecting data, and documentation. Others are more interested in reason, rationale, cause and effect, and challenging conventional beliefs.

In teams, a balance of both styles is needed to ensure thoughtful beginnings and solid completions to team actions.

3.7 Thinking Style: Divergent Versus Convergent

Convergent and divergent thinking are two poles on a spectrum of cognitive approaches to problems and questions. On the divergent end, thinking seeks multiple perspectives and multiple possible answers to questions and problems. On the other end of the spectrum, convergent thinking assumes that a question has one right answer and that a problem has a single solution.[34] Divergent thinking generally resists the accepted ways of doing things and seeks alternatives. Convergent thinking, the bias of which is to assume that there is a correct way to do things, is inherently conservative; it begins by assuming that the way things have been done is the right way. Divergent thinkers are better at locating novel ideas, whereas convergent thinkers have a more difficult time finding additional ideas. Convergent thinkers exhaust the list of possible ideas before divergent thinkers do. However, convergent thinking strengthens the ability to bring closure and to conclude problems. Divergent thinkers are good at brainstorming and introducing unusual ideas. Convergent thinkers, however, are good at judging and selecting items from a large set of possibilities.

Improvement teams often have an equal need for both styles of thinking, for example, where divergent thinking is used to find possible causes, and then convergent thinking is used to select likely key causes to be carried forward for further investigation.

3.8 Decision Style: Intuitive Versus Factual Decision-Maker

In making decisions a certain amount of personal judgment is required to be combined with the hard data available to help reach a conclusion. An intuitive decision-maker tends to rely more on feelings and unidentified experience to solve a problem, while a factual decision-maker will seek to increase confidence in a decision by seeking out and analyzing clear facts. Those health care teams associated with direct patient care understand and appreciate the need for input from intuitive and factual decision-makers. Quality patient care is associated with evidenced-based medicine (factual decision making) and clinical expertise (intuitive decision making). The best clinical decisions utilize both forms of evidence.

Quality improvement activities tend more toward the factual end of this spectrum, although there are some situations (often to do with people) where there is little hard data available, and an intuitive approach can yield good results.

3.9 Conclusion

Due to a variety of reasons including an expanding regulatory environment, the emerging and expansion of the scope of care of medical professions, insurance provider oversight, multiple levels of clinical care, legalities, and the complexity of services offered to the patient the solo practitioner has become an anachronism. All aspects of medical care now are now provided in a team-based, consultative environment. As a respected and valued profession, physical therapy services are represented on many organizational clinical, nonclinical, customer service, and regulatory committees and teams throughout the health care continuum. Doctor of physical therapy curricula are therefore tasked with not only providing to the student clinical content but also content related to team behaviors and team roles. Fruitful and effective participation in health care teams adds to the perception of our professional as viable, effective and important member of the health care team and deserving of a seat at most health care team meetings.

3.10 Review Questions

1. The most important aspect of any team is which of the following?
    a) The leadership structure.
    b) The quality of the agenda and meeting minutes.
    c) Defining the specific task or aim of the team.
    d) The number of members.
2. Team members should be chosen based on which trait?
    a) Expertise related to the specific task or aim of the team.
    b) Age.
    c) Experience.
    d) Affability.
3. Trust is an important characteristic of team members. Trust is developed among team members through which of the following?
    a) Spending time together.
    b) Socialization.
    c) When team members recognize and appreciate the unique skills of other team members.
    d) Reviewing team members' resumes.
4. The team leader's role within the team is primarily which of the following?
    a) Recording meeting minutes.
    b) Responsibility for the aims, scope, and process of the team.

c) Providing unique specialty knowledge.

d) Setting the agenda and directing the meeting.

5. The team facilitator's role within the team is primarily which of the following?

    a) Recording meeting minutes.

    b) Responsibility for the aims, scope, and process of the team.

    c) Providing unique specialty knowledge.

    d) Setting the agenda and directing the meeting.

6. Which team member role is not considered "full time"?

    a) Leader.

    b) Analyst.

    c) Consultant.

    d) Recorder.

7. In the health care arena which team member coordinates and plans discharge?

    a) Nurse.

    b) Physical therapist.

    c) Case manager.

    d) Physician.

8. What is the educational requirement for a home health aide or personal health aide?

    a) Master's degree.

    b) Bachelor's degree.

    c) High school degree.

    d) No degree required.

9. The entry-level degree for physical therapists is which of the following?

    a) Master's degree.

    b) Doctoral degree.

    c) Bachelor's degree.

    d) Associate's degree.

10. Which team member best fits the following description: "assist physician in many duties such as history taking, ordering tests, prescribing medication, making a diagnosis and prognosis, and performing limited invasive and noninvasive procedures. In most states they must be supervised or be in collaborated practice with a licensed physician"?

    a) Dentist.

    b) Physical therapist.

    c) Physician's assistant.

    d) Medical technologist.

3.11 Review Answers

1. The most important aspect of any team is which of the following?

    c. Defining the specific task or aim of the team.

2. Team members should be chosen based on which trait?

    a. Expertise related to the specific task or aim of the team.

3. Trust is an important characteristic of team members. Trust is developed among team members through which of the following?

    c. When team members recognize and appreciate the unique skills of other team members.

4. The team leader's role within the team is primarily which of the following?

    b. Responsibility for the aims, scope, and process of the team.

5. The team facilitator's role within the team is primarily which of the following?

    d. Setting the agenda and directing the meeting.

6. Which team member role is not considered "full time"?

    c. Consultant.

7. In the health care arena which team member coordinates and plans discharge?

    c. Case manager.

8. What is the educational requirement for a home health aide or personal health aide?

    d. No degree required.

9. The entry-level degree for physical therapists is which of the following?

    b. Doctoral degree.

10. Which team member best fits the following description: "Assist physician in many duties such as history taking, ordering tests, prescribing medication, making a diagnosis and prognosis, and performing limited invasive and noninvasive procedures. In most states they must be supervised or be in collaborated practice with a licensed physician."

    c. Physician's assistant.

References

[1] Mitchell P, Wynia M, Golden R, et al. Core principles and values of effective team-based health care. Washington, DC: Institute of Medicine; 2012

[2] Interprofessional Education Collaborative Expert Panel. Core Competencies of Interprofessional Collaborative Practice. Available at: www.aacn.nche.edu/education-resources/ipecreport.pdf. Accessed December 13, 2016

[3] Agency for Healthcare Research and Quality. Available at: https://www.guideline.gov/. Accessed December 12, 2016

[4] National Center for Interprofessional Practice and Education. IOM 1972 Report: "Educating for the Health Team." www.nexusipe.org/resources-exchange/iom-1972-report-educating-health-team. Accessed December 13, 2016

[5] Buring SM, Bhushan A, Broeseker A, et al. Interprofessional education: definitions, student competencies, and guidelines for implementation. Am J Pharm Educ. 2009; 73(4):59

[6] Verma S, Paterson M, Medves J. Core competencies for health care professionals: what medicine, nursing, occupational therapy, and physiotherapy share. J Allied Health. 2006; 35(2):109–115

[7] McNair RP. The case for educating health care students in professionalism as the core content of interprofessional education. Med Educ. 2005; 39(5):456–464

[8] Mickan S, Rodger S. Characteristics of effective teams: a literature review. Aust Health Rev. 2000; 23(3):201–208

[9] Pearce JA, David F. Corporate mission statements: the bottom line. Acad Manage Exec. 1987; 1(2):109–115

[10] BusinessDictionary. Available at: http://www.businessdictionary.com/definition/mission-statement.html

[11] Kirkman BL, Rosen B. Beyond self-management: antecedents and consequences of team empowerment. Acad Manage J. 1999; 42(1):58–74

[12] Bassoff BZ. Interdisciplinary education as a facet of health care policy: the impact of attitudinal research. J Allied Health. 1983; 12(4):280–286

[13] Ivey SL, Brown KS, Teske Y, Silverman D. A model for teaching about interdisciplinary practice in health care settings. J Allied Health. 1988; 17(3):189–195

[14] Hult GTM, Cavusgil ST, Kiyak T, Deligonul S, Lagerström K. What drives performance in globally focused marketing organizations? A three-country study. J Int Mark. 2007; 15(02):58–85

[15] Sundstrom E, De Meuse KP, Futrell D. Work teams: applications and effectiveness. Am Psychol. 1990; 45(2):120–133

[16] Senior B. Team roles and team performance: is there 'really' a link? J Occup Organ Psychol. 1997; 70(3):241–258

[17] Belbin R. A reply to the Belbin team-role self-perception inventory by Furnham, Steele and Pendleton. J Occup Organ Psychol. 1993; 66(3):259–260

[18] Furnham A, Steele H, Pendleton D. A response to Dr. Belbin's reply. J Occup Organ Psychol. 1993; 66(3):261–261– Retrieved November 22, 2007

[19] Fisher S, Hunter T, MacRosson W. A validation study of Belbin's team roles. Eur J Work Organ Psychol. 2001; 10(2):121–144

[20] Doyle M, Strauss D. How to Make Meetings Work: The New Interaction Method. New York, NY: Peter H Wyden; 1976

[21] Fisher R, Ury W, Patton B. Getting to Yes. 2nd ed. Chicago, IL: Random House Business; 1999

[22] Kepner CH, Tregoe BB. The New Rational Manager: An Updated Edition for a New World. Princeton, NJ: Princeton Research Press; 1997

[23] Barczak NL. How to lead effective teams. Crit Care Nurs Q. 1996; 19 (1):73–82

[24] Proctor-Childs T, Freeman M, Miller C. Visions of teamwork: the realities of an interdisciplinary approach. Br J Ther Rehabil. 1998; 5(12):616–635

[25] Freshman B, Rubino L. Emotional intelligence: a core competency for health care administrators. Health Care Manag (Frederick). 2002; 20(4):1–9

[26] Calhoun JG, Dollett L, Sinioris ME, et al. Development of an interprofessional competency model for healthcare leadership. J Healthc Manag. 2008; 53 (6):375–389, discussion 390–391

[27] Groopman JE, Prichard M. How Doctors Think. Boston, MA: Houghton Mifflin; 2007:177–202

[28] Gilligan P, Bhatarcharjee C, Knight G, et al. To lead or not to lead? Prospective controlled study of emergency nurses' provision of advanced life support team leadership. Emerg Med J. 2005; 22(9):628–632

[29] Pearce JA, Ravlin EC. The design and activation of self-regulating work groups. Hum Relat. 1987; 40(11):751–782

[30] Mills PD, Weeks WB. Characteristics of successful quality improvement teams: lessons from five collaborative projects in the VHA. Jt Comm J Qual Saf. 2004; 30(3):152–162

[31] Maple G. Early Intervention: some issues in co-operative team work. Aust Occup Ther J. 1987; 34(4):145–151

[32] Horwitz JJ. Team Practice and the Specialist. Springfield, IL: Charles C Thomas Publisher; 1970

[33] Snyder M. Preparation of nursing students for health care teams. Int J Nurs Stud. 1981; 18(2):115–122

[34] Kim KH, Pierce RA. Convergent versus divergent thinking. In: Encyclopedia of Creativity, Invention, Innovation and Entrepreneurship. New York, NY: Springer; 2013: 245–250

4 Documentation

Stephen J. Carp

Keywords: Abbreviations, discharge summary, documentation standards, electronic medical record, evaluation, legal record, legibility, letter of medical necessity, liability, malpractice, paper record, progress note

"Writing, the art of communicating thoughts to the mind through the eye, is the great invention of the world…enabling us to converse with the dead, the absent, and the unborn, at all distances of time and space."

—Abraham Lincoln

Chapter Outline

"One of the most important and lasting pieces of advice I ever received came to me on my first clinical internship. I was placed in a small community hospital and was working on the orthopedic floor. After perhaps three weeks of fairly intense clinical work my clinical instructor approached me and told me that I was performing beyond expectations and asked if I would like to take a break for a day from clinical care and observe two knee arthroplasty surgeries. Having never observed surgery I quickly said that I would love to observe the surgeries. I was told the surgeon was Dr. Becker.

"The next day I met my clinical instructor outside the operating room and changed into scrubs. In the locker room, I was met by a kind gentleman who asked who I was. He was dressed in khakis and a golf shirt. I explained that I was a physical therapy student and was provided the opportunity to observe surgery. He asked me what I expected to see and learn. He also asked about my education and my family. He told me he had three sons, two of whom were in college and one in high school. He told me that his wife, Mary, was a social worker at the hospital. After a few minutes, he stood explaining he needed to change his clothes and get to work. He laughed saying with two kids in college and one entering next year he could not afford to get fired. He emerged a few moments later in scrubs and asked me to follow him. We entered the operating room. He was the surgeon! He was Dr. Becker.

"The next five hours were amazing. Dr. Becker verbally took me through each step of the surgery from intubation to extubation. I stood at his shoulder as he identified the various anatomical landmarks. He explained the biomechanical adaptations of the prostheses. He taught me about blood loss, hemoglobin, hematocrit, and the risk of thrombocytopenia. He talked about deep vein thrombosis prophylaxis.

"After the surgery we returned to the locker room and he asked if I had any questions. I had about twenty. He patiently sat with me and answered every one. Eventually, he looked at his watch and said his wife was working late and he had to get home to make dinner. Amazing.

"As he was readying himself to walk out of the locker room I shyly asked him for advice. He stopped and looked at me. 'I have three small pieces of advice. The first is that you have been given a gift to serve the sick, impaired, and poor. The gift you have been given is the opportunity. Not many people are granted that gift. Make the most of it. Second, everyone you meet in health care will not always be nice. Treat everyone with love and respect. You never know the burden they are carrying. And third… (he smiled here), write good notes. Good note writing is the best method I know to reflect upon what I did or didn't do clinically. Reflection makes me a better surgeon. It will make you a better PT.'"

—A. Sanders, Lexington KY

4.1 Overview

The terms "medical record," "health record," and "medical chart" are used somewhat interchangeably to describe the systematic documentation of a patient's medical history, examination, evaluation, tests, measures, interventions, related communication, diagnosis, and prognosis across time within one particular health care jurisdiction. The jurisdiction may be as large as a health system or as small as a health care practitioner's office. In recent years, the adjective "electronic" has been added to convey that the storage of particular health data is on a server and available online. The development and maintenance of complete and accurate medical records is a requirement of health care providers and their places of employment and is generally enforced through the practitioner's state board requirements, the place of employment's accreditation agency's requirements, and by requirements stipulated by the insurer.

Medical records have traditionally been compiled and maintained by health care providers, but advances in online data storage have led to the development of personal health records (PHRs) that are maintained by patients themselves, often on third-party websites.[1] This concept is supported by U.S. national health administration entities and by the American Health Information Management Association (AHIMA).[2] For a number of reasons few Americans have adopted this format of medical record storage. The primary reasons continue to be security and confidentiality concerns.[1,2]

Because many consider the information in medical records to be sensitive personal information covered by expectations of privacy, many ethical and legal issues are implicated in their maintenance, such as third-party access and appropriate storage and disposal. Although the storage equipment for medical records generally is the property of the health care provider, the actual record is considered in most jurisdictions to be the property of the patient, who may obtain copies on request.

4.2 History of Medical Records

The earliest medical records date from astrologers in the Middle Ages. During that period of history, astrologers were considered practitioners of health care. Some of them, such as Nicholas Culpeper (1616–1664), the famous astrologer and physician, specialized in medical questions, but his records are lost.[3] Astrologers needed to compute the locations of the celestial bodies and to map them on a chart before they could make a medical or predictive judgment. Astrologers kept records of their consultations from at least the 15th century. The earliest surviving true medical records are Forman's and Napier's casebooks.[4] Forman's and Napier's casebooks are probably the most extensive surviving set of medical records from before 1700. Astrology and medicine were cognate disciplines. Unlike astrologers, other medical practitioners had no need to work with a pen in hand. They read the signs of disease from a patient's complexion, pulse, or urine—thus the obvious need to record findings. Surviving medical records from the Middle Ages fall into roughly three categories.

The most rudimentary were lists of the names of clients and their payments for treatments or prescriptions. These are account books and need to be understood alongside the broader trends of record keeping which developed in late medieval Europe. Narratives of cures—what we might think of as case histories—were recorded in ancient Greek medical works and the practice was revived in the 14th and 15th centuries. Some of these narratives recorded advice to patients about diet and recipes, others were framed as testimonials of successful or remarkable cures, autopsies or lessons for surgeons. These elements were expanded and multiplied in the 16th century, fueled by a growing interest among scholars in focusing on natural particulars and using observation to obtain knowledge of the natural world. As part of this trend, medical practitioners began publishing collections of cases that they called "observations."[4]

A.L. Rowse referred to Forman's records as "casebooks" in the 1974 book that popularized the astrologer's papers. This project has retained casebooks as a useful shorthand to mean "medical records." Neither term was used in the early modern period. Around 1750, doctors borrowed the term "casebook" from lawyers. In the following decades "case records" began to be kept in hospitals, signaling the promotion of systematic and objective medical practices. When studying Forman's and Napier's casebooks, it is important to remember that their records predate modern medical records.[4]

In the English context, Forman's and Napier's records are remarkably extensive and systematic. Like other medical records, whether account books or full case histories, they were designed to collect information. All of these records document a process that involved conversation, observation, judgment, and the collection of this material in a written form.

As we today believe, as Forman and Napier perhaps believed 300 years ago, quality documentation has the potential to improve patient outcomes and enhance patient safety through the permanent recording of the patient's examination metrics, the practitioner's assessment, and the patient's responses to medical interventions. Through appropriate written presentations, all members of the health care team can be apprised of all patient-related activities and assessments. Conversely, inappropriate, indifferent, or incomplete physical therapy documentation can negatively impact patient outcomes and patient safety.

The purposes of medical documentation are as follows:

- Permanently document the history of the examination, diagnosis and treatment of a patient. This information is vital for all providers involved in a patient's care and for any subsequent new provider who assumes responsibility for the patient.
- Provide an effective and reliable method of communication among the health care team members.
- Provide for a permanent, legal record of the episode of care.
- Provide data that may be used concurrently or retrospectively for clinical and behavioral research to improve the quality of care offered.
- Provide a source of data for department-specific, organization-specific, and mandated performance improvement activities to improve the quality of care offered.
- Provide a narrative explanation and rationalization to the insurer for the submission of billing and diagnostic codes.
- Assist decision making in reimbursement and utilization disputes among the provider, the patient, and the insurer. Medical records provide evidence as to what services were rendered, when and why they were rendered, and how they were rendered.
- Offer evidence in medico-legal disputes. Medical records are the single most important evidence for the provider whenever a civil, administrative, or criminal claim or other inquiry arises concerning patient care.
- Enable portability of the patient's health-related information. Today's health care environment, now features multispecialty care in multiple geographic areas including tele-health and ever-changing health care networks. This paradigm shift often requires consumers to transfer to different providers. The need for comprehensive, accurate medical records simply cannot be overemphasized as a tool for the sharing of reliable patient history and test results.

4.3 Electronic and Paper Documentation

The United States is currently investing nearly $50 billion in health information technology in an attempt to push the country to a tipping point with respect to the adoption of computerized records, which are expected to improve the quality and reduce the costs of care.[4] The portability of a patient's medical record is years behind the portability of other personal data such as financial holdings. An American traveler to Europe can, within seconds, access an ATM or internet-capable laptop and learn, up the moment, the balance in his checking account or the value of his 401(k). The same traveler, injured and in a hospital, may wait days for his European doctor to access his American medical records from his hometown primary care physician—longer if it is a weekend or holiday. A fundamental question is how best to design electronic health records (EHRs) to enhance clinicians' workflow, portability, security, confidentiality, and the quality of care. Although clinical documentation plays a central role in EHRs and occupies a substantial proportion of the clinician's time, documentation practices have largely been dictated by billing and legal requirements. Yet the primary role of documentation should be to clearly describe and communicate what is going on with the patient.

For physicians, dentists, nurse practitioners, and physician assistants electronic prescribing appears to reduce the rate of medication errors, but the other benefits of electronic records are less clear.[5] For EHRs to be universally accepted—especially with the cost of implementation—there must be research which indicates that electronic clinical documentation works effectively to improve care. Yet many questions about it persist. For example, can it be leveraged to improve quality without adversely affecting clinicians' efficiency? Will the initial and ongoing cost offset clinical gains? Will the quality of electronic notes be better than that of paper notes, or will it be degraded by the widespread use of templates and copied-and-pasted information?

For physicians, a fundamental part of delivering good medical care is getting the diagnosis right. Unfortunately, diagnostic errors are common, outnumbering medication and surgical errors as causes of outpatient malpractice claims and settlements.[3,4] Physical therapists are also impacted by the diagnosis error rate but also by the outcome measure and intervention. As indicated by current and pending pay-for-performance models, future physical therapists will most likely be reimbursed by value rather than procedures performed. Value-based reimbursement will be tied to clinical improvement. Facilitating clinical improvement involves correct diagnosing, choosing the correct outcome measure or measures, and providing evidenced-based interventions. EHRs promise multiple benefits to the physical therapist, but one key selling point is their potential for preventing, minimizing, or mitigating diagnostic errors, assisting with choosing the appropriate outcome measure tool, and assisting with choosing the evidenced-based intervention. Evidence to support the existence of such a benefit is currently lacking but intuitively the benefit seems appropriate. One can argue that computing offers enhanced evidence capabilities and content as compared with our brains, and that our brains offer enhanced clinical expertise and experience than computing. Therefore, clinical outcomes should improve with the addition of the computing power of the EHR. This hypothesis runs counter to the sentiments and claims of many health care workers and administrators who argue that electronic documentation in its current incarnation is time-consuming and can degrade diagnostic thinking—by distracting clinicians from the patient, discouraging independent data gathering and assessment, and perpetuating errors.[6,7] Future EHR functions will anticipate new approaches to improving diagnosis, choosing outcome measures, and choosing interventions. The diagnostic and interventional processes must be made reliable, not heroic, and electronic documentation will be key to this effort. Systems developers and clinicians will need to conceptualize documentation workflow as part of the next generation of EHRs, and policymakers will need to lead by adopting a more rational approach than the current one, in which billing codes dictate evaluation and management and providers are forced to focus on ticking boxes rather than on thoughtfully documenting their clinical thinking. Electronic medical records (EMRs) have tremendous potential to improve the quality and timeliness of health care offered, decrease medical errors, and add to the portability of our medical histories. ▶ Table 4.1 describes common problems identified by the users and stakeholders of the EMRs and offers potential solutions to the identified problems.

4.4 Defining Documentation Standards

A number of constituencies have historically defined documentation standards. Today, these constituencies primarily include accreditation agencies, state boards of health, insurers, state practice acts, professional associations, and malpractice and liability providers. Due to the multiple constituencies involved in determining the content of the medical record, the scope of medical record content may vary considerably between organizations, jurisdictions, clinical specialists, arenas of care, and states.

Accreditation agencies: though a number of agencies offer accreditation to health care facilities, the one with the largest umbrella of authority is the Joint Commission. Ernest Amory Codman, MD (December 30, 1869–November 23, 1940)—a pioneering Boston surgeon who made contributions to anesthesiology, radiology, duodenal ulcer surgery, orthopedic oncology, shoulder surgery, and the study of medical outcomes—is considered the founding father of the Joint Commission.[8]

Dr. Codman was an advocate of health care reform and is the acknowledged founder of what today is known as outcomes management in patient care. Dr. Codman was the first American physician to follow the progress of patients through their recoveries in a systematic manner. He kept track of his patients via "end result cards," which contained basic demographic data on every patient treated, along with the diagnosis, the treatment he rendered, and the outcome of each case, and any possible technical or clinical decision-making errors which may have occurred during the episode of care.[9] Each patient was followed for at least one year to observe long-term outcomes. It was his lifelong pursuit to establish an "end results system" to track the

Table 4.1 The future of electronic health records: how can they be improved?

Problem	Potential solution
Information from patients' previous clinical encounters and tests will soon be more readily available with electronic than with paper records. The problem of having too much information is now surpassing that of having too little, and it will become increasingly difficult to review all the patient information that is electronically available, especially during emergent situations	One virtue of computerized systems is that they can display recorded information in various formats. Designers will need to leverage the "visual affordance" capabilities of EHRs to facilitate the aggregation, trending (of a patient's weight or renal function, for instance), and selective emphasis or display of data so as to facilitate rapid judgments
"Point and click" boilerplate documentation adds little room for clinician's expertise, intuition, and conclusion	EHRs can foster thoughtful assessment by serving as a place where clinicians document succinct evaluations, craft thoughtful differential diagnoses, and note unanswered questions. Free text narrative are often superior to point and click boilerplate in accurately capturing a patient's history and making assessments
Hardware and software limitations often impact the timeliness, quality, and ease of documentation	Documentation of clinicians' thinking must be facilitated by streamlined text entry tools such as voice recognition. Exam room layouts, screen placement, hardware availability and reliability, and workflow should be redesigned to enable clinicians ease of use of EHR documentation tools
EHRs are often designed to be "episode of care" formatted. These individual episodes may be hospital-based, PCP office-based, physical therapist-office based and so forth. Due to confidentiality and security issues, formatting issues, and practical issues related to transference of data there is often little or no communication between these individual episodes of care documentation	The EHR systems should facilitate the documentation of evolving history and ongoing assessment. Rather than requiring a record to start from scratch with each new clinician encounter, electronic notes should follow an evolutionary paradigm—especially for chronic conditions. Putting this strategy into effect will require clinicians to go beyond reflex criticism of copy-and-paste methods to a search for creative approaches—based on functions such as annotation, tracking of changes, and threads—that not only enable information to be carried forward but also allow it to be continuously refined and updated. Chronology-based EHRs will require sophisticated solutions to handle access, confidentiality, security, and multiple formatting issues
Lack of adoption of a multi-clinician patient problem list. Hierarchical problem lists are often designed by individual clinicians involved in the patient's care but not universally shared among the health care team	A better approach to managing problem lists is needed. The failure to effectively integrate the creation, updating, reorganization, and inactivation of items on problem lists into the clinician's workflow has been one of the great failures of clinical informatics. Although such lists are vital for ensuring that important problems are not overlooked, clinicians will not maintain them unless they are made more useful and easier to incorporate into clinical conversations and documentation. Tools for easily reordering these lists and allowing specific providers (for instance, specialists or nonphysician staff members) to work selectively with a subset of problems are necessary features that most current EHRs lack
The processes of ordering tests and tracking results are separate from the note-taking function. This disparate nature of documentation often leads to lost or missed test results. Lost or missed test results negatively impacts care, increases safety concerns, and adds cost	EHRs should ensure failsafe communication and action in the areas of ordering tests and tracking the results. These steps are central to diagnosis, yet current systems often separate these functions from clinical note taking. Tracking tests is integral to documenting the acknowledgment and assessment of results and the subsequent actions taken and is vital to ensuring that important results don't fall through the cracks. Better tools are needed to efficiently weave results management into EHR documentation and workflow and to link laboratory results to problem lists and medications
The development of the differential diagnosis list: adding to, removing from, and confirming a diagnosis, is based on the clinician's clinical expertise, memory, and interpretation of tests and measures	Electronic systems should incorporate checklist prompts to make sure that key questions are asked and relevant diagnoses considered. Despite renewed interest in safety checklists, diagnostic checklists have so far been neither clinically helpful nor widely used. Yet human memory alone cannot guarantee that key questions will be asked and important diagnoses considered and accurately weighed. Decision support software and predictive models have also had limited use to date, but both could become important if their design were more practical and evidence based—if, for example, they automatically generated differential diagnoses that facilitated both documentation and decision making
Currently, discharge from one level of care to another is an "open-looped" system often placing the onus of follow-up on the patient: "call for an appointment in 3 weeks"; "don't forget to get your blood test in one month"; "follow-up with your surgeon next week." Placing this responsibility on the patient or the patient's family often leads to poor adherence	Electronic systems should do more to help with follow-up and the systematic oversight of feedback on diagnostic accuracy. Clinicians need a reliable, automatic follow-up system that goes beyond the provision of simple, one size fits all instructions to "return in 4 months" or "call if not better." For example, a button embedded in a note might activate automated follow-up calls after a physician specified interval. Computerized documentation could also be used to educate patients about symptoms to watch for. Automated feedback that spans patients and providers could convert our current "open loop" system, in which feedback is often lacking, to one in which outcomes can be used to systematically learn from diagnostic decisions and errors

Abbreviations: PCP, primary care physician; EHR, electronic health record.
Source: Schiff GD, Bates DW. Can electronic clinical documentation help prevent diagnostic errors. N Engl J Med 2010; 362:1066–1069.

outcomes of patient treatments as an opportunity to identify clinical misadventures that serve as the foundation for improving the care of future patients. He also believed that all of this information should be made public so that patients could be guided in their choices of physicians and hospitals. To support his "end results theory," Dr. Codman made public the end results of his own hospital in a privately published book, *A Study in Hospital Efficiency*. Of the 337 patients discharged between 1911 and 1916, Dr. Codman recorded and published 123 errors.[8]

With an interest in health care quality, Dr. Codman also helped lead the founding of the American College of Surgeons (ACS) and its hospital standardization program. The first hospital standards manual was published in 1926 and was all of 18 pages. The latter entity eventually became the Joint Commission on Accreditation of Healthcare Organizations. The American College of Physicians, the American Hospital Association, the American Medical Association, and the Canadian Medical Association join with the ACS as corporate members to create the Joint Commission on Accreditation of Hospitals (JCAH), an independent, not-for-profit organization, in Chicago, Illinois, whose primary purpose is to provide voluntary accreditation based on best evidence related to error reduction and optimum patient outcomes.[10] The Joint Commission seeks through its mission to continuously improve health care for the public, in collaboration with other stakeholders, by evaluating health care organizations and inspiring them to excel in providing safe and effective care of the highest quality and value.[11] The Joint Commission evaluates and accredits more than 21,000 health care organizations and programs in the United States. An independent, not-for-profit organization, the Joint Commission is the nation's oldest and largest standards-setting and accrediting body in health care. To earn and maintain the Joint Commission's Gold Seal of Approval, an organization must undergo an on-site survey by a Joint Commission survey team at least every three years. (Laboratories must be surveyed every 2 years.)

The states' boards of health: Each state has a board of health, which promotes healthy lifestyles in the state, assists with injury prevention, and helps to assure the safe delivery of quality health care for all citizens within the state.

Patient insurers: As the provider of reimbursement to clinicians and facilities for health care services rendered, insurers have the right to require custom items be added to the medical record to assist in documentation of care provided and the reimbursement and diagnostic codes submitted. An example of an insurer requiring specific documentation is the Medicare requirement for the HCFA 700 AND 701 forms used with Medicare Part B billing.[12] The HCFA 700 is the plan of treatment for outpatient rehab. The HCFA 701 form is an updated plan of progress for outpatient rehab. As an example of the vagaries of requirements even from the same umbrella insurer some but not all states require these forms for Medicare and Medicaid. Since Medicare and Medicaid laws vary so drastically from state to state and from Medicare intermediary to intermediary providers should contact their intermediary with specific questions.

The state board of physical therapy: Each state's board of physical therapy regulates the practice of physical therapy in the particular state and therefore, either directly in indirectly influences the documentation practices of its licensed members.

American Physical Therapy Association (APTA): The professional scope of practice for physical therapists is ever evolving. The scope of practice is defined by a unique body of knowledge, supported by educational preparation, a body of evidence, and existing or emerging practice frameworks. APTA has a primary role in determining the professional scope of practice of physical therapy.

The following documents and resources related to physical therapist (PT) scope of practice, education, and research provide a foundation for the physical therapist professional scope of practice.

4.5 APTA Resources Related to Physical Therapist Professional Scope of Practice[13]

The following resources are to documents and resources that describe the depth and breadth of the clinical practice and services of licensed physical therapists:
- Guide to Physical Therapist Practice 3.0 (http://guidetoptpractice.apta.org/)

The *Guide to Physical Therapist Practice* is the profession's definitive description of who physical therapists (PTs) are and what they do.
- APTA House of Delegates Policies Related to Practice (http://www.apta.org/Policies/Practice/)

APTA positions, standards, guidelines, and policies related to physical therapy practice as passed by APTA's House of Delegates and board of directors.
- APTA Guidelines: Scope of Practice (.pdf) (http://www.apta.org/uploadedFiles/APTAorg/About_Us/Policies/Practice/ScopePractice.pdf)

APTA guidelines outlining the various aspects of the physical therapy professional scope of practice.
- APTA Special Interest Sections (http://www.apta.org/Sections/)

There are 18 special-interest sections that provide resources in areas of expertise related to physical therapy practice.

4.6 Malpractice and Liability Insurers

Due to the litigious environment of health care, clinicians and organizations require clinical malpractice and professional liability insurance. These insurers may influence documentation standards to decrease the clinician's and organization's exposure to civil, criminal, and administrative lawsuits and actions. Malpractice insurance is a type of professional liability insurance purchased by health care professionals (and sometimes by other types of professionals, such as lawyers). This insurance coverage protects health care providers against patients who sue them under the claim that they were harmed by the physician's negligent or intentionally harmful treatment decisions. Professional liability insurance protects professionals such as accountants, lawyers, physical therapists, and physicians against negligence and other claims initiated by their clients. It is required by professionals who have expertise in a specific area because general policies do not offer protection against claims arising out of business or professional practices such as negligence, malpractice or misrepresentation.

Depending on the profession, professional liability insurance may have different names such as medical malpractice insurance for the medical profession and errors and omissions insurance for real estate agents. Professional liability insurance is a specialty coverage that is not provided under homeowners' endorsements, in-home business policies or business-owners' policies and only covers claims made during the policy period. An example of how a professional liability insurer may impact documentation standards is follows. A physical therapist is training a patient to use crutches non-weight bearing on the right lower extremity on steps without a railing and during the intervention, the patient falls and is injured. The patient subsequently files a lawsuit against the organization and physical therapist. Following resolution of the lawsuit, the insurance company investigates the injury occurrence and recommends because stair training is such a high-risk activity that two paid employees must be on the steps whenever a patient is being trained on the steps and that the fact that two paid employees were on the steps during the intervention must be documented in the progress note.

4.6.1 Organizational Requirements

Organizational owners and delegated administrators have the right to develop and mandate policy related to running the business. This includes documentation. Organizations often have unique documentation requirements manifested in custom documentation forms and formats. For instance, an organizational policy may mandate that physical therapists calculate basal metabolic indices on all patients. Or there may be a policy mandating that physical therapists document the patient's cell phone number.

4.6.2 Clinician Preference

Clinicians often have unique documentation practices based on expertise, history, education, or interpretation of evidence. Documentation templates, especially those with multiple narrative fields, are easily customized by the clinician.

With multiple constituencies influencing the content of the medical record documentation, and these constituencies varying in arenas where physical therapy services are performed, insurance type, malpractice and liability insurance carrier, state of practice, organizational prerogatives, and individual clinician prerogatives, one can easily appreciate the challenges of developing and implementing documentation templates that meet all the constituents' needs. An evaluation form thoughtfully developed by a practitioner in New Jersey may not be transferable to Pennsylvania. A form developed to meet the requirements of a patient with traditional Medicare insurance may not meet the needs of a patient insured by a Medicare advantage program. A form developed for use in a comprehensive acute rehabilitation facility may not transfer to the outpatient arena. A form developed for a patient with a neurological injury may not work well with a patient with an orthopedic injury. These are the reasons why there are no universal "physical therapy" documentation forms.

4.7 Types of Documentation Utilized by Physical Therapists

Physical therapists utilize an array of documentation tools during daily clinical activities. The types of documentation (initial evaluation, discharge summary, progress note, letter of medical necessity, etc.) will be rather standard among clinics but the forms, template, and narrative will change among clinics and clinicians. The one consistent in documentation are outcome measures and outcome instruments. Outcome measures are the result of outcome instruments. Outcome instruments are reliable and valid tests which are commonly used to objectively determine the baseline function of a patient from a particular cohort at the beginning of treatment. Outcome instruments may also be health related quality of life assessments completed by the patient/client. Both types of instruments and measure data are ubiquitous in physical therapy documentation providing important baseline, demographic, epidemiological, and postintervention information, which can be used by the therapist within the specific episode of care and retrospectively as a research instrument. Once treatment has commenced, the same instrument can be used to determine progress and treatment efficacy. Performance of these instruments, by nature of the reliability and validity testing, cannot vary from practitioner to practitioner.

Below is a list of common physical therapist documentation tools and a description of their content and indication.

4.8 Initial Evaluation

The initial evaluation is arguably the most important tool within the physical therapist's documentation toolbox. The initial evaluation typically occurs at the first therapist–patient interaction. The initial evaluation provides the clinician with the majority of data required to make a diagnosis and prognosis, and to develop a plan of care. The initial evaluation consists of six segments: data review, development of the patient–therapist collaborative alliance, examination, evaluation, diagnosis and prognosis, and plan of care.

4.8.1 Data Review

Following self-referral by the patient, colleague referral, or referral by clinical pathway, the therapist should review all pertinent available patient data. The amount of reviewable data will vary based on the arena in which the therapist is practicing. In acute care hospitals, the therapist may find a rich data mine of historical data about the patient in the health record. Episodes of care may be categorically documented with comprehensive discharge summaries written previous to changes in the level of the continuum of care. Current and historic laboratory, radiographic, and systems testing results may be just a click of a computer key away.

The Joint Commission mandated "patient hand off" between practitioners may provide another rich data source. However, in other arenas in which physical therapists work, the data mine will not be as rich or as easily accessible. Physical therapists working in the emergency department often encounter patients who are poor historians and the historical patient record may not be available. In the outpatient arena, if the patient is self-referred under a direct access provision, there may not be historical data to review other than that provided by patient memory. Often outpatient therapists ask their patients during the scheduling of the initial evaluation to bring with them to the first appointment a list of current medications, a list of current health care practitioners with whom they are regularly visiting, and a list of past medical and past surgical histories. In the outpatient pediatric setting, the only source of historical data may be a family member. If, during the data review or after the initial evaluation, the therapist feels additional data is required to complete the evaluation, to offset safety concerns, or to develop a diagnosis or prognosis, the therapist may need to actively search for data. Often this requires a call to the primary physician's office who is the repository of the historical medical record, or to a consultant.

4.8.2 Development of the Patient–Therapist Collaborative Alliance

The construct of a patient–therapist partnership in therapeutic situations is derived from theories of transference first outlined by Freud[14] and refers to the sense of collaboration, warmth, and support between the client and therapist. In further developing this concept, Bordin[15] in 1979 defined the three main components that contribute to the alliance construct as[1] the therapist–patient agreement on goals of treatment,[2] the therapist–patient agreement on interventions, and[3] the affective bond between patient and therapist. The research to date has used a variety of different tools to measure the alliance, and there has been some argument that each tool represents conceptually different, although overlapping, constructs.[14]

Several research studies and review articles using the above-mentioned alliance measures have found that a positive alliance between patient and physician is associated with positive health outcomes.[14,15,16,17] In the medical profession, trust is seen as a global attribute of treatment relationships, encompassing satisfaction, communication, competency, and privacy and has long been viewed as vital to cooperation with treatment and physician recommendations.[15,18]

It would appear from the previous research with physician practices that the alliance is positively associated with treatment outcome and could potentially be used as a predictor of treatment outcome in physical therapy settings. However, the degree to which the alliance relates to outcome in the physical therapy treatment settings is not yet clear.[12,13,14]

Though the foundation of the collaborative alliance is constructed prior to the examination, the alliance is further strengthened in scope and in depth throughout the examination, assessment, and intervention portions of the episode of care, and in fact, as the profession moves toward a primary care model encompassing a series of episodes of care, through these multiple episodes of care.

4.8.3 Examination

The examination typically occurs chronologically after the data review and the development of the patient–therapist collaborative alliance. A number of components are included in the examination and are detailed below.

- Chief complaint (CC): The CC is a one sentence statement provided by the patient briefly detailing the reason for this episode of care. The CC, because it is verbatim from the patient, is often documented in quotations (e.g., "I have back pain" or "I lost my leg due to an infection").
- History of present illness (HPI): Typically, one paragraph providing detail of the course of events of this particular episode of care. The HPI is a chronological recounting of signs, symptoms, health practitioner encounters, and tests and measures related to the current episode of care. For example, the patient was admitted to acute medical rehab after a 1-week stay at the acute hospital for bilateral total knee arthroplasties secondary to long-standing degenerative joint disease. The postoperative course was complicated by a deep vein thrombosis in his left popliteal vein requiring anticoagulation.
- Past medical history (PMH) and past surgical history (PSH): In this section, the patient, with the therapist triangulating and verifying from the data review, chronologically lists with dates, all medical and surgical events. Another method of triangulation is to relate the medical and surgical histories to physicians currently being seen and with medications (e.g., 2012 appendectomy; 2010 diagnosed with osteoarthritis of knees; 2009 diagnosed with high blood pressure; 2002 fractured right radius).
- Medications: The physical therapist documents all currently prescribed, over the counter, herbal, and illegal medications, dosages, and time/frequency of use (e.g., metoprolol 100 mg once per day in the morning; NSAIDS as needed for pain; red yeast rice herbal 1,000 mg in the morning; multivitamin in the morning).
- Alcohol and tobacco: Document the quantity of alcohol ingested and the type and frequency of tobacco products used. Example: The patient states he drinks one 4-ounce glass of red wine each evening. He denies smoking but often utilizes chewing tobacco on weekends. He has been using chewing tobacco for 10 years.
- Social and vocational history: includes information about the patient's living and employment arrangement: type of home such as apartment, house, extended care facility; number of floors; steps to enter and to floors; location of kitchen, bathroom, shower, bedroom, laundry; type of car; with whom the patient lives; marital status; previous use of social support networks; occupation; transportation to occupation; occupation's physical environment; hobbies; educational level; cultural and religious preferences.
- Systems' screening: The systems' screening is the result of a verbal interview with the patient in which the therapist questions the patient, at minimum, about the patient's integument, cardiopulmonary, musculoskeletal, and neurological systems and may include, based on the verbal history and data review, a full 10-point systems' screen. As physical therapy evolves into a primary care practitioner role, therapist needs to adapt more at reviewing and interpreting findings associated with all corporal systems. ▶ Table 4.2 provides a framework of questions the physical therapist should ask the client during a systems' review.
- Systems' review: The systems' review differs from the systems' screening in that in screening data is collected based on

verbal intake while in the systems' review; data is collected primarily from the physical examination. The systems' review is a brief or limited examination of, at minimum, the integument, cardiopulmonary, musculoskeletal, and neurological systems and may include some or all components addressed during the full 10-point systems' screening. Physical therapists must be fully aware that clinical findings outside the scope of a physical therapist's knowledge, expertise, experience, or education, as noted in the APTA Guide for Professional Conduct[19] should be referred to the appropriate practitioner.

- Tests and measures: From the information gathered (often referred to as "clinical scripts"[20,21] during the data review, the patient–therapist collaborative alliance, and the examination thus far), the practitioner begins to develop a differential diagnosis list. The differential diagnosis list is a group of hypothesized diagnoses which fits the data collected thus far. Tests and measures are thus used to eliminate, confirm, or add items on the differential diagnosis list. There is no specific or required number of tests and measures for the physical therapist to employ per patient; the number depends on the clinical decision-making ability of the therapist to narrow the differential diagnosis list. The goal, of course, is to continue to eliminate the incorrect differential diagnoses and thus only one differential diagnosis will remain, the correct one. The aim of the differential diagnosis list is to direct the physical therapist into choosing those tests and measures relevant to the particular patient and therefore avoiding tests and measures irrelevant to confirming the diagnosis.

Table 4.2 Ten-point systems' review

System	Examples
Constitutional symptoms	Unexplained weight loss, night sweats, fatigue/malaise/lethargy, sleeping pattern, appetite, fever, itch/rash, recent trauma, lumps/bumps/masses, unexplained falls
Eyes	Visual changes, headache, eye pain, double vision, scotomas (blind spots), floaters, or "feeling like a curtain got pulled down"
ENT	Runny nose, frequent nose bleeds (epistaxis), sinus pain, stuffy ears, ear pain, ringing in ears (tinnitus), gingival bleeding, toothache, sore throat, pain with swallowing (odynophagia)
Cardiopulmonary	Chest pain, shortness of breath, exercise intolerance, paroxysmal nocturnal dyspnea, orthopnoea, ankle or calf swelling, palpitations, faintness, loss of consciousness, claudication. Cough, sputum, wheeze, hemoptysis, shortness of breath, exercise intolerance
Gastrointestinal	Abdominal pain, unintentional weight loss, difficulty swallowing (solids vs. liquids), indigestion, bloating, cramping, anorexia, food avoidance, nausea/vomiting, diarrhea/constipation, inability to pass gas (obstipation), vomiting blood, BRBPR (hematochezia), foul smelling dark black tarry stools (melena)
Genitourinary	Urinary incontinence, dysuria, hematuria, nocturia, polyuria, hesitancy, terminal dribbling, decreased force of stream Genital: vaginal—discharge, pain, menses—frequency, regularity, heavy or light (ask about excessive use of pads/tampons, staining of clothes, clots always indicate heavy bleeding), duration, pain, first day of LMP
Musculoskeletal	Pain, stiffness (morning vs day long; improves/worsens with activity), joint swelling, decreased range of motion, crepitus, functional deficit, arthritis
Integumentary/breast	Pruritus, rashes, stria, lesions, wounds, varicosities, incisions, nodules, tumors, eczema, excessive dryness and/or discoloration. Breast pain, soreness, lumps, or discharge
Neurological	Changes in sight, smell, hearing and taste, seizures, fainting, seizures, headache, pins and needles (paraesthesia) or numbness, limb weakness, poor balance, speech problems, sphincter disturbance, higher mental function and psychiatric symptoms
Psychiatric	Depression, sleep patterns, anxiety, difficulty concentrating, body image, work and school performance, paranoia, lack of energy, episodes of mania, episodic change in personality, expansive personality, sexual or financial binges
Endocrine	Hyperthyroid: prefer cold weather, mood swings, sweaty, diarrhea, oligomenorrhea, weight loss despite increased appetite, tremor, palpitations, visual disturbances Hypothyroid: prefer hot weather, slow, tired, depressed, thin hair, croaky voice, heavy periods, constipation, dry skin Diabetes: polydipsia, polyuria, polyphagia, symptoms of hypoglycemia such as dizziness, sweating, headache, hunger Adrenal: difficult to treat hypertension, chronic low blood pressure, orthostatic symptoms, darkening of skin in nonsun exposed places Reproductive (female): menarche, cycle duration and frequency, vaginal bleeding irregularities, use of birth control pills, changes in sexual arousal or libido Reproductive (male): difficulty with erection or sexual arousal, depression, lack of stamina/energy
Hematologic/lymphatic	Anemia, purpura, petechia, prolonged, or excessive bleeding after dental extraction/injury, use of anticoagulant and antiplatelet drugs (including aspirin), family history of hemophilia, history of a blood transfusion, refusal for blood donation
Allergic/immunologic	"Difficulty breathing" or "choking" (anaphylaxis) as a result of exposure to anything (and state what; e.g. "bee sting"). Swelling or pain at groin(s), axilla(e) or neck (swollen lymph nodes/glands), allergic response (rash/itch) to materials, foods, animals (e.g., cats); reaction to bee sting, unusual sneezing (in response to what), runny nose or itchy/teary eyes; food, medication or environmental allergy test(s) results

Abbreviations: BRBPR, bright red blood per rectum; ENT, ears, nose, mouth, and throat; LMP, last menstrual period.

Along with standard tests and measures typically employed by physical therapists such as range of motion, manual muscle testing, sensory examination, fall risk assessment, vital signs, and palpation of pulses, the therapist should utilize outcome measures. Measuring outcomes is an important component of physical therapists practice. Outcomes are important in direct management of individual patient care and for the opportunity they provide the profession in collectively comparing care and determining effectiveness of interventions.

The use of standardized tests and measures early in an episode of care establishes the baseline status of the patient and provides a means to quantify change in the patient's functioning. Outcome measures, along with other standardized tests and measures used throughout the episode of care as part of periodic reexamination provide information about whether predicted treatment goals are being realized. As the patient reaches the termination of physical therapy services and the end of the episode of care, the physical therapist typically measures—for the final time—the outcomes of the physical therapy services. As physical therapists move from a service's provided reimbursement schema to a value-based schema, outcome measures will provide much of the basis and rationale for reimbursement.

Standardized outcome measures also provide a common language with which to evaluate the success of physical therapy interventions and to communicate with other health care practitioners and insurers. Outcome measures also provide a basis for comparing outcomes related to different intervention approaches which can be detailed in the research arena. Measuring outcomes of care within the relevant components of function, including body functions and structures, activity, and participation among patients with the same diagnosis, is the foundation for good clinical research and ultimately for determining which intervention approaches comprise best clinical practice. The Guide to Physical Therapist Practice provides information on many of the common outcomes tools utilized by physical therapists.[22]

Choosing the most appropriate outcome measures requires careful thought and consideration by the therapist. Included in the decision-making process are the patient's tolerance for testing, environmental constraints, the sensitivity and specificity of the measure, the validity and reliability of the measure, and the time it takes to perform the measure.

4.8.4 Evaluation

The evaluation—often confused with the patient examination—is a correlative thought process which only the results may be included in the formal documentation. The evaluation correlates all data obtained though the data review, interview with the patient, and examination to determine impairments, activity limitations, and participation restrictions. The documentation of the evaluation results is typically in the form of a problem list. The problem list, in an outpatient physical therapy setting, may be proprietary to the physical therapy needs. In a multidisciplinary setting such as an acute care hospital or acute medical rehabilitation facility, the problem list may contain problems identified from a number of clinical disciplines. One of the challenges of practicing in a multidisciplinary facility is the coordination of treatment for the multiple problems identified and the prioritization of the identified problems.

4.8.5 Diagnosis and Prognosis

Diagnosis

To best understand the contemporary practice of physical therapists performing the function of diagnosing, there must be a prerequisite knowledge of the concept of a disablement model. Disablement models provide benefits to health professionals through the organization of clinical practice and research activities; creation of a common language among health care professionals; facilitation of the delivery of patient-centered, whole-person health care; and provide a justification narrative of interventions prescribed based on the comprehensive assessment of the effect of illness or injury on a person's overall health-related quality of life. Disablement models need to be understood, used, and studied by physical therapists to promote patient-centered care and clinical outcomes assessment for the development of evidence-based practice in rehabilitation.[23,24,25,26]

Currently, the predominant conceptual framework of disability in health care is the International Classification of Functioning, Disability, and Health (ICF) developed by the World Health Organization in 2001 and adopted by APTA in 2008. The ICF focuses on human functioning within the context of personal and environmental factors. A diagnosis is determined by the attending physical therapist after thoughtful consideration of the results of the evaluation process. Because physical therapists are functional and movement specialists and not specialists in cellular pathology, physical therapist diagnoses tend to be related to and based on impairment, activity, and participation variables and not cellular pathology.[22] Often, the physical therapist will use as a diagnosis the preferred physical *therapist.*

Prognosis

A prognosis conveys the attending physical therapist's professional judgment related to a prediction of the functional outcomes of the intervention provided and with a time frame for accomplishment of these goals and that the functional outcome requires the input of skilled physical therapy services. When documenting prognosis, the results of the tests and measures employed during the examination should be used to support the prognosis. A prognosis is not a list of functional goals; rather it is a prediction of the eventual functional outcome of the physical therapy intervention based on the many variables associated with the episode of care including, but not limited to physical therapy diagnosis, cellular diagnosis, comorbidities, patient motivation, availability of support, cognitive status, disease progression, and so forth.

4.9 Plan of Care

Documentation by the physical therapist for the plan of care should include the following components which are elucidated below: statement of goals, statement of interventions, duration and frequency of services required to accomplish goals, anticipated discharge plans, and precautions.

4.9.1 Statement of Goals

In conjunction with the patient (and perhaps the patient's family or caregivers) the physical therapist develops a consensus list of short and long-term goals which best convey all stake-holders' understanding of the functional changes they hope the plan of care will facilitate. The physical therapist must understand that he or she cannot determine the functional goals for the patient. The physical therapist does not "walk in the patient's shoes" and cannot possibly prioritize functional goals for the patient. Just as large a mistake would be permitting the patient (or patient's family or caregivers) to unilaterally determine the functional goals. The patient, family, and caregivers lack the knowledge of pathology and intervention to fully understand which functional goals have a reasonable chance of being attained and which, with reasonable expectations, will not be obtained.

Goals are dynamic items; they should be confirmed, updated, deleted, and amended based on progress obtained through the intervention and as new or updates supported by test and measurement data is obtained. Updated goals are often termed "revised goals." Goal revision is documented in the daily progress note (see below).

Goal writing serves a number of functions. Goals are the foundation on which the interventions are based. Each goal should be relatable to a functional limitation identified during the evaluation and to an intervention. The physical therapist and the patient utilize the goals to measure functional gain. Reimbursers utilize goals to determine if progress continues to be garnered. Goals provide a motivational component for the patient and therapist.

Well-written goals include a number of common characteristics. The goals should be objective, measurable, easily understood by all stakeholders, tied to function, and have an associated time frame for accomplishment. The practice of a goal-based treatment approach to physical therapy has been a common practice for decades. This approach of evaluation to identifying problems to assessment to the development of functional goals to intervention is the cornerstone to an effective treatment approach. For this algorithm to lead to productive outcomes all aspects of the algorithm must be performed using evidenced-based guidelines (see ▶ Fig. 4.1). ▶ Table 4.3 illustrates correctly written goals. Physical therapists often write goals in the short- and long-term format. A short-term goal relates that the patient will reach the goal in the near future while a long-term goal relates that the goal accomplishment may be weeks to months away.

4.9.2 Intervention

The plan of care includes a list of interventions. Interventions are the prescribed services detailed by the attending physical therapist based on the findings of the examination, evaluation, diagnosis and prognosis, and the statement of goals. In some cases, the intervention list may be influenced or determined by other members of the rehabilitation team. For instance, for a patient who recently underwent open reduction internal fixation of a proximal femur fracture, the weight bearing status may be dictated by the expertise of the attending surgeon. As another example, the activity level of a patient who recently underwent heart transplant may be dictated by the cardiothoracic surgeon and not left to the physical therapist's expertise. Many orthopedic procedures utilize research-based clinical pathways, clinical practice guidelines, and protocols to determine physical therapy intervention.

A well-documented intervention consists of
- The patient status, which includes the physical, cognitive, and emotional factors, which may impact care; the diagnosis and prognosis; and learning barriers and remediation.
- Planned discharge disposition.
- A list of functional intervention items.

Specific exercise parameters such as the number of repetitions for each interventional item, the location, frequency and duration of the intervention, and specific precautions related to each interventional item are best left for the progress note. These variables are often impossible to determine at evaluation; only through careful therapist monitoring of the patient's performance of the intervention can these variables be realistically delineated.

4.9.3 Discharge/Disposition Planning

Discharge/disposition planning begins during the examination. In the outpatient arena, insurers do not always reimburse until 100% of the patient's functional limitations have been remediated. At discharge, if the outpatient is much improved but still lacking full function, how will the therapist ensure that the remaining impairments are remediated? If the insurer will no longer pay for skilled therapy, what are the therapist's options? Examples include: home program, referral to a fee for service interventions such as a local gym, or referral to a support group.

In the inpatient arena, discharge/disposition planning is often more complicated than in the outpatient arena. Physical therapists, because of their expertise in developing functional prognoses are beginning to assume much of the responsibility for inpatient discharge planning. Can the patient in the acute care hospital be discharged directly home? Is home care necessary and if so, which services? Should the patient be discharged to a skilled nursing facility, long-term acute care hospital, or acute medical rehabilitation facility? Should the patient be discharged home and be scheduled for outpatient PT services? Does the patient have rehabilitation potential, and if not, should the patient be discharged to a nursing home? Disposition planning on the part of the physical therapist requires a strong understanding of the requirements and opportunities of each level of care, potential out of pocket costs to the patient, clinical expertise in developing prognoses, and the ability to perform a valid and reliable evaluation. Discharge/disposition planning is one of the most important functions of being a physical therapist.

4.9.4 Precautions

Precautions are typically documented on the initial evaluation. The purpose of documenting precautions is to remind the primary physical therapist of potential safety issues but also to alert the physical therapy team (weekend, sick, vacation, bereavement

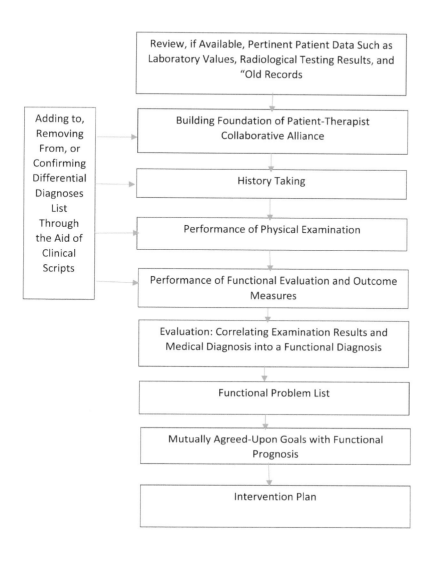

Fig. 4.1 The evaluation algorithm.

Table 4.3 Examples of incorrectly and correctly written goals

Incorrectly written goals	Reasons goal is incorrectly written	Correctly written goals
"Increase shoulder flexion range of motion to 180 degrees within 2 weeks"	Goal is not tied to a functional activity; no time frame for accomplishment	"Increase shoulder flexion range of motion to 180 degrees to permit return to work as a grocery store shelve stocker within 1 week."
"Decrease hip pain"	Not measurable; goal not tied to a functional activity	"Decrease hip pain sufficiently within 2 weeks to permit safe ambulation with cane 200 feet on level ground to access mailbox."
"Heal forearm wound within 6 weeks"	Goal not tied to a functional activity	"Within 1 week the patient will be independent in daily wound dressing changes to optimize wound healing to permit the patient to return to work as a phlebotomist"

(Continued)

Table 4.3 continued

Incorrectly written goals	Reasons goal is incorrectly written	Correctly written goals
"Patient will return to her high school track team within 1 week and set a personal best time in the 1 mile run by the end of the track season"	Goal is inappropriate	"The patient will return to full participation in high school track activities within 1 week"
"Will order brace for patient within 2 weeks"	Goal is not tied to a functional activity; goal is nonspecific	"In two weeks the patient will appropriately us a custom made hand splint for 3 hours to diminish hand neuropathic pain sufficiently to permit return to work as an elementary school teacher"

coverage) of potential safety issues. Examples of precautions include the following:

- Patient must remain nonweight bearing on the right lower extremity for six weeks.
- High fall risk as measured by Berg.
- Pancytopenia.
- Leukopenic precautions.
- Anticoagulation.
- Airborne precautions.
- Contact precautions.

4.10 Progress Note/Documentation of Visit

Following the documentation of the initial evaluation in the medical record, every patient–therapist interaction must be documented by a progress note/documentation of visit. In the outpatient arena, reimbursement is currently based on submission to the insurer of time-based and service-based codes (see chapter on reimbursement). For this reason, insurers often require a much more complex progress note in the outpatient setting as compared with the inpatient setting. Most inpatient arenas utilize a modified outpatient progress note to detail the documentation of the visit.

4.10.1 SOAP Note

Many physical therapists utilize the classic SOAP note format (an acronym for subjective, objective, assessment, and plan) (see ▶ Fig. 4.2) or a modification of the format for the progress note. The SOAP note is a method of documentation employed by health care providers to facilitate and organize the writing the progress note/documentation of visit. The SOAP note originated from the problem-oriented medical record (POMR), developed by Lawrence Weed, MD.[27] It was initially developed for physicians who, at the time, were the only health care providers allowed to write in a medical record—most other disciplines such as nursing and physical therapy did not document or documented solely on flow sheets. Today, it is widely adopted as a communication tool between interdisciplinary health care providers as a way to document a patient's progress. Versions of SOAP notes are now commonly found in EMRs and are used by providers of various backgrounds. Each encounter results in the documentation of a SOAP note.

The SOAP note is used by most health care disciplines. The length and focus of each component of a SOAP note vary depending on each encounter. For instance, a SOAP note occurring early in the episode of care may be weighted heavily on the *objective* and *assessment* portions of the note while an encounter toward the end of the episode of care my weigh heavily toward the *plan* aspect of the note.

Subjective component

This is a very brief statement by the patient—often directly quoted—describing the patient's subjective concerns related to the encounter. These concerns may be related to location and quantity of pain, perceptions of improvement or degradation of function, or any other personal comment related to the episode of care. The mnemonic below refers to the information a physical therapist should elicit from the patient related to pain before referring to the patient's "old charts" or "old carts."[27]

Onset.

Location.

Duration.

CHaracter (sharp, dull, etc.).

Alleviating/**A**ggravating factors.

Radiation.

Temporal pattern (every morning, all day, etc.).

Severity.

Objective component

The objective section of the SOAP includes information that the health care provider observes or measures from the patient's current presentation. The objective component in the physical therapy progress note often includes the following:

- Vital signs and measurements, such as blood pressure, heart rate, respiratory rate, oxygen saturation, blood sugar, temperature, weight, height, BMI.
- Findings from physical examination of corporal systems including cardiopulmonary, musculoskeletal, integument, and neurological (and any other systems relevant to the diagnosis). The functional examination is also documented in this section which includes such variables as bed mobility, transfers, gait, and activities of daily living. Lastly, the results of validated outcome measures are included here.
- Results from laboratory and other diagnostic tests already completed.
- Medication list.

Assessment

The physical therapist assessment often includes a diagnosis for the purpose of the medical visit on the given date of the note written. Further elucidation may include a quick summary of the main symptoms/findings including a differential diagnosis, a list of other possible diagnoses usually in order of most likely to

June 21, 2017

0900-1000

Subjective:

"I believe I am improving. My office co-worker reported that she thought my limp is much less pronounced than a week ago." The patient reports that she is still having pain "radiating" from her right hip to her knee when ambulating more than 100 feet. She states the pain returns to its "typical" gentle ache in her right low back after sitting down. She denies bowel or bladder dysfunction. Pain at rest 3/10; with activity 7/10.

Objective:

i. Brief re-assessment:

a. Cardiopulmonary: HR 80; BP (right arm sitting) 142/87; RR 16; O2 saturation room air 97%; blood sugar 120.

b. Musculoskeletal: No focal or patterned weakness. Strength symmetrical at 5/5 in both LE via myotomal screen L1-S2. Right hip abduction 30 degrees with "leathery" end feel. Intact sensation L1-S2 dermatomes via light touch, pin, vibration. Markedly flattened lumbar lordosis with diminished lumbar active extension.

c. Neurological: DTR's symmetrical at 2/4. Normal tone. No posturing. Negative clonus. Babinski: toes downward bilaterally.

d. Integument: Calves non-tender to palpation. Distal pulses +2.

e. Function: Independent all transfers. Ambulates without assistive device 200 feet with mild right hip compensated trendelenberg and with decreased stance phase on right.

f. Reassessment of Berg Balance Test. Score today 46 (was 41 last week)

ii. Intervention:

Fig. 4.2 SOAP note example. This figure illustrates a well-written SOAP note.

1.   Gentle (Grade II) mobilization techniques to right hip to improve articular ROM and decrease pain

2.   Stationary bicycle X 10 minutes at level 2 to improve muscular endurance and improve hip ROM

3.   Static stretching aided by contract-relax techniques by therapist into hip abduction

4.   Cold pack 20 minutes right hip sidelying with two pillows between knees.

Assessment:

Improving. Pain improved from 5/10 at rest and 8/10 with activity last week to today's scores of 3/10 and 7/10, respectively. Ambulatory distance has improved from last week of 100 feet to today of 200 feet. Berg Balance Test score also improved from 41 to 46. Expect one more week of therapy and then discharge back to local YMCA to continue exercises.

Skilled therapy is necessary to provide manual therapy and teaching activities not available at her local gymnasium.

Plan:

1.   Begin gentle hip abduction strengthening in unilateral standing (contralateral pelvis hiking) and standing on contralateral leg with ipsilateral hip active abduction at next visit. Continue manual therapy regime.

2.   Will call primary care physician's office to obtain results of hip MRI

3.   Call patient's YMCA to determine if the facility contains a stationary bike and hip abduction exercise equipment.

4.   Discharge next week if improvement continues.

Fig. 4.2 (*Continued*)

least likely. The assessment will also include possible and likely etiologies of the patient's problem. The assessment may also include the patient's progress since the last visit, and overall progress toward the therapeutic goals detailed on the initial evaluation from the physical therapist's perspective. A statement of potential disposition and date of discharge may also be included. If goals need to be restated they will be written in this section.

Plan

The plan is what the physical therapist will do to treat the patient's concerns—such as the types of interventions, frequency, duration, and number of repetitions of each exercise, precautions, planned follow up activities, and requesting additional consultations.

(SOAP commentary courtesy James Smith, DPT.)

The enlarged scope of physical therapist practice now includes disposition planning. ▸ Table 4.4 briefly outlines potential disposition options and the rationales for choosing each option.

Date, time in, time out, provider of care: since reimbursement is based on the date of service and the number of minutes of service provided, physical therapists are required to document in the progress note the date of service, the time the patient began the intervention, and the time the intervention ended. The provider of care is identified by the ink or electronic signature following the note. Many insurers now require that the name of the provider, along with the signature, be printed in non-EMRs.

Table 4.4 Potential disposition targets for physical therapy inpatient and outpatient discharges

Location of physical therapy intervention	Potential disposition	Description
Outpatient service	Home with home program	Returns home with home exercise program, instructions, information regarding diagnosis and precautions. Typical follow-up is one or two telephone calls from primary physical therapist
	Fee for service exercise program	Research has shown improved exercise adherence with a supervised, group home program.[28,29] Physical therapist makes referral to appropriate program: personal trainer, group class such as yoga, Tai Chi, aerobics, aquatics, adult day care
	Referral to another provider	Diagnoses outside the scope of physical therapy, unexpected finding, red flags, failure to improve—all may prompt referral to another provider
	Home care	Referral to home care is appropriate if the patient is certified as homebound and cannot easily attend outpatient care
Home care	Outpatient service	Patient is no longer eligible for home care services due to no longer being homebound or home care benefits have been exhausted
	Home with home program	Remains home with home exercise program, instructions, information regarding diagnosis and precautions. Typical follow-up is one or two telephone calls from primary physical therapist.
School-based physical therapy	Home with home program	Returns home with home exercise program, instructions, information regarding diagnosis and precautions. Typical follow-up is one or two telephone calls from primary physical therapist.
	Outpatient service	Patient may no longer be eligible for school-based physical therapy or the patient may benefit from equipment or services provided in a formal outpatient facility
Inpatient care[a]	Home with home care	Referral to home care is appropriate if the patient is certified as homebound and cannot easily attend outpatient care
	Home with home program	Returns home with home exercise program, instructions, information regarding diagnosis and precautions. Typical follow-up is one or two telephone calls from primary physical therapist
	Acute medical rehabilitation	Must meet criteria for admission to an acute medical rehabilitation. Criteria include meeting specific diagnostic requirements, need for multidisciplinary rehabilitation services, and ability to tolerate up to three hours of therapy per day
	Skilled nursing facility	Must meet criteria for admission to an acute medical rehabilitation. Criteria include meeting specific diagnostic requirements and having a skilled need
	Nursing home	Level of required care or socioeconomic status precludes returning to prior level of care

[a]Disposition from an inpatient facility may also be based on the patient's medical insurance requirements and allowances.

*Patient's **subjective** response to impairment or intervention:* often documented as a direct quote, this item is the patient's subjective response to his/her perception of the impact of the impairment and/or the patient's perception of the effectiveness of the intervention. The subjective response may also include a patient quote detailing current symptoms and impairments.

***Objective** component:* in this section the therapist documents a number of objective findings including reevaluation of tests and measures, intervention performed, changes in the intervention with rationale, and billing codes representative of the narrative written of the intervention. With insurers reimbursing physical therapists based on minutes of service per intervention provided, many physical therapists, along with documenting the intervention performed, also document the number of minutes the intervention was provided.

***Assessment** component:* in this section the therapist details accomplishment, deletion, addition, and amendment of short- and long-term goals. Insurers require that interventions provided require the component of a skilled therapist. Simply documenting the intervention in a narrative in the objective section of the progress note does not convey the requirement for skilled therapy. Documentation of a skilled need incorporates the type and level of skilled assistance provided to the patient, the clinical decision which resulted in the choosing of the intervention, the recording of the type and quantity of verbal, visual, and physical cues and assistance provided to the patient during the intervention process, and the functional interpretation and use of data to further rationalize the use of specific interventions as skilled therapy. These items are often placed in the assessment section.

***Plan** component:* This section details the therapist's plan for the next intervention session, changes in clinic intervention or home program, referrals, and any future plans.

Often, the final intervention session is utilized as a "reevaluation" to repeat the evaluation tests and measures utilized in the initial evaluation to assist with assessing the accomplishment of short and long-term goals. The reevaluation documented on the final progress note and the data is also utilized in the discharge summary.

4.11 Discharge Summary

Following the termination of an episode of care or the transfer of a patient to another level of care along the continuum, physical therapists write a discharge summary which becomes part of the medical record. The discharge summary provides an opportunity for the physical therapist to reflect on changes in the patient's physical and performance data (comparing the initial evaluation data with the reevaluation data). The discharge summary is typically written as a narrative. Included in the discharge summary are typically a statement summarizing the CC and HPI, a comparison of the initial evaluation and reevaluation tests and measures, a copy of the short- and long-term goals, a statement discussing goal attainment, referrals made, and, disposition. Often included in the discharge summary is a copy of the home program and any educational information provided to the patient.

4.12 Letter of Medical Necessity

The aim of a letter of medical necessity is to advocate for and obtain funding from the patient's insurance company or other potential third-party provider, for medically necessary equipment or services for a patient. The effectiveness of a funding advocacy/medical necessity letter can be greatly enhanced if a clinician understands the legal issues involved, pertinent components of a medical necessity letter, and writes the letter in a manner that lays the groundwork for the appeals process if needed (see ▶ Fig. 4.3).

Before writing the letter, confirm the following:
- The patient is covered by insurance.
- Confirm the patient's medical insurance number.
- The diagnosis is a covered diagnosis.
- The item requested is not an exclusion of the policy.

The components of a medical necessity letter include
- Identifying information: patient's name, date of birth, insured's name, policy number, group number, Medicaid number, physician name, and date letter was written.
- A statement of who you are: the patient's primary physical therapist.
- The date you last evaluated the patient.
- The diagnosis of the patient. Think carefully about what diagnoses to include (include as many as possible) as some diagnoses may be an exclusion.
- Document pertinent medical and evaluative information. Do not overburden the insurance reviewer with too much data; only include data pertinent to the equipment you are requesting.
  - Document why the requested evaluation/treatment/equipment is medically necessary. This is critical to the process. When writing about medical necessity consider the following definition of medical necessity: reasonably calculated to prevent, diagnose, or cure conditions in the patient that endangers life, causes suffering or pain, physical deformity or malfunctions, or threatens to cause a handicap or exacerbate a safety issue; and, there is no equally effective course of treatment available for the recipient which is more conservative or less costly.
- A summary statement. In this statement, try to emphasize the logical conclusion.
- Signature, professional qualifications, and contact information in case the reviewer has questions.
- Keep a copy of the letter in the patient's medical record. You/the family will need it if you/the family needs to file an appeal.

Proper salutation and dating

Ms. Mary Smith

Customer Service Associate

Reliable Insurance Company

1111 Insurance Way

Chicago IL 00000

January 10, 2017

Dear Ms. Smith,

Describe who you are, what you want, and beneficiary's name:

As an introduction, my name is Samantha Jones, and as John Doe's physical therapist at Mercy Hospital, I am requesting funding authorization for a right custom molded ankle foot orthosis for Mr. Doe. John Doe is medically insured by the Reliable Insurance Company and his policy number is 111AAA1111.

Establish your credentials, experience in the field and relationship to beneficiary:

I have worked at Mercy Hospital as a staff physical therapist since I graduated with my Doctor of Physical Therapy (DPT) degree from Benjamin Franklin University in 2002. I am currently the Director of the Mercy Hospital Prosthetic and Orthotic Clinic. Along with my DPT I am also certified as a certified Assistive Technology Professional (ATP). I also currently hold an adjunct faculty appointment at Benjamin Franklin University where I teach orthotic prescription to third year

Fig. 4.3 Example of a letter of medical necessity. In order to obtain assistive and adaptive equipment for patients, physical therapists are often required to write letters of medical necessity detailing the functional rationale for such recommendations. This is an example of a letter of medical necessity.

DPT students. I have been Mr. Doe's physical therapist for the last two years seeing him intermittently during that period of time.

Explain the beneficiary's condition, including diagnosis, or nature of injury:

Mr. Doe's original diagnosis was multiple trauma to his right leg due to a motor vehicle accident. His recovery was complicated by compartmental syndrome for which he underwent a fasciotomy. Unfortunately, due to the compartmental syndrome he developed an axontometic injury to common peroneal nerve resulting in complete loss of ankle right ankle dorsiflexion and eversion and loss of much of the sensation in his right leg and dorsum of his right foot. He was originally fitted with an over the counter orthotic but due to the unusual shape of his leg developed a number of partial thickness ulcerations- one of which developed into cellulitis requiring an inpatient hospitalization for intravenous antibiotics. After careful consideration, the Orthotic and Prosthetic Clinic has recommended a custom molded ankle foot orthosis for Mr. Doe.

Discuss the impact on the beneficiary's and caregiver's life. Note both the limitations and abilities without the requested equipment:

Because of his diagnosis and impairments John is currently required to utilize a cane to prevent falls. He is unable to wear an over-the-counter brace. His foot drop and toe drag during swing diminish his dynamic balance and exacerbates the fall risk. This is especially problematic on steps without railings. Without a properly fitted brace objective testing (Berg, Dynamic Gait Index) indicate a high fall risk.

Fig. 4.3 (Continued)

State the type of equipment and accessories being requested:

For this reason, I am requesting custom molded foot orthosis. The ordering physician will be the Medical Director of Mercy Hospital's Orthotic and Prosthetic Clinic: Dr. William Brown, Suite 414, Mercy Hospital Drive, New York, NY 00000

Describe equipment, adjustments for growth, and psychological benefits:

The custom molded ankle foot orthosis will remediate much of Mr. Doe's fall risk, increase his ambulatory endurance, aesthetically improve his gait, and diminish risk of further musculoskeletal injury due to compensation.

Describe why the device is medically necessary. Show how the requested equipment will result in an increase of function and other physical benefits:

The custom molded ankle foot orthosis is medically necessary for Mr. Doe because it will enhance his ambulatory endurance, decrease his fall risk, and decrease the risk of pressure ulcerations (as compared with an over the counter brace). Ameliorating fall risk is extremely important. Fall risk is correlated with fractures and decreased quality of life. Pressure ulcers may lead to cellulitis and osteomyelitis often requiring hospitalization and long-term interventions.

Summary and contact information

In summary, I am respectfully requesting the Reliable Insurance Company to approve the funding of a custom molded ankle foot orthosis for Mr. John Doe (policy number 111AAA1111) to remediate his fall risk and to diminish the risk of additional pressure ulcers on his leg. Two over the counter brace trials proved unsuccessful at preventing pressure ulcers. If additional questions arise I may be reached by telephone at 555 121 1212 or via email at sjones@Mercy.org. I look forward to hearing of your decision.

Fig. 4.3 (*Continued*)

4.13 Review Questions

1. The use of medical records to document clinical care dates back to which era?
    a) The Roman Empire.
    b) The Middle Ages.
    c) World War I.
    d) The Vietnam War.

2. Which of the following constituencies have not historically defined documentation standards?
    a) Accreditation agencies.
    b) State boards of health.
    c) Insurers.
    d) Local governments.

3. The "data review" is considered as a component of which part of physical therapist documentation?
    a) The initial evaluation.
    b) Letter of medical necessity.
    c) Discharge summary.
    d) SOAP note.

4. The patient therapist collaborative alliance is used to develop which aspect of the delivery of quality health care?
    a) Method of payment.
    b) Trust.
    c) Evidence-based practice.
    d) Clinical expertise.

5. Which component of the examination is typically documented as a quotation from the patient?
    a) Chief complaint.
    b) History of present illness.
    c) Medical history.
    d) Medication list.

6. When asking a patient about his or her medications which of the following types of medications should be documented?
    a) Prescription medications.
    b) Over the counter medications.
    c) Herbal and illicit medications.
    d) All of the above.

7. Which of the following statements is false about the writing of patient clinical goals?
    a) Goals should be objective and measurable.
    b) Goals, once written, cannot be amended.
    c) Goals should be time based.
    d) Goals should be functional.

8. Precautions are documented on the initial evaluation. The purpose of this documentation is which of the following?
    a) To maintain compliance with regulatory standards.
    b) To use in the event of a patient lawsuit.
    c) To remind the therapist and therapy team of potential patient safety concerns.
    d) To ensure a safe and effective intervention.

9. The acronym SOAP stands for which of the following?
    a) Subjective, Overt, Assessment, Procedure
    b) Simplify, Objectives, Accuracy, Plan.
    c) Safety, Ongoing, Addendum, Prescription.
    d) Subjective, Objective, Assessment, Plan.

10. The aim of a well-written letter of medical is which of the following?
    a) Advocacy for the professional of physical therapy.
    b) Obtain funding for medical equipment or services for the patient.
    c) Encourage patient compliance with therapy.
    d) Update the referring physician as to the care provide to date by the physical therapist.

4.14 Review Answers

1. The use of medical records to document clinical care dates back to which era?
    b. The Middle Ages.

2. Which of the following constituencies have not historically defined documentation standards?
    d. Local governments.

3. The "data review" is considered as a component of which part of physical therapist documentation?
    a. The initial evaluation.

4. The patient therapist collaborative alliance is used to develop which aspect of the delivery of quality health care?
    b. Trust

5. Which component of the examination is typically documented as a quotation from the patient?
    a. Chief complaint.

6. When asking a patient about his or her medications which of the following types of medications should be documented?
    d. All of the above.

7. Which of the following statements is false about the writing of patient clinical goals?
    b. Goals, once written, cannot be amended.

8. Precautions are documented on the initial evaluation. The purpose of this documentation is which of the following?
    c. To remind the therapist and therapy team of potential patient safety concerns.

9. The acronym SOAP stands for which of the following?
    d. Subjective, Objective, Assessment, Plan.

10. The aim of a well-written letter of medical is which of the following?
    b. Obtain funding for medical equipment or services for the patient.

References

[1] Personal Health Records. CMS. April 2011. https://www.cms.gov/Medicare/E-Health/PerHealthRecords/index.html. Accessed December 11, 2018

[2] American Health Information Management Association. Available at: https://www.ahima.org/. Accessed December 11, 2018

[3] Kassell L. Casebooks in early modern England: astrology, medicine and written records. Bull Hist Med. 2014; 88:595–625

[4] Casebooks Project (History of medical record-keeping). Available at: http://www.magicandmedicine.hps.cam.ac.uk/on-astrological-medicine/further-reading/history-of-medical-record-keeping. Accessed January 14, 2017

[5] United States Congress. American Recovery and Reinvestment Act of 2009/Division B/ Title IV Health Information Technology for Economic and Clinical Health Act. Available at: http://en.wikisource.org/ wiki/American_Recovery_and_Reinvestment_ Act_of_2009/Division_B/Title_IV. Accessed December 30, 2016

[6] Stead WW, Lin HS, eds. Computational Technology for Effective Health Care: Immediate Steps and Strategic Directions. Washington, DC: National Academies Press; 2009

[7] Croskerry P. A universal model of diagnostic reasoning. Acad Med. 2009; 84(8):1022–1028

[8] Facts about the Ernest Amory Codman Award. Available at: www.jointcommission.org. Archived from the original on 2006–05–14. Accessed February 14, 2017

[9] Mallon B. Ernest Amory Codman: The End Result of a Life in Medicine. Philadelphia, PA: WB Saunders; 2000

[10] The Joint Commission. Available at: https://www.jointcommission.org/assets/1/6/TJC_history_thru_2016.pdf. Accessed January 14, 2017

[11] The Joint Commission. Available at: https://www.jointcommission.org/the_joint_commission_mission_statement/. Accessed January 14, 2017

[12] CMS. Available at: https://www.cms.gov/Medicare/CMS-Forms/CMS-Forms/CMS-Forms-Items/CMS006595.html. Accessed January 14, 2017

[13] APTA. Available at: https://www.apta.org. Accessed January 14, 2017

[14] Greenson RR. Technique and Practice of Psychoanalysis. New York, NY: International Universities Press; 1967

[15] Bordin ES. The generalizability of the psychoanalytic concept of the working alliance. Psychotherapy. 1979; 16:252–260

[16] Hall AM, Ferreira PH, Maher CG, Latimer J, Ferreira ML. The influence of the therapist-patient relationship on treatment outcome in physical rehabilitation: a systematic review. Phys Ther. 2010; 90(8):1099–1110

[17] Jensen GM, Gwyer J, Shepard KF, Hack LM. Expert practice in physical therapy. Phys Ther. 2000; 80(1):28–43, discussion 44–52

[18] Resnik L, Jensen GM. Using clinical outcomes to explore the theory of expert practice in physical therapy. Phys Ther. 2003; 83(12):1090–1106

[19] APTA. Available at: http://www.apta.org/uploadedFiles/APTAorg/Practice_and_Patient_Care/Ethics/GuideforProfessionalConduct.pdf. Accessed January 14, 2017

[20] Rothstein JM, Echternach JL, Riddle DL. The Hypothesis-Oriented Algorithm for Clinicians II (HOAC II): a guide for patient management. Phys Ther. 2003; 83(5):455–470

[21] Baker SM, Marshak HH, Rice GT, Zimmerman GJ. Patient participation in physical therapy goal setting. Phys Ther. 2001; 81(5):1118–1126

[22] APTA. Available at: http://www.apta.org/Guide/. Accessed January 14, 2017

[23] Verbrugge LM, Jette AM. The disablement process. Soc Sci Med. 1994; 38(1):1–14

[24] Jette AM. Toward a common language of disablement. J Gerontol A Biol Sci Med Sci. 2009; 64(11):1165–1168

[25] Jette AM. Toward a common language for function, disability, and health. Phys Ther. 2006; 86(5):726–734

[26] Parsons JT, Valovich McLeod TC, Snyder AR, Sauers EL. Change is hard: adopting a disablement model for athletic training. J Athl Train. 2008; 43(4):446–448

[27] Weed LL. Medical records, patient care, and medical education. Ir J Med Sci. 1964; 462(6):271–282

[28] Forkan R, Pumper B, Smyth N, Wirkkala H, Ciol MA, Shumway-Cook A. Exercise adherence following physical therapy intervention in older adults with impaired balance. Phys Ther. 2006; 86(3):401–410

[29] Hayden JA, van Tulder MW, Tomlinson G. Systematic review: strategies for using exercise therapy to improve outcomes in chronic low back pain. Ann Intern Med. 2005; 142(9):776–785

5 Physical Therapy and Community Service

Stephen J. Carp

Keywords: Advocacy, American Physical Therapy Association Code of Ethics, community service, Good Samaritan laws, liability, political action committee, pro bono physical therapy, reflection, reflection-in-action, reflection-on-action, service learning, volunteerism

"My fellow Americans. Ask not what your country can do for you; ask what you can do for your country."

—John Fitzgerald Kennedy

Chapter Outline

1. Defining Community Service and Differentiating Service-Learning from Volunteerism
2. Benefits of Students Performing Service-Learning
3. Service-Learning and the American Physical Therapy Association
4. Examples of Service-Learning
   a) Pro Bono Physical Therapy
   b) Pro Bono Services by Setting
      1. Pro Bono Services in a Clinical Setting or Institution
      2. Pro Bono Services in the Local Community
      3. Pro Bono Services in a Different U.S. State or Jurisdiction
      4. Pro Bono Services in Other Countries
5. Non-Clinical Involvement with Professional Organizations
6. Participation in Political Action Committees and Advocacy Efforts
7. Clinical and Non-Clinical Short-Term Volunteerism
8. Final Considerations
   a) Licensure/Legal
   b) Code of Ethics and Standards of Practice
   c) Documentation
   d) Liability
   e) Good Samaritan Laws
   f) Third-party Private Payment Issues

"My parents were excellent modelers of community service. They were forever volunteering at church, at Little League, for the PTA, Meals on Wheels, and driving the sick to doctor's appointments. They took in sick relatives and cared for them. They delivered food to the hungry. For us, community service was not a performance expectation; it was a way of life.

"Therefore, community service, to me, was a natural as breathing in and breathing out. I have often heard the expression 'for every door that closes, one opens.' Perhaps a truer expression is 'for every door that opens, another opens.' As the door to becoming a physical therapist opened for me, additional doors opened to community service activities. With my physical therapist license, I now volunteer providing physical therapy services two weeks per year in Guatemala. I volunteer in pro bono (free) clinics providing physical therapy services to the poor and uninsured. I collect durable medical equipment (canes, crutches, wheelchairs) to be shipped to the poor overseas. And I do numerous community lectures on the benefit of wellness and healthy lifestyle choices.

"The ironic thing about community service—about serving those less fortunate than I am—is that I feel my meager attempts at service help me more than I help my community. Always, after returning home after performing community service, I am recharged, energized, comforted, motivated, thankful, and overall a better person than when I left my home that morning. We all have a list of mentors who have positively influenced our lives and careers. I always list community service as a mentor. What a valuable teacher she is!"

—Diane M., Roslyn, Pennsylvania

5.1 Defining Community Service and Differentiating Service-Learning from Volunteerism

In its most elegant and basic form community service is non-paid work done by a person or group of people that benefits others, the public in general, or an institution. Service-learning and volunteering are subsets of community service. Service-learning differs from volunteering in that service-learning is not always performed on a truly volunteer or altruistic basis. Service-learning is an evidenced-based teaching and learning strategy initiated by the student, faculty, or institution that integrates meaningful volunteerism with preactive determined instruction and associated reflection opportunities to enrich the learning experience, teach civic responsibility, and strengthen communities. Many universities, colleges, and high schools require community service as a service-learning activity as a graduation requirement. Volunteering is an altruistic activity in which a person or group of persons may assist an individual, group, or institution in meeting goals and aims or improving status. Unlike service-learning, volunteering does not directly impact the accomplishment of the student's career aims. Volunteering may be mandated as part of a citizenship requirement—for instance as an alternative to military service for conscientious objectors. Volunteering may be mandated as part of a legal settlement through the criminal justice system as an alternative to or in addition to incarceration or other punishment. Many professional, social, and religious groups' codes of ethics include statements encouraging community service. Lastly, in some countries, volunteering is a requirement for the receiving of social welfare benefits.

5.2 Benefits of Students Performing Service-Learning

A number of published studies define the benefits of service-learning experiences. Service-learning participation among college students resulted in significant positive effects on a number of outcome measures including academic performance (GPA, writing skills, critical thinking skills), values (commitment to activism and to promoting racial understanding), self-efficacy, leadership (leadership activities, self-rated leadership ability, interpersonal skills), choice of a service career, and plans to participate in service after college.[1,2,3] Studies involving students in school/university-supported service-learning opportunities were significantly more likely than those in the traditional discussion courses to report that they had performed up to their potential in the course, had learned to apply principles from the course to new situations, and had developed a greater awareness of societal problems. Classroom learning and course grades also increased significantly because of students' participation in course-relevant service-learning. Pre- and post-survey data revealed significant effects of participation in service-learning on students' personal values and orientations. Survey results indicate that experiential learning acquired through service appears to compensate for some pedagogical weaknesses of classroom instruction.[4] The benefits of service-learning to university students appear to take time to manifest themselves. In the cohort studied differences between those students who participated in service-learning activities related to course content as compared to students who did not participate in service-learning activities did not become apparent by midterm but rather in semester-end measures of their mastery of course content (the second midterm and the final exam).[4]

The advantages of service-learning are most apparent with indices of students' learning that entail narrative assessments of the course content. The service-learning students outperformed the non-service-learning students on the essay portion of the midterm assessment and on the essay take-home final, but not on the multiple-choice items of the second midterm. This advantage might stem from the experience the service-learning students had throughout the semester of writing narrative entries in their journals as a way of reflecting on their experiences and making the course content richer and more acceptable.[5] In any event, this finding is certainly consistent with that of other research which indicates the service-learning experiences do not appear to enhance students' mastery of factual knowledge as much as their ability to apply their knowledge in new and more real-world constructs.[6,7] These findings appear consistent with earlier works identifying the consistent use of reflective practice as a differentiating characteristic between novice and expert clinicians.[8,9,10] In summarizing their observations of the contributions service-learning might make to student learning, Eyler and Giles[2] point out that "service-learning students may not always perform better on tests of information recall at the end of a semester...but they may gain a greater depth of understanding and a greater ability to apply what they learn," and they advise us to look carefully when assessing the impact of service-learning for "qualitative differences in understanding of academic material."

Research has provided a number of principles which should be considered by faculty developing and teaching and students enrolled in professional programs related to service-learning experiences:

- Academic benefits associated with course-based service-learning were strongest for academic outcomes, especially writing skills.[4]
- The results of undergraduate service-learning on the performance of graduate and professional school admissions tests such as the graduate record examination and law school admission test were generally not significant.[5]
- Service-learning participation, especially when performed in high school or early during the undergraduate curriculum appears to have a strong influence on the student's decision to pursue a career in a service field. This effect occurs regardless of whether the student's university freshmen career choice is in a service field, a nonservice field, or "undecided."[6]
- The positive effects of service-learning can be explained in part by the fact that participation in service increases the likelihood that students will discuss their experiences with each other and that students will receive emotional support for participation from faculty.[6]
- Quantitative and qualitative research suggest that providing students with an opportunity to process the service experience with each other through shared reflection is a powerful component of successful community service and service-learning. Compared to the performance of community service activities, engaging in service-learning is much more likely to generate such student-to-student discussions.[7]
- Better than four service-learning students in five felt that their service "made a difference" and that the experience resulted in didactic learning and professional growth.[7]
- The single most important factor associated with a positive service-learning experience appears to be the student's degree of interest in the subject matter. Subject-matter interest is an especially important determinant of the extent to which the service experience enhances understanding of the "academic" course material and that the service is viewed as a learning experience. These findings provide strong support for the notion that service-learning opportunities should be Included in the student's major field of study.[7,8] Therefore, physical therapy students (and faculty teaching physical therapy students) should direct service-learning opportunities toward physical therapy-related fields.
- The second most significant factor in a positive service-learning experience is whether the professor encourages class discussion —so-called "reflection-in-action" and "reflection-on-action."[9]
- The frequency with which professors connect the service experience to the course subject matter is an especially important determinant of whether the academic material enhances the service-learning experience, and whether the service experience facilitates understanding of the academic material.[9]
- The extent to which the service experience is enhanced by the academic course material depends in part on the amount of training that the student receives prior to service participation. The experience is enhanced when students participate in planning, controlling, leading, directing, and scheduling the experience.[8,9]

- Qualitative findings suggest that service-learning is effective in part because it facilitates four types of outcomes: an increased sense of personal efficacy, an increased awareness of the world, an increased awareness of one's personal values, and increased engagement in the classroom experience.[8,9,10]
- The qualitative findings suggest that both faculty and students develop a heightened sense of civic responsibility and personal effectiveness through participation in service-learning courses.[10]
- Both qualitative and quantitative research results underscore the power of reflection as a means of connecting the service experience to the academic course material and, in the case of medical professional programs, to previous clinical experiences. The primary forms of reflection practiced were self-reflection by the participants, discussion among student participants, discussions with professors, and written reflection in the form of journals and papers.[7,8,9,10]
- Both the qualitative and quantitative findings provide strong support for the notion that service-learning courses should be specifically designed with the objective of assisting students in making connections between the service experience and the academic/clinical material.[6,7,8,9]
- Community service opens students up to numerous networking opportunities. These opportunities allow students to build social and professional relationships within their community as they contribute to the greater good of society. Along with establishing professional contacts, students learn how to develop these contacts through professional conversation, the sharing of professional experiences and aims, and through actions framed by integrity and ethics.[10]
- Lastly, community service has been shown to assist in the development of morals. Morals are a person's standards of behavior or beliefs concerning what are and are not acceptable for them to say, advocate for, do, or encourage. Morals are often developed through experiential learning. Experiences and exemplars are filed away to reemerge during periods of moral uncertainty to assist in guiding behavior.[10] When faced with a moral uncertainty, Abraham Lincoln would often relate an incident from his past as a prompt for himself or others to act in a specific, moral way.[11] Once, Lincoln was asked by an apparently lazy subordinate how Lincoln was able to write such complex but direct sermons (speeches). The subordinate admitted that his own narratives were often short, incomplete, and not direct. Lincoln, who had long-questioned the subordinate's work ethic, decided to use a moral exemplar to answer the subordinate. Lincoln's choice of exemplar was self-deprecating, informative, and nonthreatening to the subordinate, but nonetheless perceptive and instructive. Lincoln answered: "well, I guess I could write shorter and less direct sermons but when I get started I'm too lazy to stop."[12]

5.3 Service-Learning and the American Physical Therapy Association

For students enrolled in professional physical therapy educational programs an additional impetus for the performance of service-learning activities are the implicit and explicit recommendation for such activities made through the American Physical Therapy Association's (APTA's) Code of Ethics for the Physical Therapist.[13] Principles 1 and 8 directly address the ethical requirement for physical therapists and physical therapist assistants to perform service-learning:

Principle 1: Physical therapists shall respect the inherent dignity and rights of all individuals.

(*Core Values: Compassion, Integrity*)

1A. Physical therapists shall act in a respectful manner toward each person regardless of age, gender, race, nationality, religion, ethnicity, social or economic status, sexual orientation, health condition, or disability.

1B. Physical therapists shall recognize their personal biases and shall not discriminate against others in physical therapist practice, consultation, education, research, and administration.

Principle 8: Physical therapists shall participate in efforts to meet the health needs of people locally, nationally, or globally.

(*Core Value: Social Responsibility*)

8A. Physical therapists shall provide pro bono physical therapy services or support organizations that meet the health needs of people who are economically disadvantaged, uninsured, and underinsured.

8B. Physical therapists shall advocate to reduce health disparities and health care inequities, improve access to health care services, and address the health, wellness, and preventive health care needs of people.

8C. Physical therapists shall be responsible stewards of health care resources and shall avoid overutilization or underutilization of physical therapy services.

8D. Physical therapists shall educate members of the public about the benefits of physical therapy and the unique role of the physical therapist.

5.4 Examples of Service-Learning

There are five common methods of service-learning utilized by physical therapists, physical therapist assistants and students:

1. Formal, ongoing provision of pro bono physical therapy services, such as that provided by the students of the doctor of physical therapy program at the Institute for Physical Therapy at Widener (PA) University and Hearts in Motion (IN).
2. Short-term provision of physical therapy services to a needy population, such as in New Orleans after Hurricane Katrina or in hurricane-devastated Haiti.
3. Non-clinical involvement with professional organizations, such as assisting at district, state, or national meetings, providing educational in-services to a local branch of the multiple sclerosis society, or developing a fall-prevention program at a local nursing home.
4. Political action committee participation and advocacy, such as advocating for the profession to legislatures to impact the voting of proposed legislation, writing advocacy letters for a patient to an insurance company for the provision of a specific type of durable medical equipment.
5. Non-clinical short-term volunteerism, such as with Habitat for Humanity.

5.4.1 Pro Bono Physical Therapy

The term *pro bono public* is derived from the Latin meaning "for the public good." Pro bono physical therapy, in today's lexicon, refers to the provision of physical therapy services to patients at a reduced fee or no fee, depending on their ability to pay.

Physical therapists throughout the United States and around the world are answering the call to provide pro bono services to the poor, impaired, and sick who have little or no means of paying for these services or who have difficulty accessing care. Pro bono work is accomplished through free clinics providing physical therapy services to those unable to pay or those who have abutted insurance restrictions such as the Medicare cap or maximum visit number. Physical therapists working in pro bono settings may offer evaluations, assessments, consultations, interventions, teaching, and screenings. Physical therapists may provide pro bono care independently or in teams with other health care professionals. Pro bono settings may be located locally in the community, on a university or college campus that houses an entry-level doctor of physical therapy or physical therapist assistant program, or in an established health care facility such as hospital or outpatient clinic. They may also be located in an area disrupted by disease, war, terrorism, or national disaster. Pro bono clinics may also be located internationally. International locations are typically in poorer countries with limited health care providers. Sponsors and organizers of pro bono physical therapy services nationally and internationally are health care organizations such as hospitals or clinics, doctor of physical therapy and physical therapy assistant educational programs, local, state, and federal governments, nongovernment organizations (NGOs) such as faith-based groups, not-for-profits, and humanitarian aid organizations.

The APTA House of Delegates published a policy statement in 2009 titled Guidelines: Pro Bono Physical Therapy Services G06–93.[14] In an effort to meet the physical therapy needs of society, APTA encourages its members to render pro bono physical therapy services. The guidelines state that a physical therapist may discharge this responsibility by

- Providing professional service at no fee or at a reduced fee, to persons of limited financial means.
- Donating professional expertise and services to charitable groups and organizations.
- Engaging in activities to improve access of physical therapy.
- Offering financial support for organizations that deliver physical therapy services to persons of limited financial means.

5.4.2 Pro Bono Services by Setting

Pro Bono Services in a Clinical Setting or Institution

It is often easiest and most cost effective to provide pro bono physical therapy services within an existing practice setting. When located in existing clinical space there is potential access to clinical equipment; computer hardware and software including access to clinical evidence such as systematic reviews, searches, and data bases; office supplies; policies and procedures; emergency supplies and policies; and non-clinical areas such as waiting rooms, changing areas, and bathrooms. Clinical areas have been approved for licensure by entities such as state boards of health and Medicare. Most licensed clinics are Americans with Disabilities Act–compliant which alleviates many access and safety concerns. Larger clinics often have a specific budget line for charitable care which aids in approval for the use of the space as a pro bono clinic.

Pro bono services located in a clinical setting are often one of two types: a partnership between a physical therapy educational program (DPT or PTA) and the clinic, or solely staffed and directed by the clinic personnel. If run as a partnership, the clinical care is often provided by the physical therapy student supervised by the program's faculty and the clinical employees of the facility. DPT and PTA student participation in the pro bono experience may be voluntary as an adjunct opportunity to the curriculum as a community service opportunity, or mandated as a required service-learning experience as part of the curriculum. Required pro bono service-learning experiences are often embedded in courses such as clinical decision making, professional development, and clinical examination and intervention. Regardless of the organizational structure (professional program directed or partnership with a clinical entity) or location (university or clinical setting) attention must be ensured that that the mission, vision, and scope of care of the proposed pro bono service is consistent with that of all involved organizations and that all necessary administrative approvals are received. Often it is prudent to consult with legal counsel or other advisers to ensure the service is in compliance with applicable laws, accreditation requirements, and third-party agreements. The pro bono physical therapy clinic located must develop specific policies and procedures to guide decisions in this area. These documents should also receive administrative approval from the sponsoring entities. This will help ensure decisions are made with consistency and fairness.

"I graduated from a DPT curriculum that required pro bono service. There were four required pro bono service opportunities: one in orthopedics, one in pediatrics, one in neuro, and one with medically complex geriatrics. Two of the opportunities were held at the university—pediatrics and neuro—and two were held in community clinic locations—a large outpatient facility (orthopedics) and a large life care community (medically complex geriatric). In all four opportunities, we worked in groups of four and each group was supervised by a faculty member with content knowledge in the particular specialty. All the patients we evaluated and treated had exhausted their insurances or could not pay their copays. I found the pro bono opportunities rewarding for several reasons. First, how wonderful it was to see our faculty, whom we had known as academics, getting down in the trenches with us treating patients. Observing these 'experts' away from the classroom was an amazing experience. Second, we were required to write weekly reflections on what we learned and what we felt. I had never reflected before this; I was always a 'spur-of-the-moment' person. Reflecting sourced a learning method which I never even considered. Before and after each treatment, our group, including our faculty mentor, discussed the case from an evidence-based perspective which drove home the need to practice according to the known evidence. Lastly, the students and faculty utilized an online discussion board to discuss evaluation and treatment ideas."

—Anita B.

Integrated Clinical Experiences (ICEs)—also referred to as first-level clinical educational experiences, clinical practicums, clerkships, or part-time clinical experiences—provide students with an opportunity to integrate academic knowledge and skills with practical experiences while completing coursework in the professional program. ICEs, typically found very early in the professional curriculum, focus on the foundational evaluative, intervention, and clinical decision-making aspects of clinical practice, the development of professional behaviors and immersion in the clinical setting.[13] The Commission on Accreditation in Physical Therapy Education allows programs considerable latitude in configuring ICE experiences.[15,16] These experiences typically occur at local clinical sites such as hospitals or outpatient clinics. Students may perform the ICE individually or in small groups. ICE is considered a subset of clinical internship rather than a true service-learning experience.

> "My DPT program's curriculum contained a number of tracts. One of these was professional development. There was a total of four 8-week professional development courses and we were required to perform a pro bono community-service activity in each of those courses. Along with the actual performance of the service we were required to work with the community partner to develop objectives, policies, forms, and procedures associated with the activity and to complete a formal reflection of our perceptions of the opportunity. I participated in a diabetes screening activity at a local mall, foot screens at a local nursing home, body mass index screening at the local high school, and home assessment for fall risk items at a 50 + community. I remember finding six persons with elevated blood sugars. I know that diabetes is not diagnosed by one finger stick test but I felt good asking those who tested high to visit their doctors. Who knows what I may have prevented?"
>
> —Mark C.

Pro Bono Services in the Local Community

There are many opportunities for physical therapy students to perform service-learning pro bono services in the local community. These types of clinics, rather than being developed and housed in an existing practice setting can be located in non-clinical locations such as churches, community centers, schools, or universities. Pro bono services in the local community can be organized and led by professional program faculty or jointly managed by the faculty and an employee of a local physical therapy clinic or health care facility. Most of the pro bono services in the local community consist of short-term activities such as health screens. Examples of health screens within the scope of physical therapy practice include blood pressure assessment, fall–risk assessment, assistive or adaptive device inspection, and insensate foot screen for persons diagnosed with diabetes. Although participation in pro bono services such as these can be a wonderful marketing tool for one's university or practice the focus of the program should be, especially when students are involved, the service-learning aspect of the experience.

Content of the service-learning experience should always be referenced to an aspect of the curriculum. Care should also be made by the organizers to focus attention on providing a valued service to the customer and not on any secondary business gains. Additional suggestions for pro bono services in one's community include the following:

- Volunteering to provide physical therapy services one evening or half day a month at a local free clinic.
- Volunteering at special events organized by others, such as 1-day clinics for the uninsured.
- Organizing events such as free exercise classes at community centers, onsite back schools for individuals at their work site, or a booth at a county fair focusing on diabetes management and exercise.
- As with ongoing pro bono service learning opportunities, all involved organizations' administrations should be notified of the proposed opportunity. If indicated, legal counsel should be involved to advise regarding malpractice, liability, and compliance.

> "I am a DPT faculty member and I have a child with Duchenne's muscular dystrophy. I also perform research with these children. To encourage my students to learn research methods I invited them to join me in a service-learning research project. The students and I organized a weekly bowling event for the involved children and their parents. Utilizing a variety of survey tools, we measured quality of life and functional abilities of the children before and after our intervention. We also interviewed the parents to capture data about their perceptions of their child's functional status before and after the interventions. Along with assisting with data collection, my students supervised all the bowling sessions. The most surprising outcome of my research was not the change in the children or the change in their parents. The greatest change involved my students. The service-learning opportunity fostered the emergence of a heretofore undiscovered empathy toward these children and a work ethic to find interventions which can improve function. I required the students to maintain research journal reflections, review contemporary articles and present the findings in weekly journal clubs, and attend weekly debriefing sessions. Two of my DPT students from my original research cohort are now enrolled in PhD programs."
>
> —Dr. A.

Pro Bono Services in a Different U.S. State or Jurisdiction

Opportunities in other U.S. jurisdictions, except in the event of disaster relief, are usually similar to those in one's own community. Physical therapists and physical therapist assistants who practice or work in areas that border other states often have opportunities to provide pro bono services in these adjacent states. The primary implication of crossing state lines or jurisdictions for the physical therapists and physical therapist assistants involved in these opportunities is the importance of complying with licensure laws in the state where the services will be provided.

Some states have special provisions for temporary licensure, especially in the event of a disaster. Good Samaritan laws may be relevant in some situations. However, it is important to all participating faculty, students, and clinicians participating in pro bono service-learning to maintain compliance with all requirements and statutes while providing services.

Below are a number of suggestions for pro bono service-learning opportunities in other states and jurisdictions:

- Volunteering at nationally or regionally organized events such as one-day clinics for the uninsured or special events at professional conferences. Some of these nationally organized clinics arrange for liability coverage and waivers of licensure requirements for out-of-state health care providers. Make sure all potential participants check these provisions prior to volunteering.
- Providing physical therapy services as a part of disaster relief efforts in another state.
- A professional program (DPT or PTA) partnering with another professional program in another state to add additional manpower to a pro bono service-learning event.
- Providing services related to a special clinical interest such as diabetes management, fitness, or falls prevention in conjunction with a national organization.

"Though I have been practicing more than a decade I still recall my DPT professional education as one of the most energizing, empowering, and exciting times in my life. Perhaps the most sentinel event during that three-year period is when my faculty and fellow students traveled to Mississippi—to Bay Saint Louis, to provide physical therapy services at a local hospital. The hospital's staff physical therapists were overwhelmed searching for family members, finding shelter, and caring for loved ones. We traveled by minivan to Mississippi, slept in a local school, and provided much needed physical therapy services to the sick, poor, and impaired of Mississippi. We worked twelve hours per day for almost two weeks until we were relieved by students and faculty from another DPT program. I will never forget the kindness of the local populace who lost almost everything but still found time to provide a warm dinner to us each evening. I often re-read my reflections from that time and I am so proud of our service and so proud of the local therapists who permitted us to enter their hospital to serve them."

—Charles G.

Pro Bono Services in Other Countries

When considering a pro bono service-learning opportunity in another country the first decision which must be made is whether to go it alone or to partner with an agency with experience at placing physical therapy students and mentorship faculty in overseas clinics for short-term service. Many organizations (often referred to as NGOs) offer opportunities for health care professionals to provide services to underserved populations in other countries. Utmost care should be taken in choosing the partner as the quality of the programs, the local

impact of the volunteer services, and the costs to volunteers, vary greatly. Partners should have a number of years of experience in placing therapists in underserved areas overseas, be familiar with local malpractice and liability rules and laws, have a strong relationship with clinical sites, be aware of the strengths and weaknesses of potential housing, food and water sources, and transportation. There are numerous websites which provide reviews of the performance of charitable organizations, but perhaps the most effective method of choosing a partner is to network with professional programs and colleagues who have partnered in the provision of therapy services to underserved areas overseas. APTA hosts a global health and travel website which is a valuable resource for those considering overseas service-learning opportunities (http://www.aptahpa.org/?page=GlobalHealthSIG Review).

Most organizations that coordinate international volunteer programs require volunteers to cover their own expenses. Some organizations provide a stipend or discounted living and dining arrangements while others expect volunteers to make their own living arrangements and may even charge a higher fee to volunteers to further support the mission of the organization. Some organizations have specific time commitment requirements that may involve stays of several months while others allow for short visits and greater flexibility. A few organizations cast the physical therapy service-learning opportunity within a greater sphere of religious or social proselytization.

Many underserved international areas lack safe drinking water and appropriate hygiene institutions, and host a variety of water-borne, parasitic, and infectious agents. All travelers must ensure adequate protection from diseases common to the area where they plan to visit. Scheduling a visit with a physician specializing in travel medicine is an excellent method of discussing potential health risks and developing a prophylaxis plan. Service groups should also develop an emergency evacuation plan in the event of illness, natural disaster, or social upheaval. Most countries do not have similar individual social, legal, religious, and speech freedoms that are often taken for granted in the United States. Travelers should be aware of local and national laws governing both the provision of physical therapy and with living/staying in a foreign country. For information on safety related to international travel, visit the United States State Department website (https://travel.state.gov/content/travel/en.html). The site provides up-to-date travel concerns for individual countries and areas within specific countries.

There are many benefits to providing pro bono therapies to underserved populations internationally. Providing direct services to individuals can be personally rewarding through the performance of altruistic acts. International pro bono service-learning opportunities also facilitate the improvement of evaluative and clinical skills. International clinical sites tend to be poorly staffed and equipped requiring the service-learning therapist and student to enhance behavioral competencies in flexibility, prioritization, and innovation. Even though there are benefits to providing short-term clinical care in underserved areas to the student and therapist and of course, to the patient/client, health care professionals often have a greater sustained impact by providing education and consultation to health care providers, health educators and the public who live in the country rather than the provision of short-term therapy services. As an example, teaching proper handwashing procedures to a group of elementary school teachers may have an incredible long-term impact on health and wellness. Helping these individuals obtain new knowledge and skills is a service that extends far beyond the visit.

There is a story with a wonderful message about the sustainability and long-term effectiveness of international service. Members of the congregation of a small Midwestern U.S. church traveled to Haiti to provide assistance to a small village decimated by an earthquake. Originally hoping to help rebuild damaged homes, the group, primarily carpenters, was unable to find lumber, nails, or other building materials in order to perform their work. The only item they could locate was paint. Therefore, the group repainted the local church. Later they learned that the church had been repainted by similar well-meaning groups from the United States four times in the past four months. Consideration should always be given to the long-term impact of the service trip visit to the underserved area. Efforts should always be on the sustainability of one's efforts after the term of service has ended. Be reflective: Are we facilitating long-term gains to the country's infrastructure, health, or education? Or are we simply applying another coat of paint to a church wall?

"I am a third-year DPT student. Students and faculty from my program travel to Guatemala each year to provide physical therapy services to the poor. We partner with a not-for-profit organization, Fishes and Loaves. The organization has a wonderful business plan. Staffing perhaps a dozen PT inpatient and outpatient clinics in Guatemala, the organization uses DPT students and faculty to staff these clinics. Every nine days or so a contingent of students and faculty from a U.S. DPT program arrives and assumes care for those patients whose therapists have recently returned home. The organization has a wonderful U.S.-trained PT (Nancy) permanently on the ground in Guatemala who facilitates the staffing patterns, educational opportunities, and patient scheduling. With this model, sustainability is preserved; someone is always working in the clinics; the episode of care is sustained through rotating students and faculty. I was fortunate to be able to travel to Guatemala with my class during my second professional year. Supervised by Nancy and my faculty, I treated a number of diagnoses associated with a number of systems, including neurological, psychiatric, integument, cardio-pulmonary, and musculoskeletal. Now, a year past my service in Guatemala, I can honestly say that the irony of my experience in Guatemala was that as I prepared to travel to Guatemala I believed I was traveling to serve the poor, the sick, and the impaired of Guatemala. In reality, we served each other. I served them through my therapy efforts and they served me by facilitating the development of my servant's heart and by permitting me to practice my clinical skills. Rarely does a week go by when I do not reread part of my Guatemala reflections. I want to go back one day."

—Christopher P.

5.5 Non-Clinical Involvement with Professional Organizations

Physical therapists, physical therapist assistants, and students in professional programs have a unique expertise which, through partnership in service-learning opportunities, facilitates the mission of professional organizations and charitable NGOs. Those within the physical therapy profession (students, faculty, and graduates) possess a combination of professionalism, ethical standards, clinical content knowledge, local, national, and global health policy expertise, and behavioral skills which permit effective and useful interaction to professional organizations and NGOs.

The most logical place to begin researching potential service-learning opportunities for oneself as a licensed professional, for faculty, and for students in professional degree programs, is APTA. APTA is a powerful individual membership professional organization representing more than 95,000 member physical therapists (PTs), physical therapist assistants (PTAs), and students of physical therapy. APTA seeks to continuously improve the health and quality of life of individuals in society by advancing physical therapist practice, education, and research, and by increasing the awareness and understanding of physical therapy's role in the nation's health care system. APTA is organized locally by districts, by state associations, and by the national organization.

The first step toward involvement is membership. Only through membership can there be an immersion in the culture and benefits of APTA. Practicing physical therapy clinicians, educators, and researchers often look back at their professional education as the seminal professional years of their lives. APTA membership during these "growing years" is a great facilitator of future success, professionalism, and advocacy. APTA offers broad membership dues discounts to student members. APTA recognizes the financial constraints of professional students.

One of the most user-friendly places to initiate service-learning activities as a student alone or in combination with faculty designing a professional association-related service-learning activity is the APTA National Student Conclave. The National Student Conclave, held yearly, is an opportunity to network with other PT and PTA student peers and mentors while attending educational sessions specifically designed to prepare students in the professional program for a career in physical therapy. National Student Conclave (NSC) is the only national conference that's planned for students, by students, and providing students the opportunity to[17]

- *Create* lifelong relationships with fellow physical therapy students from across the country, leaders in the field, and with APTA's president and CEO.
- *Elect* the next Student assembly board of directors.
- *Engage* in innovative topics that focus on the student's future in physical therapy.
- *Contribute* to a fun, energetic, thriving environment focused on all PT and PTA students.

"I attended my first National Student Conclave as a second year DPT student. I was blown away by the networking events, the clinical presentations, and the mentorship activities. Upon my return I provided a short in-service about the NSC to our students who were unable to attend. Next year our entire class is attending! I even signed up to help plan next year's conclave."

—Ethan M.

Another effective method of service-learning associate with a professional organization is with local chapters of national organizations which advocate for a specific disease or impairment such as the National Multiple Sclerosis Society, the Alzheimer's Association, and the American Cancer Society. Local chapters welcome volunteer support, especially from licensed or student health care professionals, to assist with fund-raising, the development of educational materials, assisting with support group activities, and short- and long-term planning activities.

"While in PT school, my mother was diagnosed with multiple sclerosis. Fortunately, my mom's symptoms were mild—and continue to be mild—and she continues to work and care for our house. However, I felt I needed to do something to either directly or indirectly help her. I called my local National Multiple Sclerosis Society chapter and asked if I could join as a volunteer. The director asked about my background and I told her I was a DPT student. She mentioned a number of potential activities I could become involved with but recommended that I volunteer at the monthly MS clinic at our local hospital. The clinic is partially sponsored by the hospital and partially by the National MS Society. Though I am unable, as a DPT student, to provide direct patient care I do assist the neurologist and physical therapist with transporting the clients to the various clinic stops, guarding them during the functional examinations, and helping with wheelchair maintenance. I can't begin to describe how much I have learned. As part of my service-learning contact with my program, I am required to write a weekly reflection about my participation. Most importantly, however, I feel as though, in some way, I am helping my mom."

—Alaina S.

5.6 Participation in Political Action Committees and Advocacy Efforts

Advocacy is an activity by an individual or group of individuals that aims to influence decisions, policy, and actions within political, economic, and social systems and institutions. Advocacy can include many activities that a person or organization undertakes such as letter writing, personal discussion, media campaigning, public speaking, and financial contributions to influence and facilitate action. An advocate is someone who performs an advocacy function. Advocacy in its most humanistic form seeks to ensure that people, particularly those who are most vulnerable in society such as those impaired, disabled, poor, and sick, are able to receive equal protection and benefits under the law as healthy person.

Advocacy has been identified as a strong behavioral goal for the members of the profession of Physical Therapy. Advocacy is mentioned in a number of APTA-related documents including the APTA Guide to Physical Therapist Practice and the APTA Code of Ethics.[13] 8B in the Code of Ethics states that "physical therapists shall advocate to reduce health disparities and health care inequities, improve access to health care services, and address the health, wellness, and preventive health care needs of people." Advocacy is also a required component of physical therapist educational programs as mandated by the standards of the Commission on Accreditation in Physical Therapy Education (CAPTE).

Members of the profession of physical therapy routinely advocate on several fronts: our profession, our patients, and the rights of the poor, sick, and impaired. When therapists advocate for our profession, they advocate to insurers, regulators, and legislators about the benefits of physical therapy knowledge and outcomes. Therapists advocate against inroads from other professional and nonprofessional organizations from usurping the scope of care of physical therapy. Therapists advocate to insurance companies for honest reimbursement for activities performed. Therapists advocate for patients/clients by writing letters of medical necessity to ensure these patients/clients receive the care and equipment they are entitled to receive. Therapists advocate for the rights of the poor, sick, and impaired by encouraging legislation such as the Affordable Care Act, the Family Leave Medical Act, and the Americans with Disabilities Act.

A good advocate possesses skills which increase the success of the advocacy efforts. A skilled advocate possesses contacts and associates who will assist in the advocacy efforts. A good advocate knows his or her rights as an advocate and knows the law and the legal system. A good advocate asks many questions to stay informed about current clinical and legislative health care climate. A good advocate can identify which areas of our profession and which areas of our patients'/clients' lives can be improved upon. A good advocate has confidence that his or her advocacy efforts will be rewarded. A good advocate can write strong, professional, and nonthreatening communications. A good advocate is prepared and organized and has the time, along with the need, to advocate. A good advocate blames the process and not an organization or individual.

Dhillon, Wilkins, and Law et al[18] studied why therapists advocate and how they learned to be an advocate. The authors discovered three reasons why all therapists advocate and also that that therapists advocate based on the positions in life. Generally, all therapists advocate for personal fulfillment—a feeling that therapists are unique in their knowledge and beliefs to advocate for the poor, sick, and impaired. They feel they are also unique in their positions as movement specialists to advocate for their patient/client. Therapists also advocate because they have the unique knowledge to advocate for their patients/clients to return as functioning members of society.

In addition to the advocacy reasons above, physical therapy clinicians advocate because they feel empowered to improve an individual patient's functional level and his or her rights as a patient. Physical therapist clinicians also advocate for the professional self and the personal self. The professional self is our role as a practicing physical therapist professional and the personal self is all that is ancillary to the professional self, such as paycheck, working conditions, benefits, and other internal and external rewards.

Physical therapists, in the roles of administrators, advocate for their business and organization, and for their employees.

Physical therapy professional program faculty and those active in APTA advocate because they believe they have the specialty knowledge, experience, and wherewithal to advocate for the profession, for quality of care, for the rights associated with function of all Americans, and for concerns for the health care environment.

Most advocacy efforts—whether for a particular patient, for our profession, for the rights of groups of patient/clients, or for additional funding of specific programs—are best accomplished through written communication. In-person one-to-one communication with representatives from insurance companies and with legislators is extremely time-consuming and difficult. Advocacy is a professional responsibility of all physical therapists and physical therapist assistants. The characteristics of an effective written advocacy communication include the following:

- Think before you write.
- The letter should be no more than one page.
- Limit opinions and use facts and evidence.
- Use the correct salutation (correct salutations when addressing letters to legislators can be found online).
- In the first paragraph thank the reader for taking the time to consider your position.
- If advocating for a bill or law clearly state in your first sentence the number and name of bill you are commenting on. If advocating for services or equipment to your patient clearly state the patient's name and insurance number in the first paragraph.
- Be specific when introducing a complaint or opinion.
- Focus on one issue at a time.
- Don't only complain.
- Do not focus on past grievances.
- Consider compromise.
- Repeat major points.
- Avoid sarcasm.
- Avoid name calling.
- If representing an organization (APTA) make sure the organization agrees with your views.
- Sign your letter and include your contact information.
- Double check for spelling and grammar errors. Have an associate review the letter prior to sending.
- Wait 24 hours, re-read the letter, and reflect as to whether this is the correct action to take.
- Either fax or email your letter; mailed letters may sit in quarantine.

If wishing to advocate in person, instead of just dropping in always schedule an appointment and describe the reason for the visit to the scheduler. Always identify yourself, your position, and the reason for the advocacy effort. Ask for an appointment with the staff person who is handling that particular issue. If advocating for or against a law or bill, research the legislator's position and background about the issue prior to the meeting. Consider ideology, party, past votes, and whether the legislator is up for reelection. Do not attempt to make an appointment during a legislative recess. Advocate as part of a coalition rather than independently. It is good to have others with you—an interdisciplinary group, if possible. Practice your presentation prior to the meeting. Be prompt. Dress professionally. Have the facts clearly outlined in a hard copy to present to the staff person. View the meeting as a discussion and not a lecture. Research the ways in which a specific vote can help the legislator. Plan for not more than 15 minutes. Write a prompt thank you letter outlining the key points of the meeting and your contact information.

5.7 Clinical and Non-Clinical Short-Term Volunteerism

For the purposes of this chapter, clinical and non-clinical short-term volunteerism may be considered a service-learning opportunity if, for students, there is a relationship of the opportunity to a specific portion of the professional curriculum and for practicing clinicians, if there is a relationship between the opportunity and the further development of a clinical, behavioral, or administrative goal. As an example, a DPT student currently studying a topic related to women's health, may benefit from a weekend immersion with a DPT with a clinical specialty in women's health who is screening nursing home residents for urinary incontinence. Though the service learning only takes place over two days and has no sustainability, the experience, if coupled with a common feedback method such as a reflection paper or a systematic review of stress incontinence interventions in the female geriatric population, may prove of lasting benefit to the student. An example of a short-term volunteerism with a service-learning component may be as follows: a recent DPT graduate is considering applying for a neurological residency. The graduate observes a neurological certified specialist (NCS) for a day and then schedules a meeting with a trusted DPT mentor (a previous faculty member, a previous clinical instructor, or a current supervisor) to discuss over coffee what was observed and learned during the observation of the neurological certified specialist and to help make a decision whether or not to apply to a neurological residency program.

Short-term non-clinical volunteerism though altruistic in nature, is difficult to label as a service-learning opportunity. Many of the common non-clinical short-term volunteerism activities performed by students and graduates: religious sponsored events, Habitat for Humanity, service trips related to construction, assisting at road running or walking events benefiting charities, charity auctions and such, are not true service-learning opportunities because there is no relationship to the further development of behavioral, clinical, or administrative skills related to physical therapy.

5.8 Final Considerations

5.8.1 Licensure/Legal

Physical therapists and physical therapist assistants performing service-learning activities must comply with all civil, criminal, and administrative laws, including licensure laws, in the jurisdiction where the service is provided regardless of whether or not a fee is charged for the service. If the services are provided in another country, the laws of that particular country are in force. A few states have provisions for temporary licensure or licensure by endorsement for physical therapists in the event of a declared national or state emergency or natural disaster. Familiarizing with local laws and rules is of tantamount importance prior to initiating any service-learning activities. Lastly, any organization impacted by the participation of its members in the provision of the service-learning activities or with the receiving of the product of service-learning activities should be made fully aware of the service-learning event and provide approval for such activities.

5.8.2 Code of Ethics and Standards of Practice

Complying with APTA's Code of Ethics for the physical therapist and the standards of ethical conduct for the physical therapist assistant[13] is an ethical and legal obligation of all physical therapists, physical therapist assistants, physical therapy students and physical therapist assistant students regardless of the location or type of pro bono service learning experience. Physical therapists and physical therapist assistants are responsible for the standard of care they provide to all patients regardless of their ability to pay, where the care is delivered, and what kinds of care are delivered. Complying with APTA's Standards of Practice for physical therapy is important for the student, the faculty member, and the patient/client.

5.8.3 Documentation

Requirements for medical record documentation are no different for individuals receiving pro bono service-learning physical therapy services than they are for all other patients/clients. Documentation of evaluation, assessment, intervention, and communication management is essential regardless of a patient's ability to pay, where the care is delivered, and what kinds of care are delivered. Medical records, as in most U.S. jurisdictions, should be maintained according to the 7/21/22 rule: at least 7 years for persons over the age 21; for persons receiving service under 21 years of age the records must be maintained until the patient has reached the age of 21 and for at least 7 years, and for services provided to women who are pregnant the records must be maintained until the child reaches the age of 21.

5.8.4 Liability

The need for liability insurance protection does not change simply because the service is provided pro bono. The malpractice/liability carrier for faculty and students should be consulted prior to any pro bono service-learning efforts to determine coverage. If a physical therapist is providing physical therapy services (pro bono or charged) away from one's primary place of employment, the therapist is typically not covered by the employer provided malpractice/liability policy.

Compliance standards: All participants in pro bono service-learning opportunities should meet, at minimum, the compliance standards developed by the major accreditation and regulatory agencies such as the Joint Commission, the Council for accreditation of rehabilitation facilities, and the associated state's department of health. These records, for confidentiality reasons, should not be automatically provided to organizations associated with the pro bono service-learning opportunity but the fact that the records are available if there is a need should be communicated to all concerned parties. These should include but are not limited to[19,20]:
- A valid license to practice physical therapy in the state the pro bono service-learning opportunity will be located.
- Valid cardio-pulmonary certification.
- Immunization records.
- Tubercular screening.
- Appropriate criminal background checks.
- Medicare check.
- Medical examination by the primary care provider.

5.8.5 Good Samaritan Laws

Many states have Good Samaritan laws that provide immunity to health care providers who come to the aid of victims under circumstances requiring immediate or emergent aid or action. Good Samaritan laws do not apply to routine or non-emergent health care such as physical therapy services. Good Samaritan laws typically apply to all regulated health care providers and are usually separate from physical therapy practice acts.

5.8.6 Third-party Private Payment Issues

The routine waiving of patients' copays and deductibles does not constitute pro bono care and may be considered fraud or abuse. Deductibles and copays are part of the contract or agreement among a third-party payer, a subscriber, and the service provider. Routinely waiving these costs, even with the intent of making the service affordable to the patient, is not permitted. If a patient has a copay, the provider must, in good faith, attempt to collect it. If the debt is not collectable and the patient/client objectively documents financial hardship, further collection efforts may be waived on a case-by-case basis. In this situation, the clinician may consider the writing off of the amount owed by the patient/client to be a pro bono service. In most settings, this would be similar to writing off a "bad debt."

An exception to this requirement may apply to physical therapists who are out-of-network providers who bill the patient directly for services. In these cases, the therapist is not contractually obligated to collect any copay or deductible amounts. However, out-of-network providers who provide courtesy billing to the patient's insurance company must abide by the deductible and copay obligations for out-of-network providers required by the patient's health plan. In essence, for out-of-network providers who are directly billing the patient, the charges to the insurer (on the courtesy billing) must equal the amount the patient is paying.

Physical therapists often ask about the option of charging different fees to different patients as a way of making their services affordable. Charging different fees for the same service to different patients is discouraged. It is important to have a consistent office policy regarding the reduction of fees.

5.9 Review Questions

1. Service-learning and volunteerism are two subsets of which type of altruistic activity?
   a) Community service.
   b) Pro bono clinic.
   c) American Physical Therapy Association-mandated activities for doctor of physical therapy students.
   d) Membership in a political action committee.

2. Research indicates that service-learning activities performed by college students results in a positive effect on which of the following measures?
   a) Grade point average.
   b) Writing skills.
   c) Critical thinking skills.
   d) All of the above.

3. If a university student performs a service learning activity in the first week of an academic semester, research indicates that the benefits of the activity become apparent when?
   a) Immediately.
   b) Within 2 weeks.
   c) By midterm or by the final examination.
   d) Two years after the activity.

4. Qualitative and quantitative research studies indicate that the effects of service-learning activities may be facilitated by the use of which activity?
   a) Direct monetary payment to the student for the activity performed.
   b) Formal and informal reflection by the student on the activity performed.
   c) Notoriety and publicity for the activity performed.
   d) Ensuring that the student's participation is long-term, at least 2 years.

5. Effectiveness of college/university level service-learning activities appears to be dependent on which of the following?
   a) A hand's off approach by faculty.
   b) Strong involvement by faculty.
   c) A hand's off approach by family.
   d) Strong involvement by family.

6. The American Physical Therapy Association's Code of Ethics for the physical therapist strongly endorses service leaning via which principle(s)?
   a) Principle 1.
   b) Principle 8.
   c) Principles 1 and 8.
   d) Principle 5.

7. "Pro bono public" is from the Latin meaning which of the following?
   a) For the public good.
   b) Out of many, one.
   c) United we stand.
   d) All for one and one for all.

8. Often the easiest and most cost-effective venue for performance of pro bono service is within an existing clinical setting. The reasons for this include all of the following except
   a) The therapy equipment is available for use; there is no need to purchase additional equipment.
   b) The facility is Americans with Disabilities Act–accessible.
   c) Most likely the owners of the facility have developed emergency policies and procedures.
   d) All of the above.

9. Which of the following clinical experiences is considered service-learning experience?
   a) Integrated clinical experience.
   b) Clinical internship.
   c) Advocacy efforts as directed and encouraged by the American Physical Therapy Association.
   d) Residencies.

10. The most effective method of involvement in service-learning advocacy for the doctor of physical therapy student is direct involvement with which activity?
   a) The American Physical Therapy Association National Student Conclave.
   b) Voting in local and national elections.
   c) Donating to a political action committee.
   d) Donating to a political party.

5.10 Review Answers

1. Service-learning and volunteerism are two subsets of which type of altruistic activity?
   a. Community service.

2. Research indicates that service-learning activities performed by college students results in a positive effect on which of the following measures?
   d. All of the above.

3. If a university student performs a service learning activity in the first week of an academic semester, research indicates that the benefits of the activity become apparent when?
   c. By midterm or by the final examination.

4. Qualitative and quantitative research studies indicate that the effects of service-learning activities may be facilitated by the use of which activity?
   b. Formal and informal reflection by the student on the activity performed.

5. Effectiveness of college/university level service-learning activities appears to be dependent on which of the following?
   b. Strong involvement by faculty.

6. The American Physical Therapy Association's Code of Ethics for the physical therapist strongly endorses service leaning via which principle(s)?
   c. Principles 1 and 8.

7. "Pro bono public" is from the Latin meaning which of the following?
   a. For the public good.

8. Often the easiest and most cost-effective venue for performance of pro bono service is within an existing clinical setting. The reasons for this include all of the following except:
   c. Most likely the owners of the facility have developed emergency policies and procedures.

9. Which of the following clinical experiences is considered service-learning experience?
   c. Advocacy efforts as directed and encouraged by the American Physical Therapy Association.

10. The most effective method of involvement in service-learning advocacy for the doctor of physical therapy student is direct involvement with which activity?

a. The American Physical Therapy Association National Student Conclave.

References

[1] Astin AW, Vogelgesang LJ, Ikeda EK, Yee JA. How service-learning affects students. High Educ. 2000:144

[2] Eyler J, Giles DE Jr, Stenson T, Gray C. At a Glance: Summary and Annotated Bibliography of Recent Service-Learning Research in Higher Education. 3rd ed. San Diego, CA: Learn & Serve America National Service-Learning Clearinghouse; 2001

[3] Eyler J, Halteman B. The impact of a legislative internship on students' political skill and sophistication. Teach Polit Sci. 1981; 9(1):27–34

[4] Strage AA. Service-learning: enhancing student learning outcomes in a college-level lecture course. Mich J Community Serv Learn. 2000; 7(1)

[5] Seifer SD. Service-learning: community-campus partnerships for health professions education. Acad Med. 1998; 73(3):273–277

[6] Markus GB, Howard JP, King DC. Notes: integrating community service and classroom instruction enhances learning: Results from an experiment. Educ Eval Policy Anal. 1993; 15(4):410–419

[7] Johnson M, Maritz C, Lefever G. The mercy circle of care: an interdisciplinary, multiinstitutional collaboration to promote community health and professional education. J Phys Ther Educ. 2006; 20(3):73–78

[8] Boss JA. The effect of community service work on the moral development of college ethics students. J Moral Educ. 1994; 23(2):183–198

[9] Andrus NC, Bennett NM. Developing an interdisciplinary, community-based education program for health professions students: the Rochester experience. Acad Med. 2006; 81(4):326–331

[10] Hamso M, Ramsdell A, Balmer D, Boquin C. Medical students as teachers at CoSMO, Columbia University's student-run clinic: a pilot study and literature review. Med Teach. 2012; 34(3):e189–e197

[11] Spielberg S, Goodwin DK, Kushner T. Mr. Lincoln goes to Hollywood. Smithsonian. 2012; 43(7):46–53

[12] Lincoln A. Abraham Lincoln: Speeches and Writings Part 1: 1832–1858: Library of America no. 45. Library of America; 1989

[13] APTA. Available at: http://www.apta.org/uploadedFiles/APTAorg/About_Us/Policies/HOD/Ethics/CodeofEthics.pdf. Accessed August 10, 2018

[14] APTA. Available at: http://www.apta.org/uploadedFiles/APTAorg/About_Us/Policies/HOD/Health/ProBono.pdf. Accessed August 10, 2018

[15] Carney PA, Pipas CF, Eliassen MS, et al. An analysis of students' clinical experiences in an integrated primary care clerkship. Acad Med. 2002; 77(7):681–687

[16] Ogur B, Hirsh D, Krupat E, Bor D. The Harvard Medical School-Cambridge integrated clerkship: an innovative model of clinical education. Acad Med. 2007; 82(4):397–404

[17] APTA. Available at: www.apta.org/nsc/. Accessed August 10, 2018

[18] Dhillon SK, Wilkins S, Law MC, Stewart DA, Tremblay M. Advocacy in occupational therapy: exploring clinicians' reasons and experiences of advocacy. Can J Occup Ther. 2010; 77(4):241–248

[19] Palombaro KM, et al. A case report of a student-led pro bono clinic: a proposed model for meeting student and community needs in a sustainable manner. J Phys Ther. 2011; 91(11):1627–1635

[20] Black JD, Palombaro KM, Dole RL. Student experiences in creating and launching a student-led physical therapy pro bono clinic: a qualitative investigation. J Phys Ther. 2013; 93(5):637–648

6 The Physical Therapist as a Researcher

Melissa A. Carroll

Keywords: Background question, best available evidence, clinical research question, critically appraised topic, database, evidence-based practice, evidence hierarchy, foreground question, in-service, journal club, PIO, PICO, and PICOT, public dissemination, research agenda, research design, search engine, statistics, three-legged stool

"Every scientist, through personal study and research, completes himself and his own humanity. ... Scientific research constitutes for you, as it does for many, the way for the personal encounter with truth, and perhaps the privileged place for the encounter itself with God, the Creator of heaven and earth. Science shines forth in all its value as a good capable of motivating our existence, as a great experience of freedom for truth, as a fundamental work of service. Through research each scientist grows as a human being and helps others to do likewise."

—Pope John Paul II

Address to the members of the Pontifical Academy of Sciences (November 13, 2000). In L'Osservatore Romano (November 29, 2000)

Chapter Outline
1. Overview
2. Evidence-Based Practice within Physical Therapy Education
3. Evidence-Based Practice and Research Courses
4. Courses with Integrated EBP Competencies
5. Clinical Research Evidence Should Support Clinical Practice
   a) The Critical Appraisal Process
6. Generation of Research Ideas
   a) Research Paradigms in Physical Therapy Practice
      1. Quantitative Research
      2. Qualitative Research
      3. Mixed Methods Research
7. Funding
   a) The Foundation for Physical Therapy
   b) Federal Funding
   c) Research Budgets
8. Presentation Forums

"Eleven years ago, at my orientation for my entry-level physical therapy program, I, as a bright eyed 23-year-old woman, looked no different than my classmates. We shared similar academic backgrounds, interests and life-goals. I sat in the same classes as my fellow DPT students: anatomy, physiology, neuroscience, clinical skills, pathology, ethics and the rest. I dutifully and energetically successfully completed my internships and passed the licensure exam. Upon graduation, I was fortunate to be offered a staff physical therapist position at a large tertiary care hospital in Houston. After a year or so of clinical work I approached my supervisor and asked for additional responsibility. As a novice therapist, I was still unsure of which direction I

wished to push my career and felt that any experience would be career-beneficial. He mentioned the Institutional Review Board (IRB) at the hospital needed an additional clinical member and that during our Department's weekly Journal Club I seemed to have an excellent understanding of research design and statistical methods. Truthfully, unlike most of my classmates, I enjoyed dissecting research articles for threats to internal and external validity and considering possible alternative research design and statistical methodology. I happily joined the IRB. After a number of months of learning the history and role of the IRB process and listening to the board debate the submitted research proposals, especially related to the safety of the enrolled subjects, I was finally partnered with an oncologist to review a submitted proposal detailing a clinical trial of lifestyle changes on specific biomarkers related coronary artery disease. The independent variables included stress reduction, exercise, nutrition, education, and the use of an over-the-counter supplement. The outcome, the dependent variable, was the serum concentration of specific biomarkers of heart disease. My job, as an IRB member, was not to provide criticisms of the proposal or research design but rather to ensure, to the best of my abilities, the safety of the invited subjects. My oncologist partner and I documented our recommendations and presented them to the full board. Our recommendation was to permit the research to commence with only mild changes to the consent form.

"The process exhilarated me. I loved being on the IRB and was soon promoted to vice-chair.

"My supervisor then approached me and asked if I would consider leading a small research study within our department. Our department had never developed a research agenda and my supervisor felt that a research agenda would improve our clinical skills, teamwork, and our clinical outcomes. He also felt that being named leader would provide me with a professional challenge. I quickly agreed to his proposal. Seven therapists joined our group and we began our nascent research examining the outcomes of early mobilization in the ICU. As a first attempt we did well; our results were published in a low-impact journal, but we were published. The thrill of adding to the professional literature and advancing clinical care thrilled me. I, however, realized that as a doctor of physical therapy (DPT) I was not trained as a researcher and if I wished to perform research as part of my career goals I needed formal training. I was accepted to the PhD in Motor Control program at a large Houston university and, with a heavy heart, resigned from my staff therapist position. Leaving my supervisor (who had believed in me by his words and delegation of tasks) was especially difficult. As was his nature he was thrilled for my acceptance and offered me any assistance I required.

"I found a home in the PhD program. The didactic content of motor control was a strong interest of mine but what I found truly rewarding was working with high-level researchers in developing research proposals, writing grants, collecting data, and drawing conclusions. For my dissertation, I compared the impact of various motor learning concepts on functional activities in persons with amyotrophic lateral sclerosis. However, even after five years in the PhD program I did not yet feel comfortable to go out on my own as a researcher. I applied to and was accepted for a post-doctorate program in Chicago. I worked under the guidance of two of the best researchers I ever met. I spent much time on grant writing but also learned a great deal about statistical analysis and research design. I also formalized my future research agenda. Just last month I finally decided to take the plunge and was offered and accepted a tenure-track faculty position at a world-class research university in Houston. I am so excited that I was able to discover my passion and that I had the determination to go and get it!"

—Asa Z., Houston, Texas

6.1 Overview

Professional expectations of evidence-based practice (EBP) in health care, including suggested education and practice goals emerged through a 2003 conference of international evidence-based health care instructors.[1] This landmark conference, and subsequent publication of the Sicily statement in 2005, outlined critical competencies for all entry level health care professionals regarding EBP. Clinicians, and those responsible for training future practitioners were charged not only to contribute and advance the public dissemination of research but also to learn the effective use of technology, critical appraisal of published literature, and application of evidence and integration into practice. Therefore, adoption of EBP and active participation in research (consuming and producing) are critical components of a physical therapist's professional identity.[2,3]

Incorporating the theory of EBP into clinical reasoning is a focus of the professional physical therapy curriculum for effective patient care and management. Effective clinical practice is dependent on integration of research evidence, clinical experience, and ongoing educational training. Physical therapy education is designed to train students for professional practice. Specifically, doctor of physical therapy curricula are designed for the development of a knowledgeable, service-oriented, critical thinker who uses evidence to support independent clinical judgment in every clinical setting and circumstance.[4]

6.2 Evidence-Based Practice within Physical Therapy Education

EBP (evolved from evidence-based medicine [EBM]) is the desire to use clinical evidence to support clinical decision making. In the 1990s, at McMaster University, Gordan Guyatt, David Sackett, and Brain Hayes recognized that medical theories were not equally supported by medical facts. This initiated an educational movement to encourage the use of unbiased, valid, and generalizable evidence when addressing health-related issues.[5,6] The goal was to prompt the application of scientific medicine, through the integration and use of research evidence to inform clinical practice—challenging the current model of patient management through tradition and authority.[6] However, the quality of research evidence was called into question, leading to another major component (if not the impetus) of EBM—implementation of critical appraisal.

Considered the father of EBM,[6,7] David Sackett (1934–2015) expanded the reach of EBM and spearheaded a transition of the health care curriculum to align with the tenets of clinical epidemiology. Through training series published in the Canadian Medical Association Journal and in the Journal of American Medical Association (JAMA), a textbook publication, and invited speaking engagements, Sackett and Guyatt contributed to the international dissemination of the EBM model.[5,6] The Sicily statement, as an international consensus, recommended replacing the term medicine in EBM with the term practice, to increase the inclusivity of a behavioral change in all of health care, to an EBP model.[1,8] In the late 1990s allied health fields started to incorporate the conceptual framework of EBM and in the early 2000s, as part of the Vision 2020 statement, the American Physical Therapy Association (APTA) incorporated the goal of evidence-based physical therapy (EBPT).[9] History of EBM can be watched at http://ebm.jamanetwork.com/.

APTA supports efficient and accurate use of research evidence for patient and client management in physical therapy practice, and reiterates that evidence should not replace clinical judgment and patient values.[10] The recommended approach for clinical decision making is the full integration of scientific research, clinical expertise, and patient values. These three resources are considered the pillars of EBP—commonly referred to as a three-legged stool where each resource equally supports positive patient outcomes.[5,11] Although most practitioners agree with the implementation of EBP, the ability to teach clinical practice and reasoning informed by evidence has been a challenge.[1,8,12] The Sicily statement identified necessary curricular competencies for teaching the five steps of the EBP process,[1] simplified here as (1) ask, (2) search, (3) appraise, (4) implement, and (5) assess (see ▶ Fig. 6.1).

EBP is a behavioral science, therefore true application of evidence informing practice is a change in human activity and clinical behavior. EBP is only considered relevant when accounting for specific parameters within a patient population and clinical context, which can be affected by society and culture. Physical therapists must know, understand, believe, and apply research evidence in practice—this complete process is called translational and implementation research.[13,14] Translating published research evidence into clinical practice is a critical step of EBP however there is a distinct research-to-practice gap between publication of clinical evidence and implementation in clinical practice.[3,14]

6.3 Evidence-Based Practice and Research Courses

Physical therapy programs are responsible for ensuring that entry-level professionals are trained to be evidence-based practitioners. Expectations for implementing EBP in professional practice include integration of evidence during patient client management, efficient use of technology to find relevant and appropriate evidence, critical appraisal of published literature, interpretation of population statistics, application and assessment of evidence in practice, and evaluation of

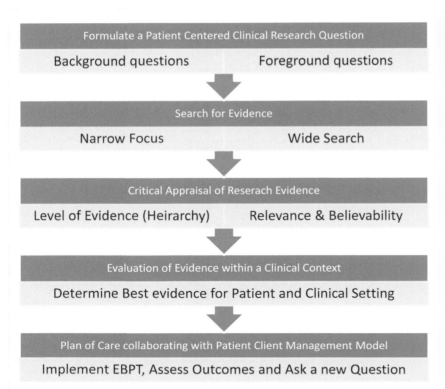

Fig. 6.1 Five steps of evidence-based practice. Evidence-based practice is the process of integrating individual clinical expertise, patient values and the best available external clinical evidence from systematic research to improve clinical decision making.

Within the figure:

Formulate a Patient Centered Clinical Research Question

Background questions — Foreground questions

Search for Evidence

Narrow Focus — Wide Search

Critical Appraisal of Reserach Evidence

Level of Evidence (Heirarchy) — Relevance & Believability

Evaluation of Evidence within a Clinical Context

Determine Best evidence for Patient and Clinical Setting

Plan of Care collaborating with Patient Client Management Model

Implement EBPT, Assess Outcomes and Ask a new Question

successful outcomes. Each of these skills can be taught separately within theoretical and didactic courses or in conjunction with clinical education.

The Commission on Accreditation in Physical Therapy Education (CAPTE) requires doctor of physical therapy programs to provide curricular content that addresses EBP for the entry level professional,[15] the content delivery is determined by each program. Standalone courses (i.e., EBP, research methods, and statistics seminars) have been developed to allow the student physical therapist to understand the foundations of EBP, research consumerism, and research production including methodology, design, quality, statistics, validity and generalizability. A few curricular models include optional participation in student research projects, capstone projects, or mandatory participation in conducting research to expose the student to the research process. Although these types of experiences have been a source of debate regarding time allotted in the curriculum, the importance of research has always been valued as an educational experience.

Skills taught within a research curriculum are critical for physical therapy practice, even when they do not explicitly relate to producing or consuming evidence. Through research, students can learn nontechnical skills such as time management, conflict resolution, and how to deal with unpredictability or ambiguity. Negotiating and defending clinical decision making, analysis of comorbidity rates, prioritizing patient problems and determining the need for physical therapy in practice are also important nontechnical competencies that can be learned from effective research courses. All research projects can have some value, even when the sample size is small; conclusions may be transferrable to a specific population or an individual clinic although it may not be generalizable to the larger population. Therefore, most research projects can still contribute to the development of interesting findings, and advancing the field, even when the research design is flawed.

6.4 Courses with Integrated EBP Competencies

Most courses within physical therapy curricula incorporate an aspect of training in EBP to ensure a full integration of evidence-based clinical decision making while learning within physical therapy practice. Developing clinical decision-making skills informed by evidence within the patient-client management (PCM) model and the International Classification of Function, Disability, and Health (ICF) from the World Health Organization should involve the use of EBPT. Each class provides an opportunity to increase exposure to the patient-client management model, ICF model, and uses a degree of EBPT, either explicitly or implicitly. As a student physical therapist, developing critical thinking skills, independent decision making and clinical judgment supported by evidence is crucial to success within clinical education. These experiences within the PT curriculum are designed to be varied as well as structured to enhance the development of EBPT skills.

Clinical reasoning in the ICF and PCM models aligns with the vision 2020 statement and the new vision of APTA. Lifelong learners and EBP practitioners should be autonomous and collaborative, determining the need for treatment and the priority of patient problems. Clinical decision making is determined by the theoretical training received in school, patient values, and the best available evidence—a combination of cognitive and psychomotor skills based on theory and evidence.[16] Several important decisions can be made with EBP related to quality assessment of patient outcomes, cost, time and expert analysis. Decisions are valued by the expected positive or harmful results based on the intervention. Patient outcomes are measured, documented and assessed for quality assurance, productivity and efficacy.

EBPT practice is defined as physical therapy practice informed by high quality, relevant, and applicable clinical evidence.[15] Implementing EBPT during patient and client management is critical to maintain a level of care that is supported by current practice and the best available evidence. Cultural variation and patient values should also influence the clinical decision-making process, whereas the evidence is weighed against the wants and needs of each client. The best available evidence is compassionate, appropriate, and considerate of each individual factor that influences the relationship between patient and clinician.

During clinical education, a student physical therapist should be able to effectively use the first three steps of the EBP model (ask, seek, and appraise). Depending on the clinical setting the clinical instructor (CI) may be modeling translational and implementation research—using appropriate evidence at the bedside and in practice. Clinical training is therefore the most realistic avenue for application of translating research into practice (step 4) and evaluation of the performance outcomes (step 5). Most student therapists, however, use CIs as their primary source of evidence—relying on authority and tradition. Although CIs are a great source to lean on for clinical expertise it is still important for the student therapist to search the literature for patient-specific evidence to support the plan of care.

As an entry-level professional, it is critical to change clinical behaviors from the tradition of authority and a "cookbook" approach to forming a plan of care, diagnosis, and therapeutic exercise to a well-supported evidence-based treatment approach. The three-legged stool of positive patient outcomes relies on (1) clinical experience, (2) patient values, and (3) best available evidence. However, as a student preparing to enter practice, and for any entry-level professional, the best two legs to stand on would be patient values and the best available clinical evidence as time and experience allows clinical expertise to develop (see ▶ Fig. 6.2).

There are challenges and benefits to the application of EBPT within clinical practice. There are innumerable sources of evidence to support or refute primary care, yet it is the duty of the practitioner to determine the best course of action. Some clinical sites will promote a dialogue surrounding the best available evidence, in the form of a journal club, in-service presentations, or just a discussion among colleagues that references current literature and new approaches. If this is not the culture of the clinical setting that you are placed, try to initiate evidence-based conversations yourself; some medical practitioners indicated an appreciation of the challenge from students as it demonstrated interest in learning and promoted forward thinking.[17] Novice practitioners, regardless of EBP culture at the clinical placement, should respectfully challenge the CIs with evidence—most are willing and wanting to learn themselves.

Patient client management and EBP sound logical to incorporate and apply to everyday practice. However, full patient loads, limited access to resources, inability to ask a relevant research question, and limited time to critically appraise research are significant barriers to implementation of EBPT. Taking an opportunity to learn how to effectively critique research evidence, having a working understanding of the best research design, and understanding the use of appropriate statistics for a research question aid in the ease of implementation during early clinical years.

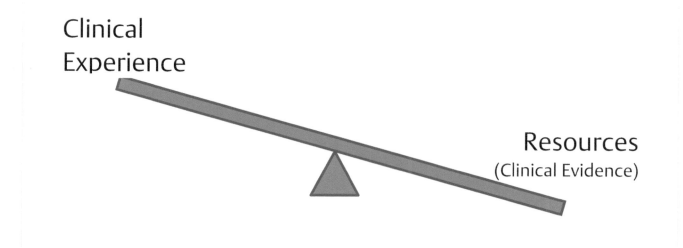

Fig. 6.2 Unbalanced experiences. Practicing physical therapists and physical therapist assistants need to appropriately balance their clinical experiences with clinical evidence as decisions are made in the clinic. Some clinical decisions are best made through clinical experience, others through resources, and others by a combination of clinical experience and resources.

6.5 Clinical Research Evidence Should Support Clinical Practice

Accessibility to research evidence can be a major barrier to the implementation of EBPT, especially in private practices that may not be affiliated with a major institution. Although an APTA membership can provide access to current research evidence, only 30% of practicing physical therapists are APTA members. As a student physical therapist and an entry-level professional, strive to be a member of APTA and use the online resources available through member sharing libraries and access to PTNow to find supporting evidence; also use your faculty and institutional library.

Evidence originates in a myriad of published literature: in journal articles, textbooks, unpublished dissertation materials, and even anecdotal evidence from authority, tradition, experience, and content experts. Each branch of the evidence can be appraised and critiqued in a way to move current practice forward. Background evidence is that which informs the who, what, where, when, and how questions. Foreground questions are then created to provide enough detail to search for evidence that is relevant, applicable, specific, and considerate of the patient in a clinical context. Asking the research question and searching for the evidence are the first two steps in making an evidence-based clinical decision[1,5] and it can be the hardest step for many practitioners.

In this respect, the use of a medical librarian is advised. Medial librarians understand the search capabilities, and limitations, of most medical databases. For example, Google Scholar, although popular and easy to use, provides search results based on the number of clicks per article—it is a search engine for articles. This process is different for databases which consider the relevance of your search terms in the results returned from each search.

Published evidence is not always the highest-quality evidence, as there are publication bias, reliability, validity, and generalizability considerations to appraise. Current evidence and journal impact factors play a role in the hierarchy of research evidence and the believability of the conclusions. Most published evidence is produced and disseminated from the research or academic sector rather than from health care researchers.[18] Some articles are published in open access journals and some undergo a peer-review process; the difference in the rigor of these publications must be considered prior to the clinician implementing the evidence.

Understanding the consumption of clinical evidence through the process of critical appraisal and healthy critique allows evaluation of the quality of research evidence and the applicability for the use with specific clients. Evaluation of research quality can make an impact on the clinical care provided. Supporting your clinical reasoning and opinions with solid resources provides an answer to those "why, what, or how long" questions that your clients may ask: *why do I need to participate in this? What are the possible benefits of this exercise intervention? How long can I anticipate feeling this pain and discomfort?*

6.5.1 The Critical Appraisal Process

Public dissemination of research through journal publication does not mean the evidence is applicable or appropriate in design, analysis, or usefulness.[19] The critical appraisal process has two primary goals: (1) to determine the validity of the study and (2) to determine the importance of the research evidence. True critical appraisal should critique the internal and external validity of a research study, discuss the logical application of evidence as compared with the level of believability, and compare the evidence with the researcher's clinical judgment. Evidence-based practitioners should also consider clinical significance when appraising literature because statistical significance does not determine effect size or magnitude of change. Several resources have been developed to assist in the methodological assessment of published evidence and evaluation of the importance to clinical practice.

Although the rigor and quality of physical therapy research has increased,[18,20] the ability to confidently make assumptions of treatment effect without bias is aided by grading research evidence.[21] Level of evidence is determined on the quality of research design and hierarchies of methodological approach. The highest level of evidence is normally pre-synthesized and pre-appraised articles, such as systematic reviews or meta-analyses. These publications allow clinicians to identify appropriate resources with confidence and provide easy, useful, and pragmatic access to current evidence.[22] Translating primary evidence to clinical practice can be challenging due to the sheer volume of published literature. For these reasons many experts within EBP recommend the use of pre-appraised and pre-synthesized evidence within everyday practice.

6.6 Generation of Research Ideas

Research ideas are generated through the identification of a knowledge gap, clinical experience, and practice controversy or conflicting published evidence.[23] Asking a clinical research question is a skill that develops with time and practice. Each researcher learns that relevant background questions and foreground questions are critical to the production of a proactive research agenda. Developing a research plan is important to the student researcher who would like to pursue a terminal doctoral degree (i.e., PhD, SciD, EdD), conduct research during clinical practice, or wants to enter an academic appointment and needs to develop a research line for rank and tenure.

One of the hardest parts of developing a research project is first developing a research question. There is also an old research adage that says, "So what? Who cares?" It sounds harsh but consider these questions at the start of any research project. Make sure that your research questions are novel, applicable, and considerate of the current knowledge gap, the patient population, and the clinical setting. It is important to figure out the purpose and goal of the research project and what type of contribution it will make to advance the field of physical therapy. APTA published a national research agenda to provide ideas for junior researchers and for funding agencies[24]; however, any patient, colleague, or administrative interaction can prompt a research question.

Clinical settings can contribute to the development of a research question, which can prompt an initial search of the literature for interesting clinical topics, quality assessment questions, diagnostic tests, prognostic factors, treatment interventions, or best patient outcomes. Each of these categories can be supported by previously synthesized and analyzed evidence, providing answers to background questions, in the form of a systematic review or meta-analysis. It is important to make sure that these synthesized data are current (within the last 3–5 years) and that they are relevant to the patient and clinical setting. Most of these documents have recommended future directions, as suggestions from the authors, this would be a great avenue to explore for the generation of new foreground questions and research ideas.

Formulating your research question can come in several forms. During the initial steps of generating any evidence-based clinical research question the "ask and search" process helps to refine the relevance and usefulness of the research project. Asking a clinical question generally can follow these formats: PIO, PICO/PECO, and PICOT. There are four types of research questions asked by health care personnel. The definitions of each assists in choosing which to use (see ▶ Table 6.1).[25]

Once the research question has been formulated, it is important to go back to the research literature to ensure that the question has not been previously or recently answered (within the last 2 years). Databases and efficient technology searches inform the direction of research projects, the best options for physical therapy research are MEDLINE/PubMed, EMBASE, PEDro, and PTNow.[26,27,28] These databases allow a researcher quick access to pre-appraised and pre-selected evidence of high quality and utility. Should there be similarities to your research inquiry, it is important to identify the research gap and answer the following questions: What still needs to be answered? Were the research assumptions met or violated? How can your research project contribute to validating the current evidence?

Table 6.1 Types of research questions: PIO, PICO, PECO and PICOT

Structural components of clinical questions		
PIO		Patient Issue/Intervention Outcome
PICO		Patient Issue/Intervention Comparison Outcome
PECO		Patient Exposure Comparison Outcome
PICOT		Patient Issue/Intervention Comparison Outcome Time
P	Who? What?	Age, sex, race, past medical history, pathology
I	What are you considering?	Intervention, diagnostic test, prognostic factor
C	How does it compare?	No comparison, control, placebo, different intervention
O	What are the goals?	Measurable and patient oriented

The literature search should include a broad scope but a narrow focus. That means that the use of Boolean logic and medical subject headings (MeSH terms) are not restricting or limiting the search and yet they are selective enough to yield results. It is critically important to search multiple databases and to also consider interprofessional evidence—seek help from medical librarians. Limiting a search to physical therapy evidence ignores the advances that may have been made by other health care professionals.

Lastly it is important to rewrite and reconceptualize the research question within the context of the current evidence. Operationally define research concepts or ambiguous terms that are important to understand the project and the contribution to advance the evidence. For example, improved function does not explain how function was measured. Does this account for range of motion, muscle strength, endurance? How does the improved function relate to the concept of physical impairment?

Once the research idea has been formalized, it is important to pick a research design that will provide an answer to the research question. During this process it would be important to evaluate if a quantitative, qualitative, or mixed methods approach would be the best research paradigm for the inquiry. Depending on the project design, formulate a research hypothesis based on the anticipated data. It is then important to define the research hypothesis and consider what statistical analysis would be appropriate for answering the research question.

6.6.1 Research Paradigms in Physical Therapy Practice

Generally, research has been divided into two primary modes of thought: quantitative theories and qualitative theories. Some generalize these paradigms as either dealing with numbers (things that can be measured and quantified) or with the process of examination and observation. Theorists are biased regarding each paradigm and beliefs regarding the best way to answer a scientific question; however, clinical research differs from bench research in how the reality of the patient must be considered. Observation of patient attitudes and perception to treatment in addition to the quantification of change, specifically related to patient improvement or decline, creates relevant research evidence for EBPT.

The scientific method created the framework for true experimental designs. Similar to EBP the scientific method has specific steps for success: (1) ask, (2) hypothesize, (3) collect data, (4) analyze, and (5) interpret. The goal is to minimize bias from the researcher and truly identify the cause-and-effect relationship of any independent variable. Although time and measurements are critically important in identifying the relationship between a manipulated variable or factor, the eventual outcome, dependent variable, can be compared for statistical significance—presence of a change or difference between the groups examined. This is the basis of quantitative research.

Quantitative Research

The scientific method, a quantitative paradigm connected to medical research, originally dictated the research approach of physical therapy practice. Quantitative research designs are considered to rely on deductive reasoning, focusing explicitly on experimental designs and a conscious effort to discover the cause and effect relationship. Within the parameters of measurement and control—considered to have developed from the method of true scientific inquiry—quantitative designs hold a high level of respect within research methodology.

Randomized control trials (RCTs), which control all confounding variables in an effort to truly evaluate the efficacy of an intervention without error, are the gold standard of determining cause-and-effect relationships. RCTs are designed to provide the efficacy of the intervention; internal validity is high because high quality RCTs control for erroneous or confounding variables. Randomization of sample sizes, tight inclusion and exclusion criteria, and protocols for treatment delivery reduce research bias but also reduce generalizability to the external environment. Although RCTs are critically important to evaluate the true value and statistical effect of an intervention; measurements and data are collected in a perfect clinical environment, which is not the reality of some patient care. Patient adherence to some intervention programs can be low[3] and therefore RCTs may not provide the best evidence for true clinical scenarios.

The use of sophisticated techniques for statistical analysis in physical therapy research has increased,[18] which enhances the use of quantitative designs like RCTs. Treatment effectiveness, which considers participant attrition during a strict protocol, can be supported through statistical analysis with an intention to treat analysis. For clinical relevance, this enhances the usefulness of RCTs as there is a prediction of the probable success of a treatment program in a clinical context.[19] Translating research evidence to clinical practice relies on applicable research conclusions that are salient to clinical decision making; therefore some quantitative research designs contribute to a research–practice gap, whereas clinicians cannot translate high methodologic, statistically significant evidence into everyday clinical practice.

Statistical significance does not mean that the evidence is clinically significant or relevant to the practice of physical therapy.[19] For this reason, clinicians have to understand why some statistical applications are used and what they determine. For example, the minimal clinically important difference (MCID), confidence intervals and effect sizes. International reporting statements have tried to encourage public dissemination that abides by useful presentation of evidence, such as the PRISMA statement or CONSORT statement.

Quasi-experimental designs have also been considered more valuable for clinical researchers. Although there may be more bias in the research design in comparison to an RCT, the reduction in internal validity is traded for greater external validity. Pseudocontrol groups, where normal treatment protocols can be administered in comparison to the new intervention protocol, are considered to be an ethical and legal alternative to withholding any treatment—as would be the need for a true control in an RCT.

Qualitative Research

In a qualitative physical therapy research design, the researcher may be the measurement instrument, with an intent to interpret patterns and themes based on patient interactions.

Qualitative processes are primarily inductive as the researcher describes a consistent phenomenon that informs a specific conclusion based on general observations.[23] Qualitative research designs are intentionally trying to triangulate data as an approach to reinforce conclusions; therefore, collecting data from several sources is critical to support a developing theory. Data, in qualitative research, are not real numbers—they are narrative or value-based codes, with the intent to provide a rich and thick understanding and description of the phenomena.

Survey designs are a common form of qualitative research in physical therapy practice.[21] Data collected is generally descriptive in nature, allowing analysis of perceptions and attitudes. Conclusions from these study designs can inform a subsequent research project or elucidate current beliefs of practice or treatment effects. This can be instrumental for understanding patient values and circumstances that may influence best clinical practice.

Qualitative research has its own limitations due to the passive nature of observation. There will always be bias in qualitative studies because of the interdependent relationship of the researcher and the participants. Pure qualitative research designs have no control group and no such thing as one reality as the investigation is completely focused on the exploration of the extraneous variables. This hands-off (no manipulation) approach is great for the opportunity to advance the field but it does not normally allow for true generalization of results as a lot of these studies are presented in case report fashion. Oftentimes the best approach is now a mixed method approach where there is a combination of observation and quantification of change.

Mixed Methods Research

Choosing between quantitative and qualitative depends on the research question which would dictate the best design to produce a relevant and useful answer. Determine the current knowledge associated with the theoretical framework related to the research question. Ask the necessary background questions and determine the gap in knowledge that will then determine the type of question that should be asked, which directs the research paradigm that answers the research question.

Viewing quantitative and qualitative designs as competitive, one superior to the other, has slowly changed in physical therapy research. Both designs have gained value and purpose within rehabilitation research for providing a global view of treatment effectiveness and patient perspectives. Knowledge is both quantitative and qualitative, each research paradigm is a combination between an epistemological and methodological approach to evidence. Research theory, psychomotor skills, quantification of standard outcomes, and observational analysis are all critical components for expert practice.[16] Therefore during the design and creation of a research project it would be pragmatic and useful to mimic the clinical environment.

6.7 Funding

Funding agencies often publish "call for proposals" (CFPs), "request for proposals" (RFPs), "funding opportunity announcements" (FOAs), "program announcements" (PAs), or "request for applications" (RFAs)—these documents are notifications of available funding oftentimes for a designated topic of inquiry. Applications for funding are most commonly, if not exclusively, submitted online. As a student researcher, you may have the opportunity to work with an advisor or faculty mentor to prepare an application for submission during school. Prior to submission it is important to read the instructions, the eligibility requirements and follow the posted deadlines. Some agencies first request that a letter of intent (LOI) is submitted; this serves as an initial review of the research idea before the opportunity to submit an application is granted.

6.7.1 The Foundation for Physical Therapy

Physical therapy research can be funded by several sources (e. g., individual awards, institutional funding, society funding, and private foundations). In 2009, APTA and the Foundation for Physical Therapy (FPT) clearly defined a separation of each organization within the bylaws of the nonprofit FPT.[2] Although APTA and the FPT are separate organizations, each work in conjunction to advance physical therapy research and provide evidence for new treatment approaches for ideal physical function.[2]

Founded in 1979, the FPT is a tax-exempt organization that can be funded by individual donations, APTA section endowments, and is supported by student fundraising—for example, the Marquette Challenge (https://foundation4pt.org/become-a-donor/marquette-challenge/). The goal of the foundation is to support physical therapy practice through scientific research by providing funds and publicly disseminating research findings. Publication bias in most available evidence is important to consider given that it is more common for positive outcomes to be published, rather than useful or pragmatic evidence.[13,29] However, the FPT publishes, disseminates, and supports new treatment approaches across the lifespan in all subspecialties, regardless of the outcome.[2] This belief emerges from the ideal that all research evidence is good and necessary evidence, especially concerning the advancement of health care.

In 2014, the FPT's strategic plan focused on research projects that increased awareness of physical therapy in society and provide supporting evidence regarding the value of physical therapy. However, supported and funded projects from the FPT range from effective physical therapy practice to a focus on geriatrics, pediatrics, orthopedics, and private practice. Opportunities for funding from the FPT may vary year to year depending on the goals of APTA,[2] and specific topics may be requested through designated funds provided by private investors.

The FPT can provide $10,000 to $40,000 for research endeavors that extend for 1 to 2 years; these projects can serve as a springboard to collect pilot data in support of an application for federal funding from the National Institute of Health (NIH). Funding from the foundation is reserved for physical therapy research; for example, rehabilitation interventions should be administered by a physical therapist, a physical therapist assistant, or supervised by a physical therapist. Application for FPT funds are critically examined and competitively awarded based on the decisions of the board of the FPT.

6.7.2 Federal Funding

The NIH can also fund research projects, research training, and career development through small grants per individual, per program, or per institution. Most commonly, research funding from the NIH is considered to be within the "R series" of grants (i.e., R01, R03, R21, and R15) and can provide a varied amount of financial support ($50,000–$275,000) for a maximum of 2 to 5 years. Successful grant application and funding is very competitive; some grants proposals require supportive preliminary data. Funding opportunities from the NIH are determined by an internal organizational structure. Each grant awarding division has a program officer responsible for the administration of funds. Program officers are great resources for training and an initial evaluation of application fitness—successful awards provide job security.

Applications for federal funding must be submitted from a recognized and accredited institution. Once submitted, the Center for Scientific Review (CSR) directs the application to an integrated review group (IRG) study section where the application is reviewed for scientific merit and scored by two to three independent reviewers. Scores range from 1.00 (best proposal) to 5.00 (worst proposal); however, the bottom half of applications may remain unscored. Scored applications are presented to an advisory council, reviewed for significance, programmatic merit, and eventually approved or denied for the disbursal of federal funds.

6.7.3 Research Budgets

Prior to submitting an application for funding, it is important to create and review a research budget. Depending on the size of the research award, consultation with an institutional grants support office is recommended. An office of sponsored projects or more experienced research collaborators may provide useful resources regarding the development of a research budget. As a researcher, it is critically important to ensure that funds are properly allocated based on the potential reward restrictions. Budgets, especially the justification for the distribution of funds, are extensively reviewed and analyzed by granting agencies; failure to follow the funding guidelines can result in application denial regardless of the scientific merit.

Discussing a detailed research budget is beyond the scope of this chapter; however, well-designed research projects should always have a well-proposed research budget. Most funding agencies are willing to clarify the funding restrictions for successful budget submissions and also provide written resources in support of the application guidelines or in the frequently asked questions.

6.8 Presentation Forums

Translational and implementation research are important terms used to identify the transition of scientific evidence from bench, to bedside and into practice.[14] There is a lot of support for the use of best evidence in clinical practice, steps 4 and 5 in the EBP process; however, it has been realized that there is a significant gap between researcher and clinician. Published research can take over a decade to be incorporated into clinical practice,[3,14] yet the theory behind translational and implementation research encourages a reduction in this lag time. One venue to enhance knowledge translation, encourage implementation of EBP, and increase exposure to research evidence is through research presentations.

Presentations of research evidence can occur within a local institution or during a wider range of dissemination on the state, regional, or national level. Regardless of the setting, research presentations should promote discourse regarding clinical relevance and contribute to ideas of immediate applicability in practice. As a student, especially one interested in research, opportunities should be sought to participate in both presenting research evidence and being a member of the listening audience. Each participatory experience has value within the training and implementation of evidence informing practice.

Dissemination of clinical research evidence through a public forum should be considerate of the impact on health care practice. Critical components of research design should be addressed, such as the patient population and specific inclusion and exclusion criteria. This allows the audience to consider who may respond well to the evidence presented. Presenters should also strive to operationally define any ambiguous topics, explain why and how clinical decisions were made, especially during examination and evaluation, and identify what led to the choice of interventions or measurement outcomes. Although clinical experts may know how to recognize relevant patient attributes during client interaction, there may be a knowledge gap regarding the consideration of all salient facts and the ability to integrate evidence during patient care—effective research presentations will explicitly provide this clinical link.

Intent to increase the amount of evidence supporting practice, research presentation forums can vary widely. Entry-level professional training during a program in physical therapy education may allow for different opportunities for a student to be engaged in primary research experiences. Standalone research-based courses may have assessment-based research presentations or capstone projects, clinical reasoning courses may have a grand rounds presentation format and some courses may have problem-based learning modules with presentations attached. Additionally, students may be invited to present an *in-service* of training during each clinical rotation. These local presentations provide great opportunities for feedback from faculty mentors, peers and CIs regarding presentation skills and translating evidence into practice.

Journal clubs are another local forum for presenting and discussing current research evidence. Oftentimes, journal clubs are informal presentations among colleagues to discuss current clinical evidence related to published clinical cases and the potential application for clinical practice.[30] The structure of a journal club can vary, including the commitment necessary from participants regarding attendance and preparation. Preparation may involve prereading the article to be able to follow the presentation and contribute to the group discussion. Participation in a journal club can increase critical appraisal skills, statistical knowledge, and understanding research designs while increasing a commitment to EBP.[30]

The most common presentation forum is a conference, which can be a local, statewide, regional, national, or international meeting. During most conferences, researchers have an opportunity to share relevant evidence through poster or platform (oral) presentations, plenary (lecture) sessions, and symposia—attendees have an opportunity to learn about cutting-edge research and clinical evidence. As an audience member, it is important to only ask questions during the presentation when it is critical to understanding the concept (i.e., what did you use to measure force production?). Each presentation will have a short question-and-answer session, which is the most appropriate place to ask questions to the presenter. Meeting with keynote speakers, dynamic presenters, or influential researchers after the presentation is a great way to network and to ask follow-up questions.

As a researcher, acceptance to present at a conference is beneficial and adds to a resume and curriculum vitae (CV). As a student researcher, having the experience to present at a conference can be viewed positively on an application to residency programs. Submission and review of a research abstract—a short summary of the project—precedes the selection to present at a conference. Some conferences require a processing fee to submit an abstract—these fees can range from $25 to $60, depending on the conference. Additionally, publication costs should be considered when applying to present at a conference. Some agencies can charge upwards of $70 to print one poster; unexpected costs can occur if there is a need to publish manuals, handouts, or pamphlets during the dissemination process. Furthermore, some conferences will not review your abstract unless you concurrently submit the conference registration costs.

6.9 Review Questions

1. During clinic one day you come across a client with a rare presentation and a challenging diagnosis. In order to effectively treat this client, you must first?
   a) Conduct an internet search to find out what the symptoms may diagnose.
   b) Gather answers to background questions regarding the symptoms by looking through textbooks and on reputable websites, like the Centers for Disease Control and Prevention.
   c) Immediately stop patient interaction and refer the client to another clinic or to a specialist.
   d) Implement a standard plan of care and hope the client improves.
2. Many of the published studies on the efficacy of physical therapy interventions are randomized control trials. For the most pragmatic and useful research design for translating evidence into practice, which of the follow modes of thought would be the best approach?
   a) Qualitative.
   b) Quantitative.
   c) Mixed methods.
   d) None of the above.
3. While searching for evidence on an outcome measure to determine functional improvement for a middle-aged client with a right total knee replacement you find the following evidence. Which would be the most appropriate article to read?
   a) Quadriceps strength postsurgical intervention in recreational athletes.

b) Endurance training for college-aged healthy adults with early osteoarthritis.

c) Incidence of reinjury post-ACL repair during noncontact sports.

d) Training programs to improve gait velocity in elderly females.

4. In your outpatient clinical rotation, it is determined that pediatric clients are nonadherent to a home exercise program. You decide to investigate ways to increase participation. Which of the following research designs would not help answer the research question?

a) Qualitative examination of the client's home environments.

b) Cohort design between successful patient participation and nonadherent clients.

c) Pediatric perspective and attitudes of rehabilitation program.

d) Randomized controlled trial of all pediatric rehabilitation programs.

5. Why does meta-analysis provide a powerful integrative tool?

a) It provides statistical methods for combining data and differentiating between comparable in previously published data analyses.

b) It provides statistical methods for combining a number of independent variables.

c) It provides methods for combining and differentiating between numerous conclusions in previously published data analyses.

d) It provides statistical methods for differentiating between the outcome measurements in previously published data analyses.

6. In meta-analysis, a correlation coefficient is one statistic which is used to calculate?

a) The sample size.

b) The effect size.

c) The variability in individual scores.

d) The standard deviation.

7. What purpose do clearly stated aims serve?

a) Aims state clearly in detail how research will be done and justify why research is being carried out.

b) Aims state clearly what the research intends to contribute and details how the research will be done.

c) Aims state clearly what the research intends to contribute and justifies the research being carried out.

d) Aims state clearly how the research will be done and what conclusions are expected.

8. Taking the idea that the more jealous someone is the more likely there are to be violent, what would the correct hypothesis be?

a) People with more violent behavior are likely to be less jealous than individuals who are less violent.

b) Jealousy is positively linked with violent behavior.

c) Greater levels of jealousy are will be associated with lower levels of violent behavior.

d) None of these.

9. "Individuals who are sleep deprived will differ significantly in their reaction time, to those individuals who are not sleep deprived." If this is the alternate hypothesis, which of the below statements would be the correct null hypothesis?

a) Greater sleep deprivation leads to a decrease in reaction time.

b) Individuals who are not sleep deprived will differ in their reaction time from those individuals who are sleep deprived.

c) Individuals who are sleep deprived will not differ in their reaction time from those individuals who are not sleep deprived.

d) Individuals who have more sleep will differ in their reaction time from those individuals who are sleep deprived.

10. Why is it important to read original articles when you are reviewing the literature?

a) To examine the validity of the conclusions.

b) To obtain an overview of methods and procedures.

c) To look for flaws in the method.

d) All of these.

6.10 Review Answers

1. During clinic one day you come across a client with a rare presentation and a challenging diagnosis. To effectively treat this client, you must first?

   b. Gather answers to background questions regarding the symptoms by looking through textbooks and on reputable websites, like the Centers for Disease Control and Prevention.

2. Many of the published studies on the efficacy of physical therapy interventions are randomized control trials. For the most pragmatic and useful research design for translating evidence into practice, which of the follow modes of thought would be the best approach?

   c. Mixed methods.

3. While searching for evidence on an outcome measure to determine functional improvement for a middle-aged client with a right total knee replacement you find the following evidence. Which would be the most appropriate article to read?

   a. Quadriceps strength postsurgical intervention in recreational athletes.

4. In your outpatient clinical rotation, it is determined that pediatric clients are nonadherent to a home exercise program. You decide to investigate ways to increase participation. Which of the following research designs would not help answer the research question?

   d. Randomized controlled trial of all pediatric rehabilitation programs.

5. Why does meta-analysis provide a powerful integrative tool?

   a. It provides statistical methods for combining data and differentiating between comparable in previously published data analyses

6. In meta-analysis, a correlation coefficient is one statistic which is used to calculate?

   b. The effect size.

7. What purpose do clearly stated aims serve?

   c. Aims state clearly what the research intends to contribute and justifies the research being carried out.

8. Taking the idea that the more jealous someone is the more likely there are to be violent, what would the correct hypothesis be?

   b. Jealousy is positively linked with violent behavior.

9. "Individuals who are sleep deprived will differ significantly in their reaction time, to those individuals who are not sleep

deprived." If this is the alternate hypothesis, which of the below statements would be the correct null hypothesis?

c. Individuals who are sleep deprived will not differ in their reaction time from those individuals who are not sleep deprived.

10. Why is it important to read original articles when you are reviewing the literature?

   d. All of the above.

References

[1] Dawes M, Summerskill W, Glasziou P, et al. Second International Conference of Evidence-Based Health Care Teachers and Developers. Sicily statement on evidence-based practice. BMC Med Educ. 2005; 5(1):1

[2] Shields RK. Above board: clear bylaws support the research mission of the Foundation for Physical Therapy. Phys Ther. 2009; 89(10):1010–1012

[3] Goldstein MS, Scalzitti DA, Bohmert JA, et al. Vitalizing practice through research and research through practice: the outcomes of a conference to enhance the delivery of care. Phys Ther. 2011; 91(8):1275–1284

[4] American Physical Therapy Association. (2004). A normative model of physical therapist professional education: Version 2004. Alexandria, VA: American Physical Therapy Association; 2004.

[5] Sackett DL, Rosenberg WMC, Gray JA, Haynes RB, Richardson WS. Evidence based medicine: what it is and what it isn't. BMJ. 1996; 312(7023):71–72

[6] Smith R, Rennie D. Evidence-based medicine—an oral history. JAMA. 2014; 311(4):365–367

[7] Stratford P. In tribute: David L. Sackett. Phys Ther. 2015; 95(8):1084–1086

[8] Young T, Rohwer A, Volmink J, Clarke M. What are the effects of teaching evidence-based health care (EBHC)? Overview of systematic reviews. PLoS One. 2014; 9(1):e86706

[9] American Physical Therapy Association. APTA vision statement for physical therapy vision 2020. Available at: http://www.apta.org/vision2020/. Accessed January 25, 2017

[10] Slavin M. Teaching evidence-based practice in physical therapy: critical competencies and necessary conditions. J Phys Ther Educ. 2004; 18(3):4–11

[11] Jewell D. Guide to Evidence-Based Physical Therapy Practice. 3rd ed. Jones and Bartlett Publishers, Sudbury, MA; 2014

[12] Bernhardsson S. Advancing evidence-based practice in primary care physiotherapy: guideline implementation, clinical practice, and patient preferences; 2015. Available at: http://liu.diva-portal.org/smash/record.jsf?pid=diva2%3A868036&dswid=popup

[13] Dijkers MP, Murphy SL, Krellman J. Evidence-based practice for rehabilitation professionals: concepts and controversies. Arch Phys Med Rehabil. 2012; 93(8) Suppl:S164–S176

[14] Jette AM. Moving research from the bedside into practice. Phys Ther. 2016; 96(5):594–596

[15] Levine D, Tilson JK, Fay D, et al Evidence based practice special interest group. American Physical Therapy Association, section on research. 2014:1–29. Available at: http://www.ptresearch.org/site/1/SIGS/EBP/EBP PT ED MANUAL FINAL 2-24-15.pdf

[16] Atkinson HL, Nixon-Cave K. A tool for clinical reasoning and reflection using the international classification of functioning, disability and health (ICF) framework and patient management model. Phys Ther. 2011; 91(3):416–430

[17] Bierwas DA, Leafman J, Shaw DK. The evidence-based practice beliefs and knowledge of physical therapy clinical instructors. Internet J Allied Heal Sci Pract. 2016;14(3):193

[18] Wiles L, Matricciani L, Williams M, Olds T. Sixty-five years of physical therapy: bibliometric analysis of research publications from 1945 through 2010. Phys Ther. 2012; 92(4):493–506

[19] Page P. Beyond statistical significance: clinical interpretation of rehabilitation research literature. Int J Sports Phys Ther. 2014; 9(5):726–736

[20] Snell K, Hassan A, Sutherland L, et al. Types and quality of physical therapy research publications: has there been a change in the past decade? Physiother Can. 2014; 66(4):382–391

[21] Page P. Research designs in sports physical therapy. Int J Sports Phys Ther. 2012; 7(5):482–492

[22] Ely JW, Osheroff JA, Ebell MH, et al. Obstacles to answering doctors' questions about patient care with evidence: qualitative study. BMJ. 2002; 324 (7339):710

[23] Carpenter C. Conducting qualitative research in physiotherapy. A methodological example. Physiotherapy. 1997; 83(10):547–552

[24] Goldstein MS, Scalzitti DA, Craik RL, et al. The revised research agenda for physical therapy. Phys Ther. 2011; 91(2):165–174

[25] Tilson JK, Mickan S, Sum JC, Zibell M, Dylla JM, Howard R. Promoting physical therapists' use of research evidence to inform clinical practice: part 2— a mixed methods evaluation of the PEAK program. BMC Med Educ. 2014; 14(1):126

[26] Moseley AM, Sherrington C, Elkins MR, Herbert RD, Maher CG. Indexing of randomised controlled trials of physiotherapy interventions: a comparison of AMED, CENTRAL, CINAHL, EMBASE, hooked on evidence, PEDro, PsycINFO and PubMed. Physiotherapy. 2009; 95(3):151–156

[27] Elkins MR, Moseley AM, Sherrington C, Herbert RD, Maher CG. Growth in the Physiotherapy Evidence Database (PEDro) and use of the PEDro scale. Br J Sports Med. 2013; 47(4):188–189

[28] Kamper SJ, Moseley AM, Herbert RD, Maher CG, Elkins MR, Sherrington C. 15 years of tracking physiotherapy evidence on PEDro, where are we now? Br J Sports Med. 2015; 49(14):907–909

[29] Ioannidis JPA. Why most clinical research is not useful. PLoS Med. 2016; 13 (6):e1002049

[30] Deenadayalan Y, Grimmer-Somers K, Prior M, Kumar S. How to run an effective journal club: a systematic review. J Eval Clin Pract. 2008; 14(5):898–911

7 Clinical Education in Physical Therapy: Past, Present, and Future

Kim Nixon-Cave

Keywords: Student, clinical instructor, director of clinical education, center coordinator for clinical education, clinical education, internship, placement, American Physical Therapy Association, The Commission on Accreditation in Physical Therapy Education, Physical Therapy Clinical Performance Instrument

Chapter Outline

1. Overview
2. Education of DPT Students in the Practice Environment
3. Physical Therapy Clinical Education
4. The Structure of Clinical Education
5. Professional Development
6. Types of Practice Settings
7. Assigning the Student to a Clinical Site
8. Clinical Sites—The Clinical Learning Environment
9. Interprofessional Clinical Education Experiences
10. Models of Clinical Education
    a) Integrated Model
    b) Independent and Separate Model
    c) Self-Contained Model
    d) Hybrid Model
11. International Clinical Experiences
12. Supervisory Approaches of Clinical Education: Traditional, Collaborative, and Cooperative Approaches
    a) The Traditional approach
    b) The Collaborative/Cooperative approach
13. The Role and Responsibilities of the Participants in Clinical Education
    a) Academic Faculty—Director of Clinical Education
    b) Center Coordinator of Clinical Education
    c) Clinical Instructor
    d) Student
    e) Patient
14. Assessment of Clinical Education Performance
15. Future of Clinical Education
16. Challenges in Physical Therapy Clinical Education: Present and Future

"I have been a Director of Clinical Education (DCE) for a large, midwestern, entry-level physical therapy program for nearly ten years. There are some days that I feel I have the best job in the entire world and other days, like today, I just want to go home, get into bed, and pull the covers over my head.

"I never planned on becoming a DCE. My love has always been pediatrics. After graduating I was fortunate to be offered a staff position in a large, teaching pediatric hospital in Chicago. Within a few years, through self-study, taking continuing education courses and two graduate courses, and with the support of my supervisor, I sat for and passed the Pediatric Certification Specialization exam. Along with treating patients I loved being a clinical instructor (CI) to interning students. I remember well the kindness and mentorship provided to me by my CIs back in the day and wanted to pass along the kindness. Soon I was promoted to the Center Coordinator for Clinical Education (CCCE) and our student program became regionally known for the quality of our curriculum.

"To my surprise I was approached by a very prestigious local physical therapy program at a local university and was asked to consider applying for a faculty position, the Assistant Director of Clinical Education. I would assist the DCE with student placement, the acquisition of additional clinical sites, perform site visits, counsel students, CIs and CCCEs, and assist in the pediatric curriculum, primarily as a laboratory assistant but also providing the occasional lecture. How could I refuse the offer to apply! I applied, interviewed, and was offered the position. Though I loved my clinical job, I jumped at the offer. Fortunately, the hospital asked me to return as a part-time clinician. Even though I accepted a full-time faculty position, I wanted to maintain my clinical skills. Ten years later I still work one weekend per month at the hospital!

"Who would have guessed that six months into my tenure as Assistant DCE the DCE would retire to become a full-time home mom and I would be promoted to DCE. This time it was I who assisted with hiring my assistant.

"My assistant and I are responsible for placing three classes of 50 students into four different clinical internships during their tenure with us. For those of you counting that is 200 placements for each cohort of students! We have placed students as close as the university hospital next door to my building and as far away as Kuwait.

"The best part of my job is seeing the excitement on the faces of our students when they return from internship. My small efforts not only provide an arena to practice the skills learned in the classroom but also provide an incredible opportunity to begin service to the poor, sick, and impaired and to stoke the inner fire of the love of our profession.

"The worst part of my job is the constant search for new sites. Each year, it seems there is more competition for existing sites as programs grow and new programs are added.

"I want to share an exemplar with the reader. Diane, a student in our program two years ago, requested an outpatient orthopedic internship for her final internship. She had already successfully completed a 12-week orthopedic internship. I felt, based upon the quality of her work and excitement in pediatrics, that she may wish to consider a pediatric internship. I told her that we had an unfilled internship position at a local pediatric hospital (my hospital!). I met with Diane and explained my thoughts. Blushingly, she said that even though she loved pediatrics she did not feel she would perform well in such a complicated and complex clinical environment. She felt that she was not as smart as some of her classmates. I rarely push my clinical site considerations onto students, but in this case, I knew Diane would do well at the pediatric hospital. Eventually she relented and accepted the placement.

"Twelve weeks after her final internship ended Diane burst into my office and with tears in her eyes gave me the biggest hug I had received since my wedding. Not only did she perform well in the pediatric hospital, she was offered a full-time position upon graduation. I do love my job!"

—Jane L., Des Moines, Iowa

7.1 Overview

The purpose of this chapter is to provide the physical therapy student with an overview of the aims and processes associated with the clinical education experience. Clinical education is a necessary and mandatory component of the entry-level physical therapy curriculum. In most physical therapy curricula clinical education encompasses almost one-third of the entire entry-level educational process. Complex, long in duration, often involving travel, requiring the development of professional partnerships with the clinical instructor (CI) and the patient, and are graded parts of the curriculum, clinical education experiences can provoke a wide range of emotions on the part of the interning physical therapy student.

Clinical education permits students to sample various arenas of physical therapy practice to help define a clinical interest (see ▶ Fig. 7.1). These experiences often also permit students to observe tangential professional opportunities and experiences such as observation of surgery, the observation of other professionals such as occupational therapists, physicians,

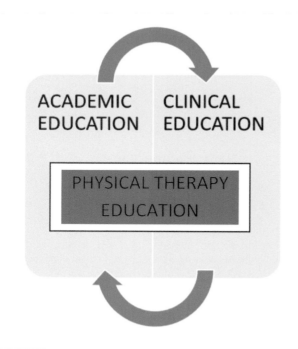

Fig. 7.1 Two components of physical therapy education. The physical therapy entry-level curriculum is anchored by two interconnected parts: the didactic academic education which occurs primarily in the classroom and online and the clinical education which occurs primarily in the physical therapy arena.

pharmacists, and speech pathologists, and to take part in formal and informal interprofessional educational experience such as clinical rounds, in-services, and meetings. Clinical education can be a sentinel event in the professional development of the student—providing an "aha" moment which forever directs the career trajectory of the physical therapist. They can be times of accelerated learning. Clinical education experiences can also be demanding, rewarding, expensive, trying, complex, difficult, worrisome, enjoyable, tense, and reflective. Clinical educational experiences provide the opportunity to work with and under the direction of skilled therapists with unique backgrounds, clinical interests, and specializations. Often these therapists become lifelong clinical and professional mentors.

The primary aim of this chapter is to provide the reader with an extensive overview of an integral part of the entry-level physical therapy program—the clinical education experience. The author also aims to provide the reader with a strong understanding of the history of the clinical education experience and how it has evolved over the past century to meet changes in the scope of care and educational standards of the physical therapy profession. A strong emphasis will be placed on defining the roles of the participants in the clinical education process and on the various assessments and outcome methodology used.

7.2 Education of DPT Students in the Practice Environment

Clinical education is an essential and required component of the physical therapy student's professional education and involves the application of the knowledge and skills learned in the classroom setting to the clinical practice arena.[1] Historically, clinical education has been referred to by many different terms, including clinical training, clinical assignments, practicum, clinical affiliation, field experience, clinical internship, and clinical experience.[1] The physical therapy education accrediting body, the Commission on Accreditation in Physical Therapy Education (CAPTE), requires that every accredited program must have a minimum number of weeks for full time clinical experiences.[2] This minimum number has changed numerous times over the course of development of the profession. The partnership of didactic classroom experiences (online or traditional) and clinical education is the standard professional curriculum algorithm in physical therapy and in most health care preparatory curricula.

Clinical education and related components have evolved over the course of the development and evolution of the profession of physical therapy. Major paradigm shifts in the profession of physical therapy have almost always resulted in major paradigm shifts in clinical education practices. Relating the history of physical therapy and its impact on clinical education practices is beyond the scope of this chapter but a brief review of the development of the profession of physical therapy in the United States is of tantamount importance to the discussion of the evolution of clinical education.

The history of physical therapy has been documented by many authors.[3,4,5] In the early 1900s, physical therapists were known as reconstruction aides. The practice of training and hiring reconstruction aides grew out of the successful work of women hired to physically rehabilitate soldiers injured in World War I. The scope of care soon enlarged to include patients with poliomyelitis, stroke, and general debility. At that time, there was no formal education—neither didactic nor clinical education—for reconstruction aides. Their education was typically on-the-job mentoring by physicians. The reconstruction aides primarily had backgrounds in physical education and massage therapy. As the profession developed and grew there was an evolution to the approach to care provided and training of therapists. In the 1950s and 1960s the care provided by physical therapists was primarily under the direction of physicians via strict oversight. During that era, the practice and education of physical therapy was technical and prescriptive. As individual states began the process of providing formal licensure to physical therapists in the 1960s and 1970s, there was a move to a formalized curriculum. The improved educational outcomes of that time led to today's practice of direct access and increased autonomy which began in the 1980s and continues to evolve today.

As the level of autonomy increased and physical therapy developed as a true profession, there were changes in the education of physical therapy students. From the certificate entry-level degree to the bachelor's degree to the master's degree to the current doctor of physical therapy (DPT) degree of the late 1990s, the depth, duration, and intensity of physical therapy education has grown to match an ever-expanding scope of care. Changes in clinical education paralleled changes in the didactic curriculum and professional practice. The next section of the chapter will focus on the evolution of clinical education of physical therapy students as well as how the roles, responsibilities, and expectations of all stakeholders involved have evolved along with the structure of clinical education.

7.3 Physical Therapy Clinical Education

Physical therapy clinical education occurs in the practice environment whereas the didactic component of educating DPT students occurs in academic institutions (traditional or online). Both aspects of the curriculum are designed to develop the students' knowledge, skills, and professional behavior.[6]

The aim of clinical education is to provide experiences and an environment which allow students to apply their didactic/academic knowledge to actual clinical practice.[7] Application of didactic/academic knowledge in the clinic may be practiced through psychomotor activities, mentored clinical decision making, developing a differential diagnosis lists, making prognoses, formulating goals, developing an appropriate intervention plan, and through clinical documentation. The clinical education experiences also provide students the opportunity to practice behavioral competencies learned in the classroom with the patient, patient's family, and other health care professionals in a clinical environment. These behavioral competencies include being on time, dressing professionally, teamwork, dedication to task, empathy, listening, kindness, compassion, and completing assignments on time.[8]

In clinical education, the application of didactic/academic knowledge and the practice of behavioral competencies is performed under the supervision of a trained CI who also acts as a professional role model. Most clinical education curricula developed by the clinical site is structured, preplanned, and outcome-oriented. However, the clinical environment—where the clinical education curriculum is carried out—is often dynamic and unpredictable. The constantly changing and unpredictable environment facilitates the development and maturation of the professional behaviors of flexibility, problem solving, teamwork, and prioritization. This type of environment cannot be fully replicated in the classroom. In summary, the clinical environment permits learning, often simultaneously, in all clinical domains: cognitive, affective, psychomotor, and spiritual. Clinical learning is an important adjunct to classroom learning.

Clinical education has developed and evolved as the profession of physical therapy developed and evolved. During the "reconstruction aide" era of physical therapy there was no formal training in the clinic or the classroom. As noted earlier, most of the physical therapists in the early years of the profession were individuals primarily with physical education and massage backgrounds who utilized their skills under the watchful and instructive eye of physicians to rehabilitate soldiers involved in World War I and patients with poliomyelitis. In 1928, the first physical therapy educational standards were developed and published by Dr. John Stanley Catilter. At this time the degree awarded was a postbaccalaureate certificate. This entry-level degree survived until the early 1980s. By 1933, the American Physiotherapeutic Association (American Women's Physiotherapy Association) and American Medical Association became involved in accrediting physical therapy educational programs.[3,5] The early standards were the "Essentials of an Acceptable School for Physical Therapy Technicians"[9] and were written primarily by physicians. These standards had a physician bias as noted by the fact that the scope of physical therapy practice and standards of care were mostly prescriptive and technical. Diagnosis, prognosis, and clinical decision making were not considered within the scope of practice of physical therapy and were therefore not taught. Most of the clinical interventions offered by physical therapist focused on massage, exercise, and modalities. Early mandated educational standards required a minimum of 800 classroom hours and 400 clinical practice hours (today known as clinical education).[10] Clinical education occurred in hospital settings. Even though the American Physiotherapeutic Association and American Medical Association were working on accreditation since the 1930s,[10] there was no formal accreditation process until 1955. In 1977, the CAPTE became the sole accrediting agency for physical therapy educational programs. CAPTE is nationally recognized by the United States Department of Education (USDE) and the Council for Higher Education Accreditation (CHEA) and has been the only recognized agency to accredit physical therapy programs since 1983.[2]

The impact of accreditation on clinical education has been minimal as compared with the didactic classroom environment, with the focus primarily on the number of hours of clinical education required by students in physical therapy educational programs, as well as the sequencing and scope of the clinical education curricula. The next section will focus on the structure of clinical education and related components, which include clinical education faculty, clinical site, resources, and the evaluation or assessment process.

7.4 The Structure of Clinical Education

The components of structure of clinical education are designed to include practice setting type, supervision model, the sequencing of the clinical experience, the lengths of the individual clinical experiences, and the student and facility assessment model. These standards are designed by a complex interaction defined by the CAPTE, the entry-level program's faculty, local practice guidelines, state practice acts, the clinical facility, and, in some cases, local clinical consortiums. The different components of clinical education are designed to provide an environment where physical therapy students can learn in an efficient and effective manner, where performance and outcome feedback is provided reliably and validly, and where patient and student safety is an utmost concern.

The physical therapy academic and clinical education experiences were originally housed in hospital-based settings but over time the academic experience migrated to the university setting and the clinical education experiences primarily to the inpatient hospital setting. Due to a number of factors over the past four decades, the clinical education experience has expanded from primarily the inpatient hospital arena to a number of diverse inpatient and outpatient arenas served by physical therapists. Reasons for this migration have not been fully elucidated in the literature but a number of factors, including the enlargement of the scope of care of the physical therapy profession, Medicare reimbursement rules associated with student workload, productivity indices, and length of stay issues may have facilitated this migration.

The structure of the clinical education experience must be a planned experience with explicitly defined outcomes. The entry-level physical therapy curriculum defines the sequence—when the experienced occurs within the curriculum, the duration of each experience (number of weeks/hours), and the types of practice setting housing the experience.[11] The clinical experience must be structured and planned and represents situated or experiential learning that occurs in a clinical practice environment and includes observation, participation and reflection.

7.5 Professional Development

Clinical education experiences are essential to the professional development of physical therapy students. Clinical education experiences should embody all domains of learning as well as practicing the translation of the core values of the American Physical Therapy Association (APTA) to the therapy clinic environment.[12] Professional development is influenced by the timing of the experience as well as the overall experience. As a novice learner, the first clinical experience is often more observational than interventional. During the first clinical experience the physical therapist is often concentrating so hard on the psychomotor aspect of what her or she is asked to perform (manual muscle test or range of motion) there is little capability to practice more advanced skills such as the development of the patient–therapist clinical alliance, empathy, therapeutic touch, the performance of systematic reviews, time management, and teamwork skills. Later clinical educational opportunities—when the student therapist is in the associative or autonomous phase of learning—provide ample opportunity to practice the more advanced skills of our profession. The student's clinical experience should focus on knowledge, skills, and psychomotor activities as well as core values of being a professional. Lee Shulman advocates that professional education needs to intertwine "habits of head (knowledge and cognitive abilities), habits of hand (technical skills), and habits of heart (ethical standards)."[13]

▶ Fig. 7.2 illustrates the journey of a physical therapy student along the continuum of entry-level student to licensed clinician to resident to fellow. Students begin their professional formation —the development of their professional identity and translatory practical knowledge—when engaged in clinical education. The clinical education of DPT students has become increasingly important to address multiple dimensions and challenges of the health care environment and the need demonstrate and extol the value of physical therapy services within the current environment of uncertainty in the health care arena.[14] Physical therapy students need to develop knowledge, clinical reasoning skills, and clinical decision techniques as they develop their professional identity. It is important that during clinical education that CIs and faculty recognize their responsibility to guide the development of the student's professional identity along with their knowledge, practical skills, and affective skills for reflective practice and mindfulness of care for their patients.[15]

7.6 Types of Practice Setting

The clinical practice setting is an important aspect to the clinical education experiences. The clinical education practice settings include acute care settings and outpatient settings and include the spectrum of the age continuum from neonatal to geriatric. Many DPT programs also offer research experiences as part of clinical education. DPT educational programs often have specific requirements for which types of clinical experiences students enrolled in the professional program must

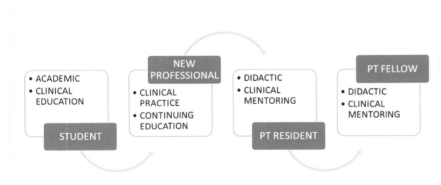

Fig. 7.2 Conceptual framework of clinical education. The progression of a physical therapist from entry-level student to expert encompasses four distinct steps: student, new professional, physical therapist resident, and physical therapist fellow. The common denominator in these four steps is the inclusion of clinical education.

complete prior to graduation. These include some or all of the following arenas: acute care hospital, rehabilitation centers (subacute and long-term), outpatient health care facilities, schools, nursing homes, wellness centers, and community-based centers. The Director of Clinical Education (DCE) develops the criteria for the selection of sites that meet the goals of the individual program and CAPTE accreditation requirements and develops a formalized contract with each facility. The number of sites "contracted" by the professional program to service the enrolled students varies according to the number of matriculated students. The number of contracted sites is typically two to four times the number of matriculated students. The high number is due to the fact that clinical sites may occasionally decline the DCE's request to take a student. Internship sites may decline students for a number of reasons including staffing issues at the facility and prior commitment to students from another program.

Each clinical education experience is designed to support the student's current level of knowledge and skills and allow the student to be successful in meeting the objectives of the experience. These experiences should allow the student to apply his didactic knowledge and skills to the clinic practice setting, bridging the connection between the academic and clinical learning environments. In designing these clinical experiences, the DCE sets goals and objectives that will allow the student to meet the learning criteria set by the academic program for clinical education as well as allow the student to practice all domains of learning (cognitive, psychomotor, affective) based on the DPT curriculum.[16]

7.7 Assigning the Student to a Clinical Site

Unlike many nonmedical internships, the physical therapy student does not determine the site of the clinical internship. The responsibility of assigning sites to students rests with the DCE. In the United States, the DCE typically chooses among a number of assignation models:

The lottery method: the lottery method is the most simplistic of the assigning methods. In its most basic form the DCE provides all students with a list of available clinical sites and background information on each site. The students are asked to study the data provided. Later, the students are asked to (metaphorically) pull a number from a hat (if there are 50 students in the class there are numbers 1–50 in the hat). Student number 1 chooses first, number 2 chooses second, and so forth. Obviously, student number one will have his or her pick of all clinical sites while student number 50 will choose last. However, during the next clinical internship cycle, the numbers are typically reversed and student 50 picks first and number 1 picks last. The advantages of the lottery method are that the DCE is completely removed from the decision-making process and cannot be accused of bias by the students. The disadvantage of this method is that the expertise of the DCE is completely removed from the process. The DCE has exceptional and intimate knowledge of each clinical site and also a unique perspective on each student's strengths, weaknesses, and needs. None of these variables are addressed when the lottery method is utilized as the method of site assignment.

DCE assignation method: in the DCE assignation method, the DCE unilaterally chooses the sites for the students. The students have no direct input in the choosing of their clinical internship sites. The advantage of this method is that students are taken out of the assignation equation which makes the assigning duties much easier for the DCE. This is also the disadvantage of this method—the students often have strengths, weaknesses, needs, and interests that the DCE is unaware of; thus, these important variables are not addressed by this method.

The DCE/student partnership method: in this method the DCE and student meet prior to the assignation of the site. The meeting agenda, developed by the DCE, features discussions about the student's perceived strengths and weaknesses, clinical interests, willingness to travel, and a review of the previous clinical education outcome measures. Together the student and DCE come to a consensus about the arena and location of the subsequent clinical site that best meets the student's needs. The advantage of the DCE/student partnership method is that this is a holistic approach utilizing both student and DCE data to make a cogent decision. The disadvantage is primarily related to use of time. Meeting with each student for perhaps 1 hour is a very large time demand on the part of the DCE.

7.8 Clinical Sites—The Clinical Learning Environment

Clinical education sites are the clinical practice environment that offers DPT students the opportunity to practice and refine their knowledge, psychomotor skills, affective skills, and overall professional behavior and development.[17] The clinical sites provide the context for clinical education and allow for situational and experiential learning. The clinical education environment occurs in a very dynamic and ever-changing clinical environment. The clinical education practice setting is an extension of the DPT curriculum for each student. There needs to be guidelines and oversight of the clinical education experience in each practice environment. This is the responsibility of the DCE. The clinical practice environment allows students to use their knowledge and skills from the didactic setting in making clinical decisions and patient management within that specific arena of clinical care. There are essential characteristics of clinical practice environment that includes the culture and structure of the learning environment.[18] The culture and structure of the clinical experience should foster lifelong learning in the students, which is role modeled by the physical therapists who supervise the students. Life learning is demonstrated in the practice environment—having an administrative structure with a supportive student program that is focused on developing the student's skills and knowledge using evidence-based approach to care. The clinical education environment is designed to "bridge the worlds of theory and practice, teaching in a real-world laboratory lessons that can only be learned through practice."[19]

The clinical education experiences in the practice environment is guided by an administrative physical therapist, often named the Center Coordinator for Clinical Education (CCCE), with oversight over the program and who can work with the DCE to ensure a quality experience for the interning student. The CCCE has clearly defined role—often elaborated in a specific job description—and dedicated time that is supported by the facility's overall administrator, allowing the CCCE the time and support to design a quality program.

The CCCE differs from the CI. Though both are employees of the clinical facility, the CCCE, in consultation with the DCE administrates the student program. Along with program design, the CCCE assigns interning students to a particular CI. The CI, with oversight from the CCCE, carries out the student experience. A clinic will have one CCCE but often many CIs. Just as the CI will meet regularly with the interning student to provide feedback, the CCCE will meet regularly with the CI to also provide feedback. Most facilities have a policy requiring CIs to have at least 18 months to 2 years of clinical experience prior to being assigned an interning student.

7.9 Interprofessional Clinical Education Experiences

The Centre for the Advancement of Interprofessional Education's (CAIPE's) definition of interprofessional education is: "Interprofessional education involves educators and learners from two or more health professions and their foundational disciplines who jointly create and foster a collaborative learning environment."[20] "The goal of these efforts is to develop knowledge, skills, and attitudes that result in interprofessional team behaviors and competence. Ideally, interprofessional education is incorporated throughout the entire curriculum in a vertically and horizontally integrated fashion."[21] A number of DPT programs have begun to include interprofessional education. The programs are designed to develop and train future health care professionals to provide evidence-based patient-centered care through interprofessional care by creating a culture of collaborative educational learning and practice. According to Buring, "the goal of IPE is for students to learn how to function in an interprofessional team and carry this knowledge, skill, and value into their future practice, ultimately providing interprofessional patient care as part of a collaborative team and focused on improving patient outcomes."[21]

Recent research has indicated that interprofessional clinical experience improves overall patient care as well as facilitates the decrease in cost of health care services due to professionals working together to provide the most appropriate care from the appropriate profession at the appropriate time. This approach allows for health care professionals to deliver high-quality patient-centered care to all patients.[22]

Clinical education experiences can occur in settings that offer interprofessional learning opportunities. Interprofessional education is an emerging trend in physical therapy clinical education. Current doctrine in all preparatory health care programs is that students, regardless the type of professional program enrolled into, will benefit from interprofessional experiences. Historically, the health care professions learned in isolated silos. This practice is counterintuitive in that in true clinical practice no practitioner acts in isolation.[23] Recent evidence has focused on moving didactic and clinical learning out of the confines of each specific profession realm to move beyond the limits of knowledge of the profession to learn about and with other professions.[24] Didactic IPE includes two or more professional programs being taught in a classroom together, thus encouraging interprofessional communication and problem solving. Didactic IPE can also include two or more professional programs partnering for clinical simulation activities, such as the use of high-frequency manikins, case studies, and standardized patients.[25] Clinical IPE includes students from two or more professional programs simultaneously interacting in the actual clinical environment. This type of learning is an interactive approach to learning within an interprofessional practice environment.[26] Interprofessional education allows for the advancement of health professional's education while learning and practicing in a collaborative team environment. Interprofessional clinical learning experiences can facilitate the professional formation of students from various professions that allows all professional health care students not only to promote good for their patient but for the public as well.[27]

7.10 Models of Clinical Education

There are four models of clinical education that are typically used to provide clinical education experiences to physical therapy students.[7,28,29,30] These experiences range from an integrated half-day per week to full-time clinical internships. Though the number of weeks of clinical internship for entry-level physical therapy programs is determined by the CAPTE, each program can determine the duration of each experience as long as the sum total of weeks meets the CAPTE requirements.[2] This is known as the clinical education model. Many factors influence the development of a program's clinical education model including the program's mission and vision statements and curricular goals.[27] Not only is the selection of the type of model determined by the program needs, but it is also influenced by the challenges that physical therapy educational programs face, such availability of clinical sites, the variations in health care environment, and the higher education environments and cultures. There is no definitive evidence that indicates that one model is better than the next nor is there a standard or uniform model for physical therapy clinical education.[28] Currently, there are various models used in clinical education for physical therapists, which are based on the philosophy and curriculum plan of the specific physical therapy curriculum as well as the changing health care and higher education landscapes. There are four models that are commonly used in the clinical education of physical therapy students.

7.10.1 Integrated Model

The integrated model is a clinical education experience that occurs during an academic term in a coordinated fashion concurrent with didactic courses.[31] This model is commonly used and familiar to faculty, students, and clinicians. The curriculum design is designed to permit students to experience the didactic and clinical education at the same time which leads substantial input from the academic and clinical environment as being responsible for the development of the student's clinical skills.[32] The integrated models of clinical education can include full-time or part-time experiences with longer full-time experiences later in the curriculum and more part-time or shorter clinical experiences earlier in the curriculum. Programs using this model find the need to have a larger number of clinical sites due to the relative brief duration of each clinical experience and the practice of not having students perform more than one clinical internship at one site. The model is designed to build on the didactic curriculum as the student progresses through the curriculum moving from simple to more complex clinical experiences. The length of this model varies depending on the curriculum plan. "The clinical experiences may consist of both part-time (< 35 hours/weeks) exposures/experiences situated earlier in the program and longer clinical experiences (> 35 hours/week), often in the final year."[16] Part-time and full-time clinical experiences are ones in which student physical therapists are in clinical environments for a minimum of 32 hours per week. Students can return after the full-time experience to additional didactic coursework. ACAPT defines part-time clinical rotations as "a clinical learning experience that is from 5 weeks long or fewer weeks in length in which student physical therapists are learning in clinical environments. Students will return to further didactic learning experiences following completion of this clinical experience."[31]

7.10.2 Independent and Separate Model

This model is not as common as the Integrated Model to DPT clinical education experiences. The Independent and Separate Model is more typically associated with medicine and dentistry clinical programs.[32] The design of the model is that the students complete all their didactic coursework/program and then move into separate and independent clinical experiences. These experiences are typically full-time internship models that usually last a year. The unique aspect of this model is that it not only occurs after completion of didactic coursework, but there is also an expectation that the student interns will obtain their professional licenses either at the end or at some point during the clinical internship.

DPT entry-level programs that that use this model for clinical education experiences employ a collaborative or shared approach for the experience. The academic structure (university) and clinical structure (facility) share equal responsibility for the development and curriculum of the clinical experience, while also partnering to ensure that students meet the entry-level requirements. Students are allowed to sit for the licensure examination during this experience when they complete the entry-level program requirements. Physical therapy programs that use this model have developed relationships with clinical facilities—students complete a year-long internship as well as receive a salary during the clinical experience. After successfully obtaining a license to practice physical therapy, the student continues at the clinical facility with the guidance and support from both academic and clinical faculty. This model requires substantial commitment from various stakeholders, including students, academic program, and clinical facility.[33]

7.10.3 Self-Contained Model

The self-contained model, common to nursing and dentistry, is unique in that the academic faculty serves a dual role as instructors within the professional program and CI in the internship facility. In nursing, the clinical faculty travel with the students to the clinical setting and function in the role of preceptors and mentors. In dentistry, many programs have large faculty practices at or near the university where the faculty practice part-time along with their academic teaching load.[34]

This is not a common model commonly seen in physical therapy education, but it is becoming more popular due to challenges in clinical education, such as availability of sites and demands within the clinical facility. This model is most easily achieved in large academic health care systems which contain physical therapy clinical sites. The clinical sites may be administered by representatives hired by the clinical facility or by the physical therapy entry-level program faculty. This model is also seen in faculty clinical practices.[35] Faculty clinical practices are usually stand-alone facilities in the university setting directed by the physical therapy faculty. These sites provide additional income to the entry-level program and provide an arena for student internships. The faculty works either exclusively within the clinical facilities or shares duties as clinician and educator within the professional program. While at the clinic they serve as CIs. This model has advantages and disadvantages to the more commonly practiced integrated model. The advantages include the typical proximity of the clinic to the academic institution, the use of faculty (who are intimately familiar with the curriculum and curricular goals) as CIs, and the academic program's control over the clinical internship curriculum. The disadvantages include the student's loss of the benefit of learning opportunities associated with travel and the loss of experiencing new and interesting clinics. Additional disadvantages are the loss of evaluative, assessment, and intervention diversity due to the fact that the CIs are typically the same faculty members who provided instruction in the didactic program. There is a loss of opportunity to work with patients across the lifespan, such as pediatrics or older adults, because most faculty practices tend to have narrow scopes of care. As a result, these self-contained models need to form partnerships with clinical facilities outside of the academic health care setting to ensure that students meet the accreditation requirements associated with diversity.[18]

7.10.4 Hybrid Model

Hybrid clinical education models are combinations of the three models previously described. The hybrid model is an alternative model and the newest model that physical therapy programs are employing for clinical education experiences.[36] This model, still in its nascent stage, stresses interprofessional education by joining students and CIs together to provide care in a patient-centered coordinated care environment.

7.11 International Clinical Experiences

Since the 1980s, there has been an increased interest in international clinical education experiences. There have been numerous studies that have examined the use of international clinical experiences in physical therapy program in various countries.[35] International clinical experiences summate the excitement and richness of travel, physical therapy clinical experience, and learning first-hand about health and health disparities in a foreign land.[37] (In recent years, to meet this need, some entry-level programs have included in their curricula international service experiences that are focused on communities that are underserved for limited time frames, such as 1 to 2 weeks. Technically, in most instances, these are considered service trips or service-learning opportunities and not clinical education.) The increased interest in international or global clinical experiences has prompted the need to determine standards and guidelines that ensure the quality of the experiences as well as determine if these experiences meet the CAPTE standards for entry-level physical therapy clinical education requirements in the United States. In October 2009, CAPTE "recognized the value of exposing students to multicultural learning experiences, both in the classroom and the clinical setting."[2] Thus, CAPTE's evaluative criteria do not preclude physical therapy students educated in the United States from obtaining a portion of their clinical experiences outside of the United States as part of their formal clinical education requirements. CAPTE expects the physical therapy entry-level program to provide the same level of supervision, quality of experience, and assessment that would be expected of any other clinical experience. In other words, "CAPTE's expectation of the clinical education component of the curriculum would remain the same for all clinical experiences, regardless of location, such that by the end of the professional program, students are able to achieve the program's goals and outcome expectations."[2] CAPTE's expectation is currently interpretable by the professional program. More comprehensive standards, especially as more U.S. accredited programs begin to look internationally at clinical internship sites, need to be discussed and enacted.[37]

Although there has been an increase in utilization of international clinical sites to meet curricular clinical education requirements, there continue to be many barriers that impact the program and the student. These include the following:[38,39,40]

- The cost and time commitment on the part of the DCE and university counsel in arranging and planning the experiences.
- There is often limited faculty support. Typically, the idea is championed by the chair or DCE and due to the legal and procedural complexity there is little opportunity for shared governance and ownership of this issue among the faculty.
- Coordinating the university calendar with the availability of international clinical site availability is often problematic.
- The cost of the experience may be prohibitive for the student and the academic program.
- Concerns that the students may not achieve the knowledge and skills for their entry-level program in the United States. The United States continues to be the only country where the doctorate is the entry-level degree for physical therapists. If the CI is not a U.S.-trained therapist there is always the possibility that the CI may have an inferior education as compared with U.S.-trained DPT therapists.
- Cultural incompetence may be an issue for the student due to the lack of familiarity with the health care system in another country as well as a basic language barrier.
- Student safety issues.

Service learning, as an alternative to international clinical education, has an increasing focus in the education of DPT students and can help to socialize students to the core values of the profession and their professional formation. However, with the increase in both international clinical experiences and international service experiences it becomes imperative that the clinical education community in the United States continue to research the costs, benefits, and outcomes of the varied available international experiences.

7.12 Supervisory Approaches of Clinical Education: Traditional, Collaborative, and Cooperative Approaches

7.12.1 Traditional Approach

Supervision of physical therapy students by the CI in the clinical setting can be described as traditional or collaborative/cooperative.[41,42] The traditional approach matches one CI to one student (1:1 model) and is the most commonly used model in physical therapy education. The traditional approach, long established in physical therapy curricula, is being challenged by alternative approaches that have been developed over the past decade. There are many complex factors that are leading to the exploration of alternative models of clinical education. These include anxiety related to evolving health care reform, the increasing number of physical therapy and physical therapist assistant educational programs competing for clinical education spots, the limited availability of clinical sites, and the accreditation standards for clinical education—especially those standards related to the commitment for students to experience patient populations across the life continuum.[43]

Strengths of the traditional approach:[41,42,43]
- Students receive individual, guided attention from the CI.
- Departmental productivity overall is not adversely impacted.
- CIs find managing a 1:1 relationship less demanding compared to other supervision models.
- Cancellation of a placement affects fewer students.

Weaknesses of the traditional approach:
- Students are dependent on one educator for their learning requirements.
- Passive dependence is fostered.
- No value is placed on peer-assisted and collaborative learning.
- Greater direct time commitment is required per educator as opposed to other models of supervision.

7.12.2 The Collaborative/Cooperative Approach

Rather than the 1:1 CI:student ratio described in the traditional approach of student supervision, the collaborative/cooperative approach permits a number of combinations of CI to student ratios.[41,44] The term collaborative and cooperative have been used interchangeably to describe alternative models to the traditional 1:1 model.

The literature reports a number of common models for the collaborative/cooperative approach to student supervision including 1:2 (one CI to two PT students) or one CI to one PT student *and* one PTA student, a 2:2, 2:3, 2:4 CI:student model, and an integrated faculty practice model where a CI supervises multiple students in a single setting to complete a clinical education experience in a specific practice area such as lymphedema, wound care, or women's health.[43,44]

The strengths of the collaborative clinical education approach include the following:[41,42,43,44]

- Promotion of teamwork/collaboration.
- Facilitation of active learning.
- Shared experience by student partners.
- The simulation of real-world collaboration.
- Collaborative reflection among the students.
- Learned interprofessional collaboration.
- Increased productivity with the students and CI all carrying a caseload.

The limitations of the collaborative clinical education approach include the following:

- Students may have different learning styles which may influence the learning experiences of the students.
- Decreased hands-on care for CI.
- Student competition.
- Students may have different levels of experience.
- Increased paperwork review for the CI.
- Availability of resources in the department for the students (e.g., computers for EMR).

7.13 The Roles and Responsibilities of the Participants in Clinical Education

As seen in ▶ Fig. 7.3, the clinical education experience includes participants from both the academic and clinical settings. Each participant has specific roles and responsibilities. The participants include students, the CI, the DCE, the CCCE, and the patient. Although each participant has different roles and responsibilities, the common goal and objective of all participants is to provide a learning environment in which the student can meet the expected entry-level physical therapist clinical and behavioral standards. Clinical education is an integral component of the student's professional development and, to be effective, must employ all domains of learning.

7.13.1 Academic Faculty—Director of Clinical Education

The DCE, formerly known as the Academic Coordinator of Clinical Education (ACCE), is the academic faculty member in the physical therapy entry-level program who directs, coordinates, and maintains the clinical education program. The DCE is the liaison between the academic program and the multiple contracted clinical practice settings. The primary responsibility of the DCE is to ensure the effectiveness of the student's clinical education experiences and that the clinical education program meets the accreditation standards as outlined by CAPTE.

The DCE is an academic faculty member who has an academic or clinical appointment with the responsibility to plan, develop, coordinate, monitor, and administer the clinical education program for physical therapy students based on the missions, goals, and objectives of the DPT program and the accreditation standards as determined by CAPTE (see ▶ Fig. 7.4). The role of the DCE is to ensure that the accreditation requirements for clinical education are met with ongoing monitoring and refinement parallel to the changes in the profession of physical therapy in particular and health care in general. The DCE works with both the academic and clinical faculty to facilitate quality clinical learning experiences by developing the goals and objectives for the student's participate in the program. The DCE also has four primary roles with associated responsibilities:

1. Liaison between the academic program and clinical education sites.
   a) In this role, the DCE is responsible for providing ongoing communication with the clinical sites to provide information about the academic clinical education program including information about the students and expectations for the clinical experience.
2. Planning, developing, coordinating, and implementing of the clinical education in both the academic and clinical environment.
   a) Develop policies and procedures for the clinical education.
   b) Develop an assessment plan and set criteria for the objectives for successful completion of the clinical education experience.

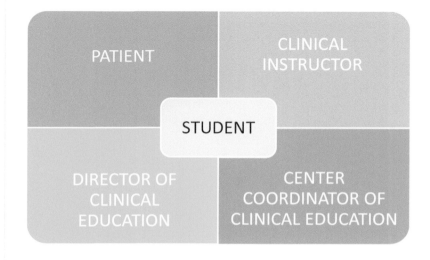

Fig. 7.3 Participants in clinical education. The clinical education portion of the entry-level curriculum focuses on the student. Four roles are integral to the student's development: the patient, the clinical instructor, the director of clinical education, and the center coordinator of clinical education.

DCE Position Description

The DCE holds a faculty (academic or clinical) appointment and has administrative, academic, service, and scholarship responsibilities consistent with the mission and philosophy of the academic program. This individual demonstrates competence in clinical education, teaching, and curriculum development. In addition, the DCE primary responsibilities are to plan, coordinate, facilitate, administer, and monitor activities on behalf of the academic program and in coordination with academic and clinical faculty. These activities include but are not limited to the following:

- developing, monitoring, and refining the clinical education component of the curriculum,
- facilitating quality learning experiences for students during clinical education,
- evaluating students' performance, in cooperation with other faculty, to determine their ability to integrate didactic and clinical learning experiences and to progress within the curriculum,
- educating students, clinical and academic faculty about clinical education,
- selecting clinical learning environments that demonstrate characteristics of sound patient/client management, ethical and professional behavior, and currency with physical therapy practice,
- maximizing available resources for the clinical education program,
- providing documented records and assessment of the clinical education component (includes clinical education sites, clinical educators, etc), and
- actively engaging core faculty clinical education planning, implementation, and assessment.

The DCE serves as a liaison between the physical therapy program and the clinical education site as part of his/her responsibilities. The DCE, in cooperation with other academic faculty, establishes clinical education site and facility standards, selects and evaluates clinical education sites, and facilitates ongoing development of and communication with clinical education sites and clinical faculty.

DCE Position Responsibilities

The DCE is responsible for coordinating and managing the efforts of the academic program and clinical education sites in the education and preparation of PT and PTA students by performing the following activities:

I. Communicates Between the Academic Institution and Affiliated Clinical Education Sites

A. Communicates news, and current information (eg, curriculum, clinical education objectives, staffing changes, and site availability) among all concerned stakeholders (eg, the academic institution, clinical education sites, clinical faculty and students) to maintain current knowledge of the educational program, the clinical education site, and health care changes affecting clinical practice and education.

B. Provides ongoing communication with clinical educators at each clinical education site to include:

- philosophy of the academic program;
- academic program curriculum and specific syllabus and learning objectives for each clinical experience and behavioral expectations that may not be addressed by learning objectives;
- policy and procedures of the academic program pertaining to clinical education;
- current materials required for accreditation;
- clinical education contractual agreement negotiated and maintained between the academic program and each clinical education site;
- dissemination of appropriate student and related information (e.g., health insurance, liability/malpractice insurance, state/federal laws and regulations such as ADA);
- collection of information about clinical education sites for use by students in their selection of or assignment to clinical education sites;
- provision of dates for each clinical education experience;
- academic program requests from clinical education sites regarding the number and type of available student clinical placements;
- coordinating student assignments (consideration might be given to items such as patient variety, health care settings and size, types of learning experiences, clinical site and student expectations, strengths/limitations of clinical experiences);

Fig. 7.4 Job requirements for the director of clinical education. The director of clinical education is a full-time member of the entry-level program academic faculty and along with teaching, scholarship, and service requirements directs the clinical education program. (Available at: http://www.apta.org/ModelPositionDescription/ACCE/DCE/PT/. Accessed October 1, 2017.)

- clinical faculty development opportunities including educational seminars and faculty availability as a resource in their areas of expertise, and;
- maintenance and distribution of a clinical education manual.

C. Communicates and oversees communication with Center Coordinators of Clinical Education (CCCEs), Clinical Instructors (CIs), and students to monitor progress and assess student performance. Provides guidance and support as required to problem solve and discuss pertinent issues with student(s), CIs, and/or CCCEs.

D. Places, supervises, and communicates with students while on clinical experiences. Responsibilities associated with these roles include, but are not limited to:

- informing students of clinical education policies and procedures;
- supplying relevant clinical education site information to facilitate students' selection of or assignment to clinical education sites (eg, learning experiences, clinical site prerequisites, housing availability);
- providing a process for students to assess their performance and satisfaction;
- preparing clinical rotation assignment schedules and coordinating information dissemination to clinical education sites;
- assisting with educational planning, behavior/performance modification, remedial education, referral to student support agencies (financial aid counseling as required), and;
- arranging for periodic and or impromptu visits/communication to students, clinical education sites and clinical faculty as needed to problem solve, support, and discuss pertinent issues with student(s), CIs, and/or CCCEs.

E. Evaluates each clinical education site through student feedback, on-site visits, and ongoing communications and routinely shares this information with academic and clinical faculties. Provides feedback to clinical educators concerning their effectiveness in delivering clinical learning experiences based on student feedback and through direct observations.

II. Clinical Education Program Planning, Implementation, and Assessment

A. Performs academic responsibilities consistent with the Commission on Accreditation in Physical Therapy Education (CAPTE), and with institutional policy.

- Coordinates and teaches clinical education courses and other related course content based on areas of content and clinical expertise.
- Directs effort and attention to teaching and learning processes used throughout the curriculum (eg, management and education theory, adult learning).
- Monitors and documents the academic performance of students to ensure that they successfully achieve the criteria for completing clinical learning experiences.
    - Reviews and records student evaluations from CIs and determines the final grade for all clinical education courses in the curriculum.
    - Utilizes intervention strategies with CIs, CCCEs, and students who excel or demonstrate difficulties while on clinical education experiences or require learning strategies where a disabling or learning condition is present.
    - Develops remedial experiences for students, if necessary. Confers with the appropriate faculty (clinical and academic), the Program Director, Dean, Administration and other individuals where applicable.

- Provides direct input into curriculum design, review, and revision processes by:
    - Collecting and organizing pertinent information from clinical education sites and students and disseminating this information to faculty during curricular review processes in a timely manner.
    - Preparing reports and/or engaging in discussions with faculty on student progress in clinical education.
    - Keeping faculty informed about the clinical education program, pertinent policies and procedures, and changes influenced by accreditation.

Fig. 7.4 (*Continued*)

- Coordinates and/or provides leadership for a Clinical Education or Program Advisory Committee consisting of area clinical educators, employers, or other persons, where feasible.
- Participates in academic program meetings, institutional governance, and/or community service activities as appropriate to the mission of the academic institution.
- Develops and implements a plan for self-development that includes the participation in and enhancement of teaching, delivery of physical therapy services, and development of scholarly activities (eg, scholarship of teaching, application, integration and discovery). {Refer to CAPTE Position Paper on Scholarship Expectations [PT Criterion 2.2.4.2], December 2000}
- Functions as a faculty member in other job responsibilities as delegated by the Program Director/Chair or as required by the academic institution, Dean or other Administrator.
- Monitors the changing health care delivery system and advises the Program Director and faculty of changing trends and potential impact on student enrollment, instruction, curriculum design, clinical education, and equipment needs.
- Develops and administers information and education technology systems which support clinical education and the curriculum.
- Participates in regional, state, and/or national clinical education forums, clinical education related activities, and programs designed to foster clinical education (eg, Clinical Education Consortia, Clinical Education Special Interest Group (SIG) of the Section for Education, Chapter Clinical Education SIGs, and APTA Education Division activities).

B. Manages administrative responsibilities consistent with CAPTE, federal/state regulations, institutional policy, and practice setting requirements.

- Administers a system for the academic program's clinical education records which include:
    - current database of clinical education sites;
    - current information on clinical education site and clinical faculty;
    - status of negotiated clinical education agreement between the academic program and clinical education site;
    - utilization of clinical education sites;
    - reports on the performance of students in clinical education, and
    - reports on clinical site/faculty performance in clinical education.
- Acts as an intermediary among the appropriate parties to:
    - facilitate the acquisition of clinical education agreements;
    - administer policies and procedures for immunization, preventive health care practices, and for management of student injury while at clinical sites, and
- ensure liability protection of students (and faculty if required) inclusive of professional, governmental, institutional, and current risk management principles.
- Assists the Program Director in the development of a program budget by providing input on items related to the clinical education program and overall program budget.
- Manages fiscal allocations budgeted for clinical education.
- Develops, implements, and monitors adherence to policy and procedures for the clinical education component of the curriculum.
    - **Clinical Site Development**
    - A. Develops criteria and procedures for clinical site selection, utilization, and assessment (eg, APTA Guidelines for Clinical Education).

    - B. Establishes, develops, and maintains an adequate number of clinical education sites relative to quality, quantity and diversity of learning experiences (i.e., continuum of care, commonly seen diagnoses, across the lifespan, health care delivery systems, payers, cultural competence issues) to meet the educational needs of students and the academic program, the philosophy and outcomes of the program, and evaluative criteria set by CAPTE.

    - C. Provides clinical education site development opportunities through ongoing evaluation and assessment of strengths and areas needing further development or action (eg, in service training, discontinue student placements).

Fig. 7.4 (*Continued*)

c) Education of the students, clinical, and academic faculty about clinical education and the specific goals and objectives of the DPT program.

d) Coordinate, monitor, and assess clinical education placement assignments for students.

e) Evaluation of the student's clinical performance in collaboration with the clinical instructor to assess if the student is meeting the course objectives.

f) Evaluation of the clinical site to ensure that the clinical experience and clinical instructors meet the accreditation requirements.

3. Clinical education site development.

a) Develop and maintain partnerships with clinical sites to meet the accreditation requirements and goals and objectives of the academic program.

b) Selecting clinical learning environments that demonstrate characteristics of sound patient/client management, ethical and professional behavior, and currency with physical therapy practice.

c) Facilitate and foster open and reciprocal communication between the academic program and clinic.

4. Clinical faculty development.

a) Develop and assess the developmental needs of the clinical faculty.

b) Provide education and support to clinical faculty.

7.13.2 Center Coordinator of Clinical Education

The Center Coordinator of Clinical Education (CCCE) is typically a licensed physical therapist employed and designated by the clinical facility. However, in the current health care environment the CCCE can be a physical therapist assistant, hospital or clinical administrator, or another health care professional such as an occupational therapist, speech and language pathologist or pharmacist. The role and responsibilities of the CCCE are primarily administrative but the CCCE can also function in the role of a clinical instructor for students. The primary roles and responsibilities of the CCCE are to serve as a liaison between the academic program and the clinical facility, to develop, implement, and coordinate the clinical education curriculum, to monitor the effectiveness of the clinical education curriculum through benchmarked outcome measures, and to provide education and guidance to the CIs.

The following is a list of the role and responsibilities of the CCCE, but it is not all-inclusive:

- Direct, organize, coordinate, supervise, and evaluate the clinical education program within the clinical facility.
- Maintain communication with academic liaison, the DCE, and program faculty regarding availability of clinical education.
- Support, educate, and evaluate the clinical instructors to ensure a quality clinical education experience for the students.
  - Assign CIs for each clinical placement, evaluating each CI's readiness and preparedness to serve as a CI.
  - Organize, coordinate, direct, evaluate, and supervise the activities of the clinical instructors and students assigned to the clinical site.
- Develops a clinical education program that supports both the students and CIs.
  - Determine the clinical site's readiness to accept students.

- Identify, organize, and coordinate the specific learning experiences available at the clinical site.
- Facilitate open and reciprocal communication between the academic program and clinic.
- Maintain communication with DCE, program faculty, CI, and student during the clinical education experience.
- Ensure that the students have an opportunity to meet the criteria and objectives for successful completion of the clinical education experience.

7.13.3 Clinical Instructor

The CI is an essential component of the clinical education program and experience. The CI is the role model for the student and is responsible for the day-to-day experiences of the student during the clinical education rotation. The CI is also responsible for completing the complex student assessment of performance, the clinical performance instrument (CPI) at midterm and at the scheduled end of the internship experience. The CI, by manipulating the clinical education curriculum is the physical therapist that helps the interning student bridge the gap between the academic and clinical environment. The CI facilitates the complex relationships between the student and the CI and between the student and the patient. During the internship, the CI contributes to the professional formation of the student in the cognitive, psychomotor, affective, and spiritual domains of learning.

The role of CI is multifaceted requiring many skills and qualifications to ensure a successful clinical experience for the student.[17] The CI's role "encompass varied and diverse behaviors that include facilitating, supervising, coaching, guiding, consulting, teaching, evaluating, counseling, advising, career planning, role modeling, mentoring, and socializing."[17] The CI is typically a physical therapist employed by the clinical facility and has at least 1 year of clinical practice. The physical therapist should demonstrate effective professional behavior and possess good communication, professional, teaching and interpersonal skills.

The following is a list role and responsibilities of the CI, but it is not all inclusive:

- Demonstrate effective communication skills, instructional skills, supervisory skills, and evaluation skills.
- Carry out the clinical education curriculum with the assigned student.
- Instruct, mentor, supervise, and evaluate the physical therapy student in the clinical education setting.
- Communicate with the CCCE and student before and during the clinical experience to provide information about the clinical site, expectations of students, and site requirements.
- Plan and provide appropriate clinical learning experiences for the students based on the student's level in the academic program and previous clinical experiences.
- Communicate expectations, assignments, and objectives to the student.
- Provide appropriate supervision and guidance to the student throughout the clinical experience.
- Perform evaluation of the student's clinical performance at midterm and final using the CPI.
- Demonstrate clinical competence and legal and ethical behavior that meets or exceeds the expectations of members of the profession of physical therapy.

To assist the CI in meeting the roles and responsibilities of the position, APTA has developed a training program, the Credentialed Clinical Educator Program to support, prepare, and educate CIs to work with students in the clinical practice settings.[45] The training program is voluntary and has been found to be effective in training CIs to provide a quality clinical education experience for students.

7.13.4 Student

Students are the central focus of the clinical education experience and thus are an essential member in the process. Students have the responsibility to be an active participant in the internship experience. The student is the functional link between the academic program and the clinical site and the improvement in student performance in all domains of practice is the primary outcome measure of the experience. Though the clinical education experience is considered a planned learning experience, the student must take active responsibility to facilitate a positive outcome. The student's responsibilities in their role in the clinical education experience include the following:

- Provide assistance to the DCE in the site selection process.
- Develop with the DCE personal goals and objectives for the specific clinical experience and share these with the CI.
- Prepare for the clinical experience by researching the scope of care of the clinical practice and reviewing the CPI from the previous clinical experience.
- With approval of the DCE, contact the CCCE at the internship site with a letter of introduction. Inquire about dress, specific policies, necessary items to bring to clinic, the performance of mandatory competencies, and such.
- Meet with the DCE to jointly reflect on past clinical internship performances.
- Develop the ability to practice in a reflective manner. Students need to develop reflective practice that includes applying knowledge and skills.

7.13.5 Patient

An understated element in the clinical education process is the patient. Though there are many learning opportunities afforded the student in the clinical education environment—observation of other disciplines, observation of assessments and interventions, written assignments, attendance at staff meetings and clinical conferences, participation in in-services, opportunities for reflection, written and oral feedback, and research—the primary learning tool in clinical education is the patient.

From an ethical and legal viewpoint, the patient must consent to treatment and with regard to clinical education, the consent to treatment must include evaluation, assessment, and treatment by a student supervised by a licensed therapist. The patient should be made aware that the primary treating therapist is a student but that the student will be continually supervised by a licensed therapist. Conventional wisdom states that patients should not be "cherry picked" for students based on the patient's behavioral attributes; students should learn through interacting with all types of patients. However, patients are often chosen for the student based on diagnostic criteria, complexity, comorbidities, and age to provide the student with a full spectrum of experiences or to assist with specific remediation. At the end of the episode of care, the patient should be thoroughly thanked by the student and the CI for participating in the student's clinical education.

7.14 Assessment of Clinical Education Performance

Assessment in clinical education primarily focuses on four key stakeholders: the student, the CI, the CCCE, and the DCE, and one environmental variable, the clinical site.[46] Assessment of the student is both formative and summative based on the student's clinical competency and skills in the clinical education experience. APTA has developed a voluntary validated standardized instrument, the physical therapy clinical performance instrument (PT-CPI) that guides the assessment of the student performance during clinical education experiences.[47] The PT-CPI is completed at the midterm (formative) and end of the experience (summative) by the CI, often with input and counsel from the CCCE. The instrument was initially developed and implemented into practice in 1997 and revised in 2006 primarily due to changes in the physical therapy scope of practice and to update it to an electronic version.[19]

Although the PT-CPI is a voluntary instrument, the majority of the physical therapist education programs in the United States and Canada utilize it.[18] The PT-CPI permits the CI to assess the student's performance based on predetermined outcome criteria. Discussion of the PT-CPI at the internship midterm and end provides data points to the student and CI which fosters performance reflection on the part of both parties. If the CI so chooses, the student may be asked to also complete the PT-CPI which provides student the ability to self-assess his performance during the clinical experience. The CPI is now a web-based instrument that requires training for all users to ensure that the instrument is used correctly and as intended.[19,48]

A number of voluntary DCE performance assessments have been developed by the ad hoc consultant group on the development of ACCE/DCE performance assessments and are available as a resource for use by physical therapist and physical therapist assistant academic programs.[49] Assessing DCE performance can be used to support promotion, tenure, workload, and professional development through clarification of the roles and responsibilities of the ACCE/DCE.[50]

These assessments are designed to obtain performance feedback on the unique leadership, administrative, and managerial functions of the DCE. The set of assessments includes tools for the academic administrator, faculty, CIs, CCCEs, students, and DCE self-assessment. Although the assessments are copyrighted, programs may choose how they wish to distribute these assessments (e.g., paper, web-based, database format) and the frequency with which they wish to use these assessments.

Performance data about the DCE, Assistant DCE, and co-DCE from evaluator groups remains with the participating academic program and is not shared with APTA. These forms include the following:[49,51]

- ACCE/DCE performance assessments for self and academic administrators.
- ACCE/DCE performance assessments for CIs and CCCEs.
- ACCE/DCE performance assessments for faculty.
- ACCE/DCE performance assessments for students.

7.15 Future of Clinical Education

The necessity to improve and update clinical education in physical therapy is related to a number of factors. Clinical advancement in health care in general and physical therapy in particular is happening at a dazzling rate. Clinical education must continue to evolve to incorporate these advancements. Along with the advancement in clinical care the changes in health care administration, global health initiatives, reimbursement patterns and health policy are also evolving at a rapid pace. Knowledge of these advancements is the background music of physical therapist practice. The clinical education internship experience, under the mentorship of the CI, is the optimum arena to practically learn about these advancements and to incorporate their tenets into clinical practice. Lastly, the scope of care of physical therapy has grown substantially over the past decades. Content such as vestibulopathy, women's health, computer-based learning tools, and computer-guided adaptive equipment were not even considered when physical therapy curricula, as recently as 20 years ago, was developed. Clinical education must continue to assimilate into its curricula opportunities for the students to experience these novel technologies and content.

There are several issues and challenges that will impact clinical education and its future. The discussion of these issues is beyond the scope of this chapter, but below are some of the issues and challenges that academic programs and clinical sites will need to address to ensure quality clinical education experiences for DPT students in the future.

In 2016, APTA formed a task force, the best practices for physical therapist clinical education task force, which was charged with looking at the current state of clinical education and to make recommendations to the APTA board of directors to identify best practice "for physical therapist clinical education, from professional level through post professional clinical training, and propose potential courses of action for a doctoring profession to move toward practice that best meets the evolving needs of society."[52] The task force outlined those recommendations in a 2017 report to APTA's House of Delegates. The report, the clinical residency and fellowship education on entry-level clinical education, provided a discussion of a number of challenges which our profession will face over the next decade with regard to clinical education. Perhaps the number one challenge relates to the availability of clinical sites for clinical education. As the number of entry-level programs increases there will be increased competition among programs for the use of these sites. Additional competition for these sites will come from the increasing numbers of residency and fellowship programs. The national study of excellence and innovation in physical therapist education provided discussion related to the future of technology in clinical education.[53] "Technology," as discussed in the report, includes clinical medical technology and ancillary technologies which may improve the outcomes of clinical education as a learning tool. As the use of technology increases in all aspects of DPT education (smart classes, clinical simulation, apps), there is opportunity to enhance the clinical education program and the student's experience by using available technology. Examples include the use of databases and electronic programs not only to provide clinical resources to interning students at a distant site, but also to maintain and manage student information and progression as well as to manage the overall clinical education program. Many of these databases already exist at the university level and technology will permit, and the portability and access for the students and CI/CCCE to use at distant sites. Live technology such as Skype can enhance the effectiveness and time management of the DCE by providing an alternative to travel to visit interning students. Educational tools already permit entry-level coursework to be taken online rather than in the standard classroom setting. This permits curricular committees to shift some coursework from busy, on campus semesters to semesters when the students are on clinical internship.

7.16 Challenges in Physical Therapy Clinical Education: Present and Future

In summary, there are a number of challenges that currently affect clinical education and the future of clinical education. Some of these challenges include the following:

1. *Availability of clinical settings.* DCEs have faced for several years the difficulty of finding and maintaining quality clinical sites. There are many reasons that are purported to be the reason for the availability of sites, one being that proliferation of DPT programs and clinical residencies and fellowships. This issue is expected to worsen before it gets better.
2. *Issues of underutilization of clinical sites.* As the competition for clinical site utilization grows our profession needs to identify and use clinical sites which are underutilized due to location, type of specialized practice, cost for students to participate, and the limited number of CIs.
3. *Residency programs.* In medicine, hospitals with residency programs are reimbursed by Medicare at an accelerated rate as compared with hospitals without residency programs. The accelerated payment rate is an enticement to develop medical/surgical residency programs. Currently, there is no accelerated payment rate for facilities which possess physical therapy residency programs and thus no enticement to develop such programs.
4. *Competition for specialized clinical sites.* There are increasing numbers of DPT programs which set requirements for students' clinical education experience (e.g., acute care, rehabilitation, pediatric, or orthopedic experiences). The competition for the clinical sites is especially heated between DPT programs when the DPT programs are in proximity to one another.
5. *Regulatory issues.* There are a number of laws, standards, and guidelines, such as those related to the Americans with Disability Act, Medicare, Joint Commission, Commission on Accreditation of Rehabilitation Facilities, and HIPPA that directly impact the student's clinical education experience by limiting or prohibiting interning students from working with specific cohorts of patients.

7.17 Review Questions

1. The position title of the person who is an academic faculty member and also directs the doctor of physical therapy clinical education program is which of the following?
   a) Student.
   b) Patient.

c) Director of clinical education.

d) Center coordinator for clinical education.

2. The position title of the person who is not academic faculty member and also directs the doctor of physical therapy clinical education program at the clinical site?

   a) Student.

   b) Clinical instructor.

   c) Director of clinical education.

   d) Center coordinator for clinical education.

3. The position title of the person who is not academic faculty member and also directs at the internship site, on a daily basis, the interning student in the doctor of physical therapy clinical education program is which of the following?

   a) Student.

   b) Clinical instructor.

   c) Director of clinical education.

   d) Center coordinator for clinical education.

4. The position title of the person who is not academic faculty member and must also consent to treatment by the interning student is which of the following?

   a) Student.

   b) Patient.

   c) Director of clinical education.

   d) Center coordinator for clinical education.

5. The type of clinical experience students matriculating in doctor of physical therapy curricula is which of the following?

   a) Clinical internship.

   b) Residency.

   c) Fellowship.

   d) Postdoctoral studies.

6. An early clinical experience, typically occurring in the first year of the professional curriculum, is part-time, and whose aim is to provide early exposure to clinical care is which of the following?

   a) Integrated clinical experience.

   b) Residency.

   c) Fellowship.

   d) Post-doctoral studies.

7. Most entry-level doctor of physical therapy programs utilize which tool for the assessment of their interning students?

   a) Physical therapy clinical performance instrument.

   b) The Berg balance scale.

   c) ACCE/DCE performance assessments for self and academic administrators.

   d) CCE/DCE performance assessments for students.

8. The primary challenge impacting today's directors of clinical education is which of the following?

   a) Too many clinical sites.

   b) Too few clinical sites.

   c) Poorly trained clinical instructors.

   d) Poorly trained center coordinators for clinical education.

9. The most commonly utilized ratio of clinical instructor: student is which of the following?

   a) 1:1.

   b) 2:1.

   c) 1:2.

   d) 1:4.

10. The independent and separate model of clinical education is utilized primarily by which professional programs?

    a) Physical therapy and occupational therapy.

    b) Veterinary medicine and physical therapy.

    c) Nursing and speech pathology.

    d) Dentistry and medicine.

7.18 Review Answers

1. The position title of the person who is an academic faculty member and also directs the doctor of physical therapy clinical education program is which of the following?

   c. Director of clinical education.

2. The position title of the person who is not academic faculty member and also directs the doctor of physical therapy clinical education program at the clinical site?

   d. Center coordinator for clinical education.

3. The position title of the person who is not academic faculty member and also directs at the internship site, on a daily basis, the interning student in the doctor of physical therapy clinical education program is which of the following?

   b. Clinical instructor.

4. The position title of the person who is not academic faculty member and must also consent to treatment by the interning student is which of the following?

   b. Patient.

5. The type of clinical experience students matriculating in doctor of physical therapy curricula is which of the following?

   a. Clinical internship.

6. An early clinical experience, typically occurring in the first year of the professional curriculum, is part-time, and whose aim is to provide early exposure to clinical care is which of the following?

   a. Integrated clinical experience.

7. Most entry-level doctor of physical therapy programs utilize which tool for the assessment of their interning students?

   a. Physical therapy clinical performance instrument.

8. The primary challenge impacting today's directors of clinical education is which of the following?

   b. Too few clinical sites.

9. The most commonly utilized ratio of clinical instructor: student is which of the following?

   a. 1:1.

10. The independent and separate model of clinical education is utilized primarily by which professional programs?

    d. Dentistry and medicine.

References

[1] Moore ML, Perry JF. Clinical Education in Physical Therapy: Present Status/Future Needs. Alexandria, VA: American Physical Therapy Association and the Section for Education; 1976

[2] The Commission on Accreditation in Physical Therapy Education. Available at: http://www.capteonline.org/home.aspx. Accessed October 10, 2017

[3] Professionalism Module 2: History of Professionalism in Physical Therapy. APTA Online Learning Center. APTA.org. Accessed October 10, 2017

[4] Johnson MP, Abrams SL. Historical perspectives of autonomy within the medical profession: considerations for 21st century physical therapy practice. J Orthop Sports Phys Ther. 2005; 35(10):628–636

[5] Neumann DA. Polio: its impact on the people of the United States and the emerging profession of physical therapy. J Orthop Sports Phys Ther. 2004; 34 (8):479–492

[6] American Physical Therapy Association. Available athttp://www.apta.org/uploadedFiles/APTAorg/Educators/Clinical_Development/Education_Resources/PTClinicalEducationPrinciples.pdf. Accessed October 12, 2017

[7] Edwards I, Jones M, Carr J, Braunack-Mayer A, Jensen GM. Clinical reasoning strategies in physical therapy. Phys Ther. 2004; 84(4):312–330, discussion 331–335

[8] Jarski RW, Kulig K, Olson RE. Clinical teaching in physical therapy: student and teacher perceptions. Phys Ther. 1990; 70(3):173–178

[9] Johnson SL. Medical education in the U.S. and Canada: data for academic year 1935–1936. JAMA. 1936; 107(9):661–692

[10] Gwyer J, Odom C, Gandy J. History of clinical education in physical therapy in the United States. J Phys Ther Educ. 2003; 17(3):34

[11] Shepard KF, Jensen GM. Handbook of Teaching for Physical Therapists. 2nd ed. Boston: Butterworth-Heinemann, 2002

[12] Hayward LM, Charrette AL. Integrating cultural competence and core values: an international service-learning model. J Phys Ther Educ. 2012; 26(1):78

[13] Dyrbye LN, Harris I, Rohren CH. Early clinical experiences from students' perspectives: a qualitative study of narratives. Acad Med. 2007; 82(10):979–988

[14] Black LL, Jensen GM, Mostrom E, et al. The first year of practice: an investigation of the professional learning and development of promising novice physical therapists. Phys Ther. 2010; 90(12):1758–1773

[15] Hayward LM, Black LL, Mostrom E, Jensen GM, Ritzline PD, Perkins J. The first two years of practice: a longitudinal perspective on the learning and professional development of promising novice physical therapists. Phys Ther. 2013; 93(3):369–383

[16] Strohschein J, Hagler P, May L. Assessing the need for change in clinical education practices. Phys Ther. 2002; 82(2):160–172

[17] Frost JS. Preparation For Teaching In Clinical Settings. In: Jensen G, Mostrom E. Handbook Of Teaching and Learning for Physical Therapists. 3rd Edition. Elsevier Butterworth Heinemann, St. Missouri. 2013. 124-144

[18] Ellen Wetherbee PT, Buccieri KM, Jean FitzpatrickTimmerberg PT, Stolfi AM. Essential characteristics of quality clinical education experiences: standards to facilitate student learning. J Phys Ther Educ. 2014; 28:48

[19] Roach KE, Frost JS, Francis NJ, Giles S, Nordrum JT, Delitto A. Validation of the revised physical therapist clinical performance instrument (PT CPI): version 2006. Phys Ther. 2012; 92(3):416–428

[20] Goldman J. Centre for the Advancement of Interprofessional Education (CAIPE). J Interprof Care. 2011; 25(5):386–387

[21] Buring SM, Bhushan A, Broeseker A, et al. Interprofessional education: definitions, student competencies, and guidelines for implementation. Am J Pharm Educ. 2009; 73(4):59

[22] Lawlis TR, Anson J, Greenfield D. Barriers and enablers that influence sustainable interprofessional education: a literature review. J Interprof Care. 2014; 28(4):305–310

[23] Bridges DR, Davidson RA, Odegard PS, Maki IV, Tomkowiak J. Interprofessional collaboration: three best practice models of interprofessional education. Med Educ Online. 2011; 16(1):6035

[24] Carpenter J. Interprofessional education for medical and nursing students: evaluation of a programme. Med Educ. 1995; 29(4):265–272

[25] Bradley P. The history of simulation in medical education and possible future directions. Med Educ. 2006; 40(3):254–262

[26] Panel IECE. Core Competencies for Interprofessional Collaborative Practice: Report of an Expert Panel. Washington, DC: Interprofessional Education Collaborative; 2011

[27] Jensen GM, Mostrom E. Handbook of Teaching for Physical Therapists-E-Book. Philadelphia: Elsevier Health Sciences; 2012

[28] DeClute J, Ladyshewsky R. Enhancing clinical competence using a collaborative clinical education model. Phys Ther. 1993; 73(10):683–689, discussion 689–697

[29] Jensen GM, Gwyer J, Shepard KF, Hack LM. Expert practice in physical therapy. Phys Ther. 2000; 80(1):28–43, discussion 44–52

[30] Ladyshewsky RK, Barrie SC, Drake VM. A comparison of productivity and learning outcome in individual and cooperative physical therapy clinical education models. Phys Ther. 1998; 78(12):1288–1298, discussion 1299–1301

[31] http://acapt.org/

[32] Holtman MC, Frost JS, Hammer DP, McGuinn K, Nunez LM. Interprofessional professionalism: linking professionalism and interprofessional care. J Interprof Care. 2011; 25(5):383–385

[33] Moore A, Morris J, Crouch V, Martin M. Evaluation of physiotherapy clinical educational models: comparing 1: 1, 2: 1 and 3: 1 placements. Physiotherapy. 2003; 89(8):489–501

[34] Huddleston R. Clinical placements for the professions allied to medicine, part 2: placement shortages? Two models that can solve the problem. Br J Occup Ther. 1999; 62(7):295–298

[35] McCallum CA, Mosher PD, Jacobson PJ, Gallivan SP, Giuffre SM. Quality in physical therapist clinical education: a systematic review. Phys Ther. 2013; 93(10):1298–1311

[36] Holaday SD, Buckley KM. Addressing challenges in nursing education through a clinical instruction model based on a hybrid, inquiry-based learning framework. Nurs Educ Perspect. 2008; 29(6):353–358

[37] Kollar SJ, Ailinger RL. International clinical experiences: long-term impact on students. Nurse Educ. 2002; 27(1):28–31

[38] Rodger S, Webb G, Devitt L, Gilbert J, Wrightson P, McMeeken J. A clinical education and practice placements in the allied health professions: an international perspective. J Allied Health. 2008; 37(1):53–62

[39] Celia Pechak PT, Mary Thompson PT. International service-learning and other international volunteer service in physical therapist education programs in the United States and Canada: an exploratory study. J Phys Ther Educ. 2009; 23(1):71

[40] Pechak CM. Survey of international clinical education in physical therapist education. J Phys Ther Educ. 2012; 26(1):69

[41] Pajak E. Approaches to Clinical Supervision: Alternatives for Improving Instruction. Hoboken: Wiley-Blackwell Company; 2000

[42] Kilminster SM, Jolly BC. Effective supervision in clinical practice settings: a literature review. Med Educ. 2000; 34(10):827–840

[43] Holloway E. Clinical supervision: a systems approach. Sage. 1995

[44] Driscoll J. Practicing Clinical Supervision: A Reflective Approach for Healthcare Professionals. UK: Oxford University Press; 2007

[45] APTA Credentialed Clinical Instructor Program.(CCIP). www.apta.org/CCIP. Accessed October 30, 2018

[46] Task Force for the Development of Student Clinical Performance Instruments, American Physical Therapy Association. The development and testing of APTA clinical performance instruments. Phys Ther. 2002; 82 (4):329–353

[47] Buccieri KM, Schultze K, Dungey J, Kolodziej T. Self-reported characteristics of physical therapy clinical instructors: a comparison to the American Physical Therapy Association's Guidelines and Self-Assessments for Clinical Education. J Phys Ther Educ. 2006; 20(1):47

[48] American Physical Therapy Association. Available at: http://www.apta.org/PTCPI/. Accessed October 1, 2017

[49] American Physical Therapy Association. Available at: http://www.apta.org/Educators/Assessments/ACCE/DCE/GuidelinesandAssessmentsforClinEd/. Accessed October 1, 2017

[50] American Physical Therapy Association. Available at: http://www.apta.org/PTCPI/Web/. Accessed October 2, 2017

[51] American Physical Therapy Association. Available at: https://www.apta.org/uploadedFiles/APTAorg/About_Us/Policies/BOD/Education/ClincialEducationSitesPart1.pdf. Accessed October 2, 2017

[52] American Physical Therapy Association. Available at: http://www.apta.org/Educators/TaskForceReport/PTClinicalEducation/. Accessed October 2, 2017

[53] Jensen GM, Hack LM, Nordstrom T, Gwyer J, Mostrom E. National study of excellence and innovation in physical therapist education: part 2-A call to reform. Phys Ther. 2017; 97(9):875–888

8 A Student's Perspective of Clinical Education

Sabrina L. Martha

Keywords: American Physical Therapy Association, APTA Clinical Site Information Form, Center Coordinator for Clinical Education, clinical education, clinical instructor, Clinical Performance Instrument, clinical site, Commission on Accreditation in Physical Therapy Education, critically appraised topic, Director of Clinical Education, integrated clinical experience, student physical therapist

"Talent is God given; be humble. Fame is man-given; be thankful. Conceit is self-given; be careful."

—John Wooden

Chapter Outline
1. Introduction to Clinical Education
2. Clinical Education Internships
   a) The Placement Process
   b) Choosing a Site
   c) APTA Clinical Site Information Form
   d) Preparing for Clinical Education Internships
   e) Requirements for Clinical Education Internships
3. Expectations and Requirements During Clinical Education
   a) How Much Am I Expected to Handle?
   b) What is an in-Service?
   c) Additional Assignments
   d) CI Expectations
   e) CI–Student Relationship
4. Evaluation and Assessment of Student Performance in the Clinic
   a) The Clinical Performance Instrument
      1. How Do I Use the CPI?
      2. Weekly Planning Forms
5. A Student's Perspective: Challenges and Surprises
   a) My First Clinical Education Experience
   b) Inpatient Versus Outpatient Experience
   c) What Surprised Me about Clinical Education
   d) What I Would Do Differently

"I arrived early for my first clinical internship. I was assigned to intern at a large skilled nursing facility in rural Maine. I volunteered for this site because I have an aunt living nearby (I could live rent-free!) and my family often spent our vacations with my aunt. The department secretary told me that my clinical supervisor had not yet arrived and I was directed to the cafeteria to have a cup of tea and wait for her.

"I sipped my tea. Writing this first-person account was difficult because I did not want to sound prideful or over-confident. Arriving for my first clinical internship I was nervous, of course, but deep down I had performed extremely well thus far in the professional program and also had performed well during my integrated clinical experiences. I was not afraid of the experience in front of me. I was not afraid of performing manual muscle tests, sensory examinations, neurological examinations, writing goals, developing a plan of care, or talking with other health care persons. I felt comfortable with my abilities. However, an unusual anxiety gnawed at me. I was concerned that I had been given an incredible opportunity—to serve in a humanistic way those who were sick, impaired, and poor. Families were entrusting me with their loved ones' care. What greater opportunity (and challenge) is there! My skills could determine if my patient walks again or never walks again, if he is ever able to dress himself or will require a family member to help don his pants, if he is transferred to a nursing home versus returning home again, if his wound heals or if he may require potential amputation, if he is forced to endure a life-long history of low back pain or enjoy pain-free movement.

"As I sat in that waiting room sipping my tea and preparing for my first clinical internship, this is what was going through my mind. I watched my clinical instructor walk into the cafeteria and with a broad smile offered her hand to me. I whispered a silent prayer."

—Kathy B., Baltimore, Maryland

8.1 Introduction to Clinical Education

My name is Sabrina Martha and I am a recent graduate of a doctor of physical therapy (DPT) program associated with a large, urban-based university in Philadelphia. As a student physical therapist (SPT), I completed 42 weeks of full time clinical education (CE), divided into four separate clinical experiences at four different sites over the course of my three years in the DPT program. I often reflect on my clinical education experience.

What Is Clinical Education?

Clinical Education (CE): The length of professional DPT programs is about three years. Eighty percent of the curriculum includes classroom and lab study, while the remaining 20% is focused on clinical education. On average, PT students spend 27.5 hours on their clinical education over the course of the program.[1]

During my first year as a DPT student I, like most DPT students, felt that my educational and clinical experiences were unique unto me. Later, as my interaction with my fellow students at my program and other programs grew and matured, I learned of the commonality of our paths, experiences, successes, and challenges prior to and while matriculated in the DPT program. I learned that the Commission on Accreditation in Physical Therapy Education (CAPTE), an accreditation agency particular to physical therapy and physical therapy assistant educational programs, is very proactive in developing standards which all programs must follow.

These universal standards are very explicit, making the similarities between programs much more common than the individual differences. All programs must follow the accreditation standards; how they follow them is each program's decision.

School was challenging. School was fun. I felt incredibly lucky to be able to pursue my dream to help others by becoming a physical therapist. I still feel this way. My program began in summer session two with two courses—physiology and teaching/learning for a combined total of 7 credits. The rationale for my program to only offer two classes in the abbreviated summer semester was to permit the incoming students to gradually become familiar with doctoral education, to provide free time for the students to learn our new city (most of us traveled from afar to Philadelphia to attend the program), and time and opportunities for us to get to know our classmates. Our program was considered a lock-step program, a term originally unfamiliar to me but I soon learned that the term "lock-step educational program" indicates that all students are in the same classes at the same time save for electives and clinical internships. Classroom bonding among students is especially important in professional programs due to the rapidity of the information delivered and the need to study in groups. Most students estimate that in the first professional year 50% of all studying is done in group situations. Strong interpersonal relationships among students are an important prerequisite to the trust needed for group studying.

After a brief 7-week summer session we began the fall semester in earnest with 18 credits. Classes were 4 days per week with Fridays off. "Off" is a relative term; we used Fridays as catch-up and study days. I quickly felt overwhelmed. I learned the difference between undergraduate and graduate education. The amount of information and the pace it is delivered in graduate school dwarfs that of undergraduate school. Eighteen credits of coursework were scheduled for my fall semester. Fall semester included anatomy lecture and cadaver lab. Anatomy lecture and dissection required much for the novice doctoral student to assimilate—psychologically, cognitively, and from a psychomotor viewpoint (the actual dissection techniques) on its own. Add four additional classes, and one can quickly appreciate why I spent most free hours in the library and coffee shop. At the start of the semester, the Director of Clinical Education (DCE) from my university (see ▶ Table 8.1) introduced my class to the process for clinical education. The DCE is a faculty member who directs all student clinical internship activities. For a student simply trying to find the school bathroom, the thought of actually evaluating

and treating a patient seemed incomprehensible. My first clinical internship would not begin until the following summer, after I completed my first full year of coursework for the program.

My program did require integrated clinical experiences (ICEs) beginning in our first fall semester. ICEs are observational experiences in which DPT students formally travel to local clinics to observe therapists providing therapy services. The "integrated" aspect is that these experiences are tied to the content delivered at the same time to the students in the professional program. For instance, if we were learning wound care we would observe, via an ICE, a therapist treating a patient with a wound. Or, if we were learning about neurological testing, we would be scheduled to observe a therapist performing a neurological examination. Though not nearly the scope of a true clinical internship, the ICEs permitted us, to a small extent, see our future as therapists. ICEs provided a welcomed initiation into the clinical world.

8.2 Clinical Education Internships

8.2.1 The Placement Process

The decision of which DPT program to attend was important to me. With the consideration of spending the next 3 years of my life—full time—in a program, I wanted to make the correct decision. Along with investigating the implicit and explicit curricula and meeting with the admission's director, I reviewed policies on placement for clinical education. Realizing that clinical internships comprised almost 25% of the professional curriculum, I wanted to maximize my opportunity to intern at the top clinics nationally. The procedures used by doctor of physical therapy programs to assign students to their clinical internships, to my surprise, varied greatly. I learned there were three primary methods by which the DCEs assigned clinical internships. The first method is a lottery. In the lottery system, the program would provide the students with a list of available clinical sites. Each student would then be randomly assigned a number, 1 to 50, and the student assigned "1" would pick his clinical site first, followed in order by students 2 to 50. This is an excellent system if the student is assigned an early number (he or she could choose the prime clinical sites) but the downside of the system is for those students assigned numbers 45 to 50 who often were required to travel great distances for a nondesirable clinical site. The lottery system would be replicated for each of the four clinical internships. The second method is where the DCE would simply assign a student to a specific clinical site. The students would arrive at school one day to see a list posted on a bulletin board detailing where she would be spending the next 12 weeks of her life. This method is the easiest for the DCE to control but obviously leaves the student's wishes completely out of the decision-making algorithm. There is no negotiating. There is no discussion. My program utilized a third method. Our DCE provided our class with a list of clinical sites. Since our program was large and well-established, the list had perhaps 250 clinical locations listed. My 49 classmates and I would each prioritize our top five clinical sites. The DCE would then do her best to provide each student with one of their top choices. My DCE also gave us the option of staying in Philadelphia or traveling anywhere in the country for the clinical internship. If we wished to remain local we could be required to drive up to 1 hour to the clinic. We learned that a "contract" with the clinical

Table 8.1 Who's who in clinical education?

Title/Position	Description of role
Director of Clinical Education	Responsible for planning, coordinating, facilitating, administering and monitoring activities on behalf of an academic program and in coordination with academic and clinical faculty[2]
Center Coordinator for Clinical Education	Responsible for coordinating activities and assignments for students at a clinical site[3]
Clinical Instructor	Responsible for direct supervision of the student during clinical affiliation in accordance with APTA standards of practice[4]

Abbreviation: APTA, American Physical Therapy Association.

site to provide student internships was not always a contract. Emergencies happened at the clinical site. Employees resigned. Practices were sold. More than once one of my classmates was set to travel to a distant clinical site and days before the start of the clinical internship the site would cancel. The DCE would then frantically search for a replacement site which met the student's needs. This is a terrible time for the student and DCE. Fortunately, this situation only occurred to a few of my classmates over the course of our four clinical internships.

Of great importance, and this is true for most programs, students are responsible for all travel and housing costs associated with clinical placement. For example, some of my classmates chose to travel to California from the east coast. These students were responsible for all travel costs, locating housing, and organizing transportation to/from their site. Some stayed with friends or family members, some found random roommates on the internet and some lived alone. Most of my classmates chose Philadelphia for two of the clinical internships to save money and traveled for two. Potential DPT students, when considering school loans, may wish to consider budgeting for the costs of the clinical internships. Most DPT programs, including mine, mandated at least one of the four clinical internships be at an outpatient site and one be at hospital-based inpatient practice. Entering DPT school students often are fairly confident in which arena of physical therapy they may want to specialize but in truth, one never knows until one experiences the particular arena as a clinician. Entering the DPT program many of my classmates were quite sure they wanted to work in outpatient orthopedics. I was surprised how many ended up specializing in acute care or inpatient medical rehabilitation.

8.2.2 Choosing a Site

The list of potential clinical sites my classmates and I received prior to each clinical internship experience contained locations throughout the United States, with a majority in Pennsylvania, New Jersey, New York, and Delaware. About 25% of possible sites were located in Pennsylvania and of this number perhaps half were in or near Philadelphia, with the remaining half scattered across the state. Programs with national reputations tend to have a large number of potential sites at the best health care facilities in the nation, while smaller, parochial programs tend to offer sites near to campus. Many students ask about international clinical sites. My program offered a number of international experiences with the caveat that the clinical instructor (CI)—the therapist supervising the interning student—graduated from a U.S.-accredited DPT program. The philosophy of our DCE is that only in the United States is the doctoral degree the entry-level degree to become a physical therapist and she did not want us being instructed by a foreign-trained therapist practicing with a lesser degree. In some countries, physical therapists are only required to have an associate's degree.

When first presented by our DCE with a list of potential clinical sites and a request for each of us to prioritize our top five choices for our first clinical internship I quickly became overwhelmed. There were so many variables to consider. In addition, we were nearing midterms and our thoughts were on simply doing well with the testing and not on where we wished to spend the summer months. Still, questions arose:

How far am I willing to travel? How will I commute to the clinic? Will I need a car? Should I travel out of state? Do I want to begin in an outpatient or inpatient setting? How can I afford renting a place out of state? How do I even find a place to live out of state? When will I know where I am placed? These are all questions that my classmates and I nervously discussed while considering our options.

One of the things I love about our profession is the flexibility and potential to move around to different settings and to pursue a specialty. One could live in pretty much any U.S. town or city and be within easy driving distance of a therapy clinic—freestanding, school based, or hospital based. As a first-year student, I had no idea what I wanted to do but it was wonderful to know I had options with regard to the arena of therapy and the location of the arena. For clinical education, my biggest priority was to be able to stay close to my family in Philadelphia. I chose five sites that were close or at most an hour commute from my home. For some of my classmates this was not the case and they preferred to travel to see a new city and have a new experience. Some were like me in that they wanted to be close to home, but home was not near Philadelphia. In these cases, when our list didn't have what someone was looking for, our DCE met with these individuals to discuss and work with them on potential opportunities. Students were not expected to coordinate or find a clinical internship on their own but our DCE was willing to consider adding clinical sites to our contract list based on student recommendations. After submitting my choices, I quickly became wrapped up in midterms, getting through the fall semester, and then finals.

8.2.3 APTA Clinical Site Information Form

The American Physical Therapy Association (APTA) Clinical Site Information Form (CSIF) is a dynamic online database consisting of a collection of information that helps to facilitate student placements and assess the learning experience and practice opportunities available to students.[5] As students we were required, at the end of each clinical internship experience, to complete the CSIF form. The form requests basic information, such as details of student transportation to and from the clinical site, housing opportunities, required dress code, learning opportunities, and student schedule. For example, if there are opportunities for the student to experience cardiac or vestibular rehabilitation or women's health initiatives. Is there a wound care clinic? Does the facility utilize an electronic medical record? Are there opportunities to observe surgery? Information is also requested about interaction with other health care professionals, patient population typically seen (pediatrics, geriatrics, neurological), and categories and types of diagnoses treated. The form also requests CI demographic data including educational and clinical background. The CSIF is a great resource to review proactively to assist students preparing for clinical internship in prioritizing site selection (if that is the method the program uses for assigning clinical sites) or to gain a better understanding of what to expect and plan for before arriving at the site. A link is provided at the end of this chapter with information on how to access this tool.[5]

8.2.4 Preparing for Clinical Education Internships

Personally, I didn't consider much about my first clinical placement until winter break arrived. I was too immersed in schoolwork to consider much of anything! With my strong fall semester grades, I was becoming more confident in my ability to successfully complete the professional program and was becoming excited about transitioning my didactic skills into the clinic. I met with our DCE at the start of fall semester to review the internship process and review my long-term career goals and personal preferences for clinical settings. I learned that I received my third choice—an outpatient setting near my home—for my first clinical internship. My program's first clinical internship was six weeks in duration with the remaining three internships each 12 weeks in length. With 1 year of classroom education and a number of ICEs, I felt somewhat comfortable entering the clinic.

My initial clinical internship responsibility was to contact my CI (see ► Table 8.1). I sent a letter introducing myself and inquiring about information regarding the site that was relevant to me. I was excited to learn more about the setting, my CI, my schedule, what types of patients I would be seeing, and what a typical day was like. My DCE was responsible for sending an information packet out to each CI at each clinical site with the necessary insurance information for students to practice, as well as an outline of the coursework the program covered to date. The packet provided my CI with insight into what coursework and lab experience I had been exposed to by the time I started in their clinic. Often, clinics have contracts with a number of DPT educational programs. As mentioned previously, all programs must teach to the mandated accrediting standards of CAPTE but are free to arrange the information and experiences in a way best suited to the program's mission and vision. For this reason, a CI must provide a different internship experience and curriculum to interning students from different programs because each student has been educated using a unique program-developed curriculum. Only prior to the final clinical internship, when all didactic information has been completed, are all DPT students from all programs essentially equal in educational content.

In my letters to my CI prior to the assigned internship, I introduced myself, provided information regarding my personal background and clinical and classroom experience, and inquired if there was anything I could provide or do ahead of time prior to starting the internship to facilitate my readiness. CIs, along with supervising students, are also practicing clinicians. Do not always expect an immediate reply to your contact. Sometimes a follow-up letter or email can prompt a response.

8.2.5 Requirements for Clinical Education Internships

Each clinical facility may have certain requirements prior to the student's arrival at the internship site. For example, my final clinical internship site required that I go to location off the hospital campus for an orientation to the clinical site, system, and facility. I was also required to have a photo ID taken. In terms of dress code, many outpatient facilities require business casual, but some specifically requested students wear khakis. In one of my outpatient sites the male therapists were required to wear dress shirts and ties. Inpatient settings' dress codes are highly variable. Some sites require business casual attire, some scrubs, and some laboratory coats. Hence, it is important to touch base with the CI prior to beginning the internship.

Two of my sites required that I provide proof of receiving a flu vaccine prior to beginning the internship. Fortunately, my program required a comprehensive list of competencies be completed prior to being assigned to our first clinical internship site, and utilized an online database to organize the completion of the competencies and dates when those that are time sensitive had to be retaken. As an example, we were required to provide the program with proof of a yearly physician evaluation. Included in ► Table 8.2 is a list of the requirements I had to fulfill as a student. Several oversite and accrediting agencies list a number of compliance items which must be completed prior to the clinical internship. Because these vary among jurisdictions the list included in this table may not be appropriate for all students. At our program orientation held prior to the start of classes we were introduced us to these requirements. This was helpful in allowing the students to begin collecting all required competency data early, as once we were in classes full time I found it very difficult to schedule. Failure to maintain one's competencies would result in an internship being delayed or canceled.

8.3 Expectations and Requirements During Clinical Education

8.3.1 How Much Am I Expected to Handle?

A common concern my classmates shared prior to the first clinical experience was about the expectations of our CI. A few of my classmates had extensive experience working in clinics as an aide or a clerical person and their perceptions were extremely helpful. Most of us did not have as much. Nonetheless, common questions were, "how much will my CI help me?" and "will I be on my own with patients?"

CIs' responsibilities and expectations change depending on the student's level of progression in the professional program. For instance, for the first clinical internship, the level of expectations and the responsibilities provided to the DPT student are very narrow in scope. Most of the expectations and experiences

Table 8.2 Student requirements for clinical education

Health requirements	Certification/Background check requirements
Physical examination	CPR for health care providers
Drug test	Basic first aid
PPD	OSHA certification
T-dap	HIPAA certification
Flu shot	**Criminal background checks:**
Vaccination and/or titers for measles, mumps, rubella, and varicella	Child abuse clearance
	Elder abuse clearance
	FBI fingerprint clearance
	OIG clearance
	State background check

scheduled revolve around observation or the performance of very basic evaluation and intervention techniques. By the final clinical internship, CIs fully expect the student to be practicing at entry-level criteria (the skills utilized by novice licensed physical therapists). The DCE provides students with the standard expectations set by APTA or students in the first, second, and final years of the professional program. This document provided me with a strong understanding of my CI's expectations. During my orientation at each clinical site I found it helpful to review the APTA document with each CI at the start of my clinical. For example, my second clinical internship was at a skilled nursing and long-term care facility. According to published expectations, I was expected to handle 50% of my CI's caseload by the end of my time there. At the start of the clinical internship, my CI mentioned that her current full caseload was about ten patients per day. So, for me, I worked toward seeing five to six people per day, and sometimes could see more. It was helpful to have a number to plan for and work toward.

▶ Table 8.3 provides a breakdown of expected caseload requirements known as "rating scale anchors." Your CI will be familiar with these and the table outlines the requirements.

8.3.2 What is an In-Service?

An in-service is an educational presentation about a relevant topic that students are required to complete while in the clinic. Typically, the in-service is in the form of a 30- to 60-minute PowerPoint presentation about a topic of interest to the employees of the internship site. In many cases the subject and content are the responsibility of the student with CI input. I was required to prepare one for each clinical experience for my school. I had to submit proof of its completion to my DCE back at the university. Depending on the clinical site and length of the internship, students are typically required to provide one or two in-services. The CI will provide the site's in-service requirements to the student at orientation.

The audience for the in-service may vary. For two of my outpatient experiences, I presented to fellow physical therapists. For my second clinical experience, the one at a skilled nursing facility (SNF), I presented to a group of residents living at the facility. In-services are usually provided toward the end of the internship. With my classmates scattered throughout the United States for our clinical internships, we often reached out for each other via social media for ideas on what to do for in-services. I also found that some of the student DPT pages I followed on Facebook shared helpful ideas. I have included a list of my in-services in ▶ Table 8.4.

8.3.3 Additional Assignments

Depending on the type of clinical setting and your CI's expectations, additional assignments may be required of the interning student. For my first clinical, I was required to provide an in-service and a weekly critically appraised topic (CAT) on various topics and present it to the PT staff at weekly meetings. These CATs were a great way for myself and the team I was working

with to review and discuss recent research and incorporate the latest techniques into our plan of care with patients. A CAT is another great idea for an in-service idea. I have included a resource at the end of the chapter that outlines the steps to writing one.[7]

Table 8.3 Rating scale anchor definitions[6]

Rating scale anchor	Anchor definition	My goal for each clinical internship
Beginning performance	• A student who requires close clinical supervision 100% of the time managing patients, with constant monitoring and feedback, even for patients with simple conditions • Student does not carry a caseload	
Advanced beginner performance	A student who requires clinical supervision 75–90% of the time managing patients with simple conditions, and 100% of the time managing patient with complex conditions	Clinical 1
Intermediate performance	• A student who requires clinical supervision less than 50% of the time managing patients with simple conditions, and 75% of the time managing patients with complex conditions • Student is capable of maintaining 50% of a full-time physical therapist's caseload	Clinical 2
Advanced intermediate performance	• A student who requires clinical supervision less than 25% of the time managing new patients or patient with complex conditions and is independent managing patients with simple conditions • The student is capable of maintain 75% of a full-time physical therapist's caseload	Clinical 3
Entry-level performance	• A student who is capable of functioning without guidance or clinical supervision managing patients with simple or complex conditions • The student is capable of maintaining 100% of a full-time physical therapist's caseload in a cost-effective manner	Clinical 4
Beyond entry-level performance	A student who is capable of functioning without clinical supervision or guidance in managing patients with simple or highly complex conditions, and can function in unfamiliar or ambiguous situations	

Table 8.4 Examples of in-services

	Clinical I	Clinical II	Clinical III	Clinical IV
Setting	Outpatient orthopedic	Skilled nursing facility	Outpatient orthopedic	Outpatient women's health care
Project type	PowerPoint presentation/CAT	Presentation and pamphlet	PowerPoint presentation/CAT	PowerPoint presentation/CAT
Topic	ODI and patient outcomes	What is CVA?	Gait speed as a predictor of adverse outcomes in older individuals	The effects of hormones on pain and plan of care
Audience	Staff/PTs/PTAs/PT aide	Residents/patient with stroke/CVA	PT/OT/management	PT/OT/SLP/management

Abbreviations: CAT, critically appraised topic; CVA, cerebral vascular accident; ODI, Oswestry disability index.

Critically Appraised Topic: A standardized summary of research evidence organized around a clinical question, aimed at providing both a critique of the research and a statement of the critical relevance of the results.[7]

For my final clinical internship, I was required to perform two in-services. I could choose the topic of my first in-service but my CI provided me with guidelines for the second. My choices were to perform a case study on a patient I was treating, assist my CI in a lecture to the first year DPT interning students (there were four of us at this particular clinic site, all from different programs), or compose an informational brochure for patients regarding PT-related care relevant to this clinical site. I chose to assist my CI with a presentation on *Women's Health and Physical Therapy* to first-year DPT students.

Several of my classmates were given required-to-complete daily or weekly assignments related to the setting in which they were practicing. For instance, one student was provided with two clinical diagnoses daily. Overnight, she was expected to develop an evaluation algorithm for both diagnoses in flowchart format and provide those, first thing in the morning, to her CI. Another student was given a number of clinical topics during the course of his internship and he was required to develop an annotated bibliography for each topic. These assignments can seem tedious at times, especially when working so hard during the day, arriving home exhausted and then working at the computer for another hour or two. My advice is to always keep open communication lines with the CI. If the student feels underutilized or feels completely overwhelmed, the relationship with the CI should be one which permits honest communication.

8.3.4 CI Expectations

I found my CIs had varying styles of practice and personalities. This made my experience very interesting and enhanced my learning experience, but I found it challenging to adapt to their different styles of teaching. Some of my CIs were hovering nearby during all my evaluations and interventions. Initially, I felt I was under a microscope—constantly being assessed and fearful of making a mistake. Eventually, I developed a level of

acceptance for this method of oversight. On another internship my CI preferred to allow me to practice independently and trusted me to come to her with questions. That level of freedom also took me quite a long time to accept. Feedback techniques also vary among CIs. Some prefer to provide ongoing feedback—often in front of the patient—while others scheduled formal feedback sessions, typically at the end of each day. Even with this variability I always felt that if I needed assistance or counsel, my CI was near and always available. I never felt alone.

I found the most difficult aspect of the clinical internship experience was the development of my clinical decision making. I once read that physical therapists make over 3,000 clinical decisions in any given 8-hour work day. Do I provide this patient with a walker or cane? Is this patient safe to get out of bed with an ejection fraction of 27% and a hemoglobin of 7.2 g? Is the wound I am examining venous or arterial in origin? Does this person, in order to treat him safely, need an MRI? There are so many variables to consider in each clinical scenario. There is no method of incorporating this variability into the classroom setting. I certainly found that making the correct clinical decision and having faith in that decision was most challenging to me.

As my CIs and I developed and matured our professional relationships I felt that my CIs' level of trust in me to be safe and do no harm to my patients grew. Over time, and as I proved myself to be a safe, effective, and evidence-based therapist, they encouraged me to mentally experiment, consider options, expand the scope of my practice, and take initiative. They told me that clinical education is a time to build my clinical expertise (experience) and to lean on what I have learned but to be open to other networks, evidence, colleagues' opinions, and resources. Through my four clinical internship experiences I was never belittled by my CIs. I did receive criticisms and suggestions and learned to take them openly and not defensively. I learned by observing the relationship of another student and his CI that the two worst things that can befall a student intern are failure to maintain safety of the patient and becoming defensive when suggestions are offered by the CI. These two errors are nearly unforgivable. I received my share of criticisms but I realize that my CIs wanted me to be a good therapist. We learn more by our difficulties than our successes. By no means did any CI expect me to know everything as a student. In cases where a patient was more clinically complex, my CIs were supportive and helped me with ideas and solutions I may not have thought of on my own. I often found myself asking my CI questions, and reaching out to professors and fellow students throughout each internship for advice. I learned the utmost importance of having colleagues and mentors. Medicine is too much for one person. There must be a team. Some great resources that I used to ask questions and problem-solve were my classes' social media page on Facebook and PT-related content on Twitter. APTA also has a clinical summaries reference site that includes information and recommended plan of care for various diagnoses and conditions.[8]

8.3.5 CI–Student Relationship

As I now begin my full-time practice (I graduated from my DPT program last year), I realize I am most certainly a mix of all my CIs. I have taken with me all their best advice and pointers, leaving behind anything that didn't work well for me. All DPT students eventually develop his or her own clinical philosophy and best practices we feel work best for us and our patients. Part of this is knowledge garnered through well-developed research studies and part of it is through experience. The CI may have a different treatment philosophy or practice algorithms than what the student has been taught or developed. This isn't a bad thing. I tried to use my time to consider differences, try out new things or recommendations, and see what felt best for me.

As an example, I had a CI who practiced based heavily on the McKenzie theory of low back pain of evaluation and intervention. My educational program did not have a heavy focus on this method and I felt it was a bit foreign to me. My CI encouraged me to treat my patients however I felt best, but did encourage me to focus on learning as much as I could about this particular method. She provided me with a textbook and numerous articles. Lastly, she scheduled me to observe a McKenzie-certified therapist as he evaluated and treated a patient. I now use this technique often with my patients.

One of the greatest challenges of being a student was having to constantly report back to someone, especially as I become more comfortable toward the end of each clinical experience. I empathized with this request; I was working under my CI's professional license and she needed to know what I was doing. I often struggled with the desire to want to practice independently and not have to answer to anyone. There were many times where I wished my CIs were not looking over my shoulder, but then many times I was happy they were. I now realize that even though I was "filled to the brim" with research knowledge I was still a novice with regard to experience. I needed to be watched.

One of my CIs told me that I am excellent at accepting constructive criticism. I truly felt that I needed to use my clinical education experiences to learn, understand what I could work on, and professionally grow. Was it easy to ask for and reflect on these criticisms and constantly receive feedback? It wasn't for me. Sometimes it was hard to hear or difficult and exhausting to go home and think about what I could do to be better the next day. Feedback, positive and negative, has been instrumental in my becoming a good PT. I now think of each of my CIs as dear friends and amazing colleagues. They took time from their daily lives, their work, and their families to make me a better person and therapist. I am truly thankful for the time and patience they gave me to grow.

8.4 Evaluation and Assessment of Student Performance in the Clinic

8.4.1 The Clinical Performance Instrument

The Clinical Performance Instrument (CPI) is an electronic-based program used to assess the student's performance in the clinic. In the classroom the faculty utilize a variety of assessment tools to determine competency: quizzes, exams, essays, papers, presentations, and competencies. In the clinic, the CPI is the definitive tool. The student and the CI complete the CPI assessment online. Students are required to complete this two times—once at mid-term and then again at the scheduled end of the internship. Reviewing the content in the CPI is a formal sit-down meeting in person between the student and CI. The midterm CPI provides the students with a progress report and indicates where the student is performing at or above expectation and where the student needs to improve. The reason why the student also completes the CPI is to encourage the student to reflect upon his or her progress to date. The ability to reflect is a tenet of self-improvement.

For my first internship, I found completing the CPI to be monotonous and time consuming. It was my first time, and I wasn't sure what to write about or how to rate myself. An important lesson I learned from my first clinical was to keep lines of communication open with my CI regarding my performance throughout the clinical. Ask for feedback. Ask about what you are doing well and what you can work on. For my first midterm CPI, I remember feeling a little discouraged after meeting with my CI. I wasn't doing poorly. As a matter of fact, he said I was right on track for where I needed to be and I received positive input. What I wasn't prepared for was the constructive criticism. I am naturally sensitive, but I was under the impression that everything was going very well based on concurrent feedback received from patients, my CI, and staff. I am amazed at my naïveté now that I can reflect on my first internship. Who in the first clinical internship cannot improve? Of course, there were about a million things I could improve upon! I was new to the profession and only had only one year completed in the professional program. The most important recommendation he made for my remaining time in that clinic was to be more confident and take the lead with more patients. At the time, I was unsure of what was expected and how much I should do. Also, I was nervous to take the lead. I knew where to focus for the remainder of my time though, and concentrated on stepping up my game. For the final CPI, I was where I needed to be, and was thankful for the mid-term feedback I received.

How Do I Use The CPI?

There is a free online training course provided through APTA that outlines details and instructions on how use and interpret the CPI. I have provided a link to a document with instructions at the end of the chapter.[9] There are 18 performance criteria that describe important aspects of professional practice for an entry-level physical therapist. These criteria are grouped into two aspects of practice: professional practice (items 1–6) and patient management (items 7–18). Once students are registered by the DCE in the CPI, I encourage students to log in and review these performance criteria and their descriptions prior to the internship. The CPI lists a number of performance criteria which the student is expected to meet. The criteria are from the cognitive, psychomotor, and affective domains (see ▶ Table 8.5).

When students log into the CPI, they will find examples of items that fall under each category to help with self-appraisal. Below is an example of the rating scale used for each performance criteria. At the start of each internship, students should know where they need to be by the end of the internship based on the rating scale anchors (see ▶ Table 8.3).[6] At the mid-term review, if I felt I was not where I needed to be, I placed the marker half way between the appropriate anchors, to demonstrate that I was still working toward my goal. Even if I felt I had already reached my expected level for certain categories, my tendency was to rate myself lower, allowing myself room and space for improvement in all areas after receiving my CI's feedback (see ▶ Fig. 8.1).

Additionally, after my first clinical, I found it helpful to write specific examples for each CPI performance criteria down as they occurred in the clinic. I kept a notebook detailing encounters with patients, so that I was not struggling for specific instances when I sat down to complete my midterm and final CPI assessment. ▶ Table 8.6 includes examples I used to describe my progress toward fulfilling the performance criteria in the CPI. Students are often asked by the CI or center coordinator for clinical education to complete the CPI as a vehicle for self-reflection. This table provides examples of student reflections as prompted by the performance criteria.

Weekly Planning Forms

A great way to avoid any surprises regarding performance in the clinic during CPI reviews is to use weekly planning forms. My DCE encouraged the students to incorporate this form into planning meetings with the CI to assist with maintaining open lines of communication. Two of my sites required the use of planning forms. The format of the form may vary. Even if it is not required to utilize one, I urge all DPT students on internship to do so. Students and the CI can create one or they may use the one outlined in ▶ Fig. 8.1. After the planning discussion, both parties, the CI and student, should date and sign it (see ▶ Fig. 8.2).

Table 8.5 Performance criteria for CPI

Patient management	Professional practice
Clinical reasoning, screening, examination, evaluation, diagnosis and prognosis, plan of care, procedural interventions, educational interventions, documentation, outcomes assessment, financial resources, direction and supervision of personnel	Safety, professional behavior, accountability, communication, cultural competence, professional development

Table 8.6 Examples for performance criteria in CPI

Performance criteria	CPI content/example
Cultural competence	*I have tried to be sensitive to Mrs. Smith's cultural beliefs, ensuring that all her treatments take place in a private room or with curtains drawn to be respectful of cultural beliefs regarding privacy.*
Plan of care	*I consistently check in with patients to assess their progress with exercise I provide in the clinic and progress their plan of care accordingly. For example, I have recently incorporated closed-chain activity to Mr. Thompson's plan of care, as he demonstrates improved stability, strength and endurance.*

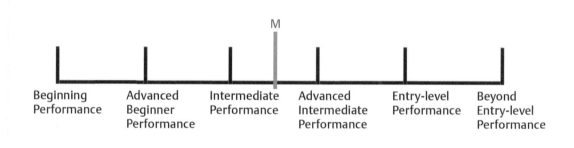

Fig. 8.1 Rating scale for CPI.[6] The rating scale was designed to reflect a continuum of performance ranging from beginning performance to "beyond entry-level performance." Student performance should be described in relation to one or more of the six anchors. For example, consider the rating on a selected performance criterion (*M*). (Reprinted from "Physical Therapist Clinical Performance Instrument: Version 2006," with permission of the American Physical Therapy Association. Copyright 2006 American Physical Therapy Association.)

Weekly Planning Form Student Name: _____ CI Name: _____ Week: _____	
Three things that went well this week:	1. _____ 2. _____ 3. _____
Three things you would like to improve on:	1. _____ 2. _____ 3. _____
Three Goals for Next week:	1. _____ 2. _____ 3. _____

Fig. 8.2 Example of a weekly planning form.

Each week I set behavioral and clinical goals for myself and asked my CI to review them, and offer comments based on his or her experience. Often the CI amended the goals and, more often than not, the amendments were appropriate. Each week, prior to reviewing my new weekly goals, we discussed the previous week's goals and whether or not I accomplished them. If I did not, we discussed possible reasons for the lack of compliance. ▶ Table 8.7 provides examples of goals I set for myself on my final clinical as a third-year DPT student. The internship was in a women's health and lymphedema setting. CIs often ask interning students to write specific learning goals for each week of the clinical internship. This beneficial activity prompts reflection, provides discussion points with the CI, forces the student to practice goal writing, and re-enforces the need to transition from a spoon-fed to self-directed learner.

Table 8.7 Examples of goals for clinical education

Week	Goal
1	Become familiar with EMR system and reduce use of abbreviations and spelling errors when writing notes
2	Practice myofascial release technique to head and neck with CI to improve technique and body mechanics for use with current patient caseload with h/o cervical cancer presenting with cervical spine impairments
4	Perform full initial evaluation on pregnant female, with proper adjustments made for positioning for physical exam
8	Have 50% of in-service draft complete to show to CI for input and feedback

Abbreviations: CI, clinical instructor; EMR, electronic medical record.

8.5 A Student's Perspective: Challenges and Surprises

8.5.1 My First Clinical Education Experience

Below is a short narrative of my first clinical experience. I decided to include the narrative in this chapter because I feel a first-person account of a first clinical experience may be beneficial to the novice DPT student. I had little in the way of practical knowledge of my first clinical experience and I feel, in retrospect, I would have benefited by such a narrative.

I was very nervous for my first clinic day. My clinic was in the middle of Philadelphia in an area that had a questionable safety reputation. Personal safety is something I would recommend thinking about when identifying potential clinical sites. Some areas of larger cities can be intimidating, especially for those students not familiar with big-city life. I grew up in New York City, so this was the least of my worries. My concerns were primarily *What if my CI does not like me? What if I do not like my CI? What if we do not see eye-to-eye on certain things? What if I hurt someone? Why did I ever think I could do this?* Pretty much any confidence I had before this seemed to disappear as soon as I stepped through the door.

The clinic was a located in a corner building at the intersection of two busy streets. The clinic was owned and operated by a national chain (something we are seeing much more of in health care) and was operated by a "site manager" who reported to corporate. The neighborhood was well-kept but obviously quite poor. Storefronts advertising "Checks Cashed" and "Cash Paid for Gold" were omnipresent. A small grocery store was next to the clinic which proved opportunistic for me to purchase lunch.

On entering, the clinic was very small. My most recent ICE was at a 700-bed tertiary care hospital with a therapy office the size of a small stadium. By the front door were three waiting-room chairs. A receptionist sat behind a small counter typing into her computer. I later learned she doubled as the physical therapy aide. Two therapists hustled about treating patients. I soon learned that one was the site manager and the other a newly hired DPT from a neighboring program. The site manager was my CI.

On my first day, I met the staff and was told to place my purse in a small desk in the therapy office. I was given a small desk with a laptop. I would have preferred that the new therapist was my CI; he seemed as nervous as me. The site manager appeared intimidating. He was all motion—texting, answering telephone calls and never standing still. I learned that his job—treating a full case load, being responsible for the operations of the clinic, and attempting to meet corporate's revenue and expense goals—was not my career path. My CI, Rob, toured the facility with me. Rob then sat me at my desk and directed me to a corporate URL with a list of mandatory competencies I was required to complete prior to seeing patients. There were perhaps 15 lengthy modules. Completion of the modules took perhaps three hours and encompassed such things as patient safety, confidentiality, infection control, safe patient handling, documentation, corporate policies, and the use of the electronic medical record. Most of the content, save for the corporate

policies, were familiar to me due to similar training I received during my first year in the DPT program. I completed some initial trainings on the first day for safety, HIPAA, and company policies. At 11 o'clock my CI sat with me to review the operating processes and work flow in the clinic. He also asked me about my previous clinical experience. He seemed a bit taken aback that all my previous clinical experiences were observational; I had never worked as an aide. Later I learned that CIs like students with experience. Experienced students require less teaching and in high-volume clinics such as this one, the CI teaching students takes much time away from patient care.

One of the most important things he asked me was how I learn best. Historically, I learn best by first watching and then practicing. We had an understanding and this discussion helped set the path to my success during this clinical. For example, during the first week I focused on getting comfortable taking patient history. By then it was lunch and we walked next door to the grocery store for lunch. The grocery store, owned by a tiny but energetic woman named Maria, was a bodega. Maria, from Guatemala, daily made absolutely the best food. Her corn tortillas and salsa verde were the best I have ever had. I must have gained five pounds on the internship. Now, a year later, my husband and I, for a treat, visit the bodega for lunch.

The rest of my first day was spent observing my CI. He was an amazing history taker. For all his energy and scatteredness when we first met, when in the presence of a patient, he was calm, empathetic, caring, and able to garner an incredible amount of information from the patient. A year later I still try to emulate his technique. At the end of the first day Rob announced to me that I would be assigned my first patient the next morning. The patient, a gentleman named Bernardo, had a diagnosis of a recently fractured distal fibula (ankle fracture). Rob asked me to develop an evaluation algorithm for the next morning. Rob asked me to arrive at the clinic by 7:30 a.m. and we would review the algorithm prior to Bernardo's scheduled arrival at 8:00 a.m. Rob would sit with me during the initial evaluation but would primarily observe. By the second day I felt comfortable trying by myself. I appreciated that my CI respected my learning style and I found it helpful to have this conversation with each of my CIs at the start of each clinical.

To this point, I had completed the basics and foundation we need as PTs (anatomy, physiology, and neuroscience) and knew how to be safe. However, I had a long way to go. When my CI asked me to perform McMurray's special test the next morning on Bernardo I didn't have a clue. The limited knowledge of DPT students, especially on the first and second internships, is always problematic for the DPT student and the CI. This led to an important discussion reviewing what courses I had so far, but also what I felt my strengths and weaknesses were. I told my CI that I could measure range of motion and perform manual muscle testing, but had not had any musculoskeletal coursework yet. We joked about my lack of exposure to musculoskeletal skills in a fast-paced outpatient orthopedic setting, but he also took time to teach me some skills throughout my time, and I was glad that he and I had this honest discussion.

Now, don't get me wrong, my CI was great, but the first few weeks, I felt intimidated by him. He would constantly quiz me and put me on the spot, with questions ranging from, "what are contraindications for ultra-sound?" to "give me an eccentric exercise for the hamstrings." All fair game, but at the time I was already a nervous wreck and just trying to keep my head above water. He also mentioned on my first day, that I would be expected to put together a weekly CAT and present it to the staff in the weekly staff meeting. In addition, I would be required to perform an in-service at the end of the clinical. My first thought: "lucky me." My second: "what exactly is an in-service?" I may have gone home and cried.

Midway through my clinical, I realized two things. First, my CI was just trying to help me boost my confidence. He challenged me to try new things and think through difficult questions. He showed me not to doubt myself and realize that yes, I had a long way to go, but knew more than I gave myself credit for. Second, I realized that I too could ask questions. He understood, as I do now, that the joy is in the process and not the outcome. A great therapist is not judged on her outcomes; there are too many variables in medicine to have a perfect score. There will be failures. But we must have a perfect score in self-improvement—being a self-directed learner. Success is in the preparation, not in the outcome.

This was my time to learn as much as I could and get different perspectives. If I wasn't sure of something, I started to ask. I asked my CI, the other therapist, and my patients tons of questions. One of the best things about being a student PT is that you get to practice and get your hands wet, but you're exposed to new therapists, colleagues, and patients in different settings, and all with different thoughts, skills, and experiences. Clinical education was an opportunity for me to listen, absorb, and take this shared knowledge with me to begin my career.

The other therapist, Albert, the new graduate, was a nervous Nellie. He was always asking Rob questions and, to me, seemed afraid to even use the bathroom. He worked incredibly hard, was kind to everyone, and always had his nose in a book. Rob constantly praised him to me telling me that one day he was going to be an expert clinician. I thought to myself that if nervous Albert was on the pathway to success and I, with two years less education than he, was performing okay in this clinic, perhaps there was hope for me.

This clinical flew by. I loved my patients. There is nothing better than watching your patients improve, reach their goals, and then get a thank you for your help. *My* help! This was the very first time I had patients directly asking me questions regarding their care and thanking me when they reached a milestone. I treated patients with varying diagnoses including rotator cuff tears, back pain, headaches, knee and hip pain, ankle sprains, and more. I enjoyed the variety of patients I worked with in all my outpatient experiences. As my confidence grew and I was able to safely demonstrate my clinical skills, Rob began to withdraw from me and allow me to practice with a bit more independence. I greatly appreciated his confidence. He was never the most verbal in his praising but I could tell he was pleased with my performance.

By the end, I was excited for my second year of PT school to increase my knowledge and skills, apply it to what I learned in the clinic, and learn the answers to questions I was still uncertain of during my first clinical.

8.5.2 Inpatient Versus Outpatient Experience

Prior to the DPT program I had only been in a hospital once: to visit my sister who had had an appendectomy. All my observation hours and volunteer work for PT school were in outpatient settings, and I was very nervous to be in an inpatient setting. The primary reason for my anxiety was the acuity of the patients.

After my first clinical internship in the small outpatient clinic where I treated relatively healthy persons with primarily impairments of the musculoskeletal system I was assigned for my second (and longer) 12-week internship in a SNF. An SNF (the abbreviation is often pronounced "sniff") is an inpatient facility which provides lower-level rehabilitation services to very sick persons. The patients are too sick to go home but too well to be in the acute care hospital. Patients in the SNF typically receive two hours of physical therapy per day along with skilled services from nursing, occupational therapy, and speech pathology. Patients typically spend 2 weeks or so in the SNF and then are sufficiently well to go home. Though the patients were not as sick as those in an acute care hospital these people were still in a hospital setting. In reviewing the facility's website and the CSIF I learned that the hospital's population was predominantly geriatric. This setting was completely new and different than my first clinical. On a call with my new CI the week before starting, she gave me a brief overview of what to expect and mentioned that I would follow a shorter schedule my first couple of days due to a bout of Norovirus sweeping through the facility. I flashed back to pathophysiology trying to remember what it was and came up blank. Maybe we didn't cover it, but more than likely we did and my brain was still organizing and sorting all the information it absorbed from my second year. I quickly learned what it was, and quickly realized that I would soon be researching a number of terms and diagnoses.

On the phone with my CI I shared the type of experiences I had so far, and asked if there was anything she recommended I prepare or review before beginning. She provided me with very helpful information including some of the comorbidities and diagnoses of her current caseload. For example, I would be working with individuals with schizophrenia, encephalopathy, stroke/cerebral vascular accident, dementia, chronic obstructive pulmonary disease, emphysema, amputees, wounds, and diabetes. Wow! Much different than sprains, strains and fractures. I spent some time reviewing these conditions and my notes from class before starting.

Whether in a hospital or SNF, the daily flow of patients is much different compared to outpatient settings. Personally, I am very organized and like to have a set schedule. This was challenging to achieve in the SNF and, as I later learned, in my first professional job, in an acute care hospital. In the outpatient arena, patients schedule their appointments and arrive on time (mostly!) ready to be seen. In the inpatient arena, there are so many variables, which makes scheduling therapy visits challenging. On any given day when I would try to see patients for physical therapy, patients could be eating a meal, receiving another treatment, be leaving for a medical appointment, have family or friends visiting, be asleep or lethargic, or be having a reaction to a medication that would affect their performance in physical therapy. The skilled facility in which I interned was housed in a life-care community and the patients in the skilled nursing unit were free to enjoy many of the events organized for the residents of the life-care community. The SNF's philosophy was to have therapy work around the patient's schedules. With this unique arrangement, there were times when the patient was enjoying the life-care activities. My most favorite reasons for having to continuously rearrange my day were because my patients were in music class, playing in the weekly volleyball tournament (wheelchair volleyball), playing cards, playing Bingo, getting their hair done because the stylist or barber was in that day, or had bell-choir practice. If you learn nothing from this chapter, please learn this: 1. Do **not** interfere with bell choir practice. 2. Attend the choir's final performance. You and your patient will smile.

Interning in a SNF was a huge adjustment for me. Some of these patients were very ill with many functional mobility limitations which resulted in major physical and emotional challenges. Many of the patients I treated were at high fall risk due to their primary diagnoses. My treatment goals for them were relatively low level, especially considering the population I treated during my first outpatient internship. On my first clinical I was trying to prepare a long-distance runner with Achilles tendonitis for the Philadelphia Marathon and a baseball player with a muscle strain to rehabilitate his shoulder in time for spring practice. Now, I was helping someone walk safely ten feet and not fall. As a therapist, I have learned that I cannot judge individual's treatment goals. Every goal is equally important. Every goal deserves my best effort. Having been in the outpatient clinic and working with high-level athletes I initially felt that I would be bored and perhaps not challenged by teaching an elderly person with a neurodegenerative disease how to transfer into the bathtub safely. This was my naiveté and ignorance. What challenges I encountered in the SNF and what joy I felt when I helped my patient accomplish his goals. A patient told me: "I would have never been able to return home to my dear wife if not for your efforts. Thank you." There were tears in his eyes. This was a humbling experience.

One thing that doesn't change, no matter what setting you are in, is to treat each patient as an individual, rather than a person with a diagnosis. What worked best for me was to listen to what my patients were saying. If their goal was to be able to sit up to visit with their grandchildren for two hours, then that's what we worked on. If their goal was to be able to transfer in and out of their son's car to attend their niece's birthday party next month, then that's what we worked on. Maybe the goal was to be able to wheel themselves to their friend's room down the hall for a visit. Many of the people I worked with went from being completely independent to completely dependent for daily activities and basic functional mobility. This is a very important concept to realize prior to interning in a skilled facility or acute medical rehabilitation hospital. As PTs we can greatly impact these individuals' quality of life.

8.5.3 What Surprised Me about Clinical Education

One of my biggest concerns for each internship was always whether I could handle what was expected of me. The biggest surprise for me was how quickly my CIs permitted me to treat my patients autonomously. I'll share a vivid memory from my third internship, which was in an outpatient orthopedic setting. My third internship was after my second year of the DPT program. Though I had an outpatient internship experience already I was now a full year away from that experience. My hope was to ease back in to the outpatient arena and maybe spend a couple days shadowing and asking questions. This was not the case. On my second day, when my CI asked me if I wanted her in the

room for my first evaluation that day, I am sure my face dropped. I felt totally panicked. Could I do it? Yes. Did I do it? Yes. Did it go smoothly? No way. Did my patient know it didn't go smoothly? Probably not.

When I say it didn't go smoothly, I mean that I felt disorganized and inefficient. We are introduced to so many tools in the classroom and I often found that by the time I would get the patient's history, there wasn't much time for a full physical and functional exam. I walked out of the room to get something, and my CI was waiting for me. I was nervous to tell her I didn't think it was going well. She probably saw I was overwhelmed and gave me a great piece of advice. She told me that if I am ever feeling confused or flustered during the initial evaluation, just excuse myself from the room and say that I need to grab something. Just go back in with a pillow, towel or goniometer when you're ready, your patient will not know. Take a step out of the room, take some deep breaths, clear your head, and ask yourself, "what am I looking at?" Then pick 1 or 2 things to go back in to look at and move on. Sometimes, you won't have all the answers on the initial exam, especially as a student, when everything is new. A small success breeds confidence. Confidence enables clear and organized thinking.

Therefore, do not be surprised when your CI wants you to jump in and start treating on your own sooner rather than later. Honestly, it's a great way to learn and you become more comfortable as the weeks go by. During my third clinical, I carried the following cheat sheet with me to be more efficient with initial evaluations. Please use this if you find it helpful in directing the flow of things.

Initial Evaluation: Key Points for History Taking ⓘ

Chief complaint? Right side neck pain.
  Mechanism of injury? MVA. Patient was driving and was hit by another car.
  Onset of injury? 3 months ago.
  Overall, is pain better/worse/the same? Worse.
  Description of pain? Achy/throbbing.
  Constant or intermittent? Intermittent.
  Radiating symptoms? Yes. Numbness and tingling to second and third digit that is intermittent.
  Pain Pattern—when is your pain better/worse? Better in a.m., worse in p.m.
  Red Flags? (Accident? Night sweats/weight loss?) No.
  Aggravating factors? Driving, sitting at desk.
  Relieving factors? Heating pad. Lying down.
  Goals? No pain. Get back to lifting weights.

8.5.4 What I Would Do Differently

The year since graduation has offered me the opportunity to reflect upon my years in the DPT program and, as any good professional does, I asked myself to list what I did well and what I could improve upon. First of all, I would be more confident in my abilities. Everything was new to me as a student. I too often questioned my worthiness to be a physical therapist followed by examining the situation literally and realizing that my problem was simply lack of knowledge which could be remediated through studying and learning. I wish I had more confidence to trust my instincts regarding my clinical decision making. Rather, I doubted my abilities or ran to my CIs for assistance. Too often my lack of confidence resulted in anxiety and near panic. I wish I had the ability, as I do now, to take a few deep breaths, relax, and have faith in myself that the correct answer will come to me.

During my final clinical, my CI often asked if there was anything that I wanted to review or practice with her. If I chose an intervention and wasn't sure of my technique, I would demonstrate on her and she would give me feedback. For example, my CI used myofascial release often for certain patients, and I hadn't tried to use it to this point. She demonstrated on me so I could better understand how the technique should feel, and then I would practice on her, adjusting based on her input.

Looking back, I should have asked all my CIs for additional hands-on practice, feedback, and recommendations on other techniques. Seeking their expert opinions and skills would have improved my confidence and my outcomes with patients. One of the most important things to remember as students on clinical internships is that this is the time to learn. We all must transition from spoon-fed learners to self-directed learners. From kindergarten to the final clinical internship, others are providing us content knowledge and feedback. The day the final clinical internship ends is the day students stop receiving content knowledge from others and the responsibility for education falls to the student. Use this last opportunity to be taught wisely and often. Take advantage of the skills possessed by your CI. Do not rush through this opportunity.

My clinical education strongly shaped how and where I would like to practice. I remember sitting in classes and labs, practicing guarding or walking with fellow classmates pretending they had impairments. My first time working with someone who had a real impairment was completely different and eye opening. I learned so much in the classroom, but the hands-on experience with patients is where most of my learning occurred. Clinical education is the best time to learn, ask questions, practice, and figure out where your strengths, weaknesses, and passions are in our field.

8.6 Review Questions

1. The faculty member who directs the clinical internship experiences for the doctor of physical therapy students is known by which title?
   a) Director of clinical education.
   b) Clinical coordinator of clinical education.
   c) Chair of the doctor of physical therapy program.
   d) Clinical instructor.
2. The clinic employee who supervises the student during the clinical internship is known by which title?
   a) Director of clinical education.
   b) Clinical coordinator of clinical education.
   c) Chair of the doctor of physical therapy program.
   d) Clinical instructor.
3. The clinic employee who supervises all the clinical instructors is known by which title?
   a) Director of clinical education.
   b) Clinic coordinator of clinical education.

   c) Chair of the doctor of physical therapy program.
   d) Clinical instructor.
4. The Clinical Performance Instrument used to assess physical therapy student performance on clinical internship was developed by which entity?
   a) Medicare.
   b) The American Physical Therapy Association.
   c) The American Medical Association.
   d) Each individual clinic has its own form.
5. The Clinical Performance Instrument has how many performance criteria?
   a) 12.
   b) 14.
   c) 18.
   d) 20.

8.7 Review Answers

1. The faculty member who directs the clinical internship experiences for the doctor of physical therapy students is known by which title?
   a. Director of clinical education.
2. The clinic employee who supervises the student during the clinical internship is known by which title?
   d. Clinical instructor.
3. The clinic employee who supervises all the clinical instructors is known by which title?
   b. Clinic coordinator of clinical education.
4. The Clinical Performance Instrument used to assess physical therapy student performance on clinical internship was developed by which entity?
   b. The American Physical Therapy Association.
5. The Clinical Performance Instrument has how many performance criteria?
   c. 18.

References

[1] APTA. Physical therapist (PT) education overview. Available at: http://www. apta.org/PTEducation/Overview/. Updated October 2015. Accessed January 8, 2017

[2] Model Position Description for the ACCE/DCE. PT program. Available at: http://www.apta.org/ModelPositionDescription/ACCE/DCE/PT/. Updated November 6, 2012. Accessed January 25, 2017

[3] Reference Manual for Center Coordinators of Clinical Education. Available at: https://www.rehabmedicine.umn.edu/sites/rehabmedicine.umn.edu/files/coordinatorreference.pdf. Published 2001. Accessed January 25, 2017

[4] Clinical Education Handbook for Clinical Faculty Doctor of Physical Therapy Program. Available at: https://cph.temple.edu/sites/chpsw/files/imce_uploads/ClinicalFacultyHandbook_2016.pdf. Updated June 2016. Accessed January 27, 2017

[5] Clinical Site Information Form (CSIF) Web. http://www.apta.org/CSIF/. Updated 9/15/2016. Accessed January 25, 2017

[6] Physical Therapist Clinical Performance Instrument for Students. Available at: http://www.med.wisc.edu/files/smph/docs/departments/physicaltherapy/clinicaleducation/dpt_acedemic_curr_cpi_1.pdf. Published June 2006. Accessed January 26, 2017

[7] Sadigh G, Parker R, Kelly AM, Cronin P. How to write a critically appraised topic (CAT). Acad Radiol. 2012; 19(7):872–888

[8] Clinical summaries APTA. Available at: http://ptnow.org/clinical-summaries. Published 2016. Accessed January 26, 2017

[9] PT CPI Web instructions for a student. Available at: http://www.academicsoftwareplus.com/files/PT%20CPI%20Web%202.0%20Instructions%20for%20Student.pdf. Updated January 21, 2014. Accessed January 26, 2017

9 Resources for Career Development

Laurita M. Hack

Keywords: Advocacy, American Physical Therapy Association, American Physical Therapy Association Code of Ethics, clinical decision making, clinical expertise, clinical practice guidelines, clinical reasoning, expertise model, fellowship, licensure, patient values, physical therapist, physical therapy, residency, specialization

Chapter Outline

1. Introduction
   a) Evidence-Based Practice
   b) Expertise Model
2. Improving Competence in Patient Care
   a) Career Development
   b) Continued Competence
3. Practice Development
   a) Patient Circumstances
   b) Practice Administration
   c) Advocacy
4. Responsibility to Society
   a) Professional Obligations to Patients and Clients
   b) Professional Obligations to Society
5. Conclusion

"The American Physical Therapy Association (APTA) is your professional association.

Professional associations consist of groups of people from the same profession who gather together electronically, in person, via common documents, and through organized activities to enhance the profession as a whole and the members individually. Doctor of Physical Therapy faculty are always working toward transitioning students from being spoon-fed learners to self-directed learners. Membership in APTA is a wonderful first step to toward this goal.

"Leaders and members of professional associations are student-friendly and want to mentor incoming physical therapists. Who better to mentor you about physical therapy than the organization leaders who altruistically donate their time to the association?

"Beyond networking opportunities and learning more about a career field, students can also benefit from these aspects of professional associations:

1. Professional opportunities. Professional associations often have listservs where employees from companies looking to hire post open jobs. These listservs are a starting point and students can be confident that the posted jobs are credible.
2. Conferences. Students can attend association-sponsored conferences at a discounted rate and hear from experts. APTA hosts multiple conferences yearly. These conferences often contain educational presentations and workshops, networking events, vendors displaying the newest technology, and opportunities to develop and practice professional behaviors. Potential employers are often impressed by the professional motivation of the conference attendee.

3. Information dissemination. Membership will bring important information that will be available to the student through the association website and various publications. Students will receive information about research and innovative clinical practices, administrative and legal updates, emerging technology, certifications, fellowships and residencies, position papers, and updated and proposed business practices. APTA membership also brings to the student various search engines to aid in research, systematic reviews, literature searches, and general updates.
4. Codes of ethics. Within the first days of entering a professional program students are taught that credibility and trustworthiness are essential professional behaviors. Students, for any number of reasons, must understand and practice the APTA Code of Ethics in order to know what is considered best practice and what is expected behavior in our profession.
5. Updates on policies. One piece of legislation can impact a profession. A section of the APTA website is devoted to updating members about these changes.
6. Advocacy. APTA leads advocacy efforts for the profession and for its professionals. APTA keeps members notified of all advocacy efforts."

—Emmanuel Esposito, San Antonio, TX

9.1 Introduction

Becoming a physical therapist means entering a profession and assuming the responsibilities and obligations that members of a profession have to their patients and to society. These responsibilities and obligations occur at two levels. First, every physical therapist must put the needs and welfare of his or her patients first. Our patients must be able to trust that the physical therapists they seek out for care have the knowledge, skills, and behaviors needed for that care.[1] Second, the profession of physical therapy has an obligation to improve the welfare of society.[2]

All of us strive, or should strive, toward being the best we can be. But, how do we figure out how to do that? There are two well-established frameworks that we can use to help answer this question. One is the evidence based practice framework and the other is the model of development of expertise in physical therapy.

9.1.1 Evidence-Based Practice

Much has been written about an approach to practice called evidence-based practice.It was developed and is widely accepted on the premise that practitioners need efficient and effective ways to continually improve their competence. Evidence-based practice is defined as the integration of
- Our own well-developed *clinical expertise.*
- An understanding of and a value for each *patient's own values.*

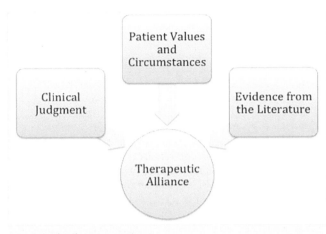

Fig. 9.1 The therapeutic alliance.

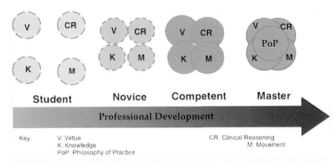

Fig. 9.2 Development of expertise in physical therapist practice.

- An understanding of and a value for each *patient's own circumstances.*
- The *best research evidence* available about our question.

The integration creates a *therapeutic alliance* (see ▶ Fig. 9.1).[3,4]

Each of these four terms defines an area for continued development across a therapist's career.

- *Clinical expertise* refers to the ability of the clinician to blend his or her skills and experience to make good clinical judgments in a timely clinical fashion.[3,4,5] While entry-level education provides a basis for clinical decision making, the constant variability and complexity of clinical practice offer continued challenges that require growth in this skill.
- *Patient values* refer to the preferences that each patient, and often the patient's family, brings to the clinical encounter. These preferences can arise from cultural or religious norms, from personal attitudes and beliefs, or from the patient's prior experiences and knowledge. While we all want to respect our patients, we need constant vigilance to stay aware of our own biases and how these can interfere with patient-centered care.[3,4,6]
- *Patient circumstances* refer to the situation in which the patient finds himself or herself. This could refer to the location of care, to the resources available to provide the care, including funding for the care, or to the resources for the patient to deal with the short and long-term sequelae of the illness or trauma. The constant changes in the health care system mean that patient circumstances are also constantly changing, requiring that therapists stay aware of these changes in the health care system, including payment mechanisms.[3,4,7]
- *Best research evidence* refers to the information that underlies our care, and that arises from the basic sciences but primarily from clinical research to help us answer specific questions about our patient care. This constitutes the area that we most commonly think of when we consider the need for continuing professional development, as science is constantly updating what we need to know and at such a volume it seems almost impossible to maintain competence.[3,4,8]

9.1.2 Expertise Model

There is a body of research studying the development of expertise in physical therapists. This work has resulted in a model of the development of expertise across time in practice.[9,10] This research has demonstrated that in physical therapy, expertise is composed of four elements: clinical reasoning, knowledge, virtue, and movement. When these four elements have reached a mature level of expertise, they merge into a unified philosophy of practice. It is hypothesized that, as shown in the figure, students entering the profession come with rudimentary mastery in each of these areas and over time, with experience and intentionality, develop a stronger and more cohesive mastery (see ▶ Fig. 9.2).

Each of these four elements also provides an area for continued development across a therapist's career.

- *Knowledge:* Experts have a multidimensional knowledge base, including specialty knowledge, with patients at the base, focusing on practical knowledge arising from reflective practice.
- *Clinical reasoning:* Experts begin their clinical reasoning in collaboration with the patient, focus their decision making on function and movement, and welcome challenges that lead to innovative solutions.
- *Movement:* Experts used movement, their own movement, and the movement of their patients in all aspects of patient care, from prevention to examination to treatment to long-term management.
- *Virtue:* Experts focus on working collaboratively with the patients to problem solve, not projecting blame or judgment about the patient's behaviors. They see patient advocacy as a vital part of their professional role and have an inner drive to continue to learn.

These two models provide us then with some excellent guidance for areas that will need continued development across the physical therapist's career.

The American Physical Therapy Association (APTA) provides many resources to assist us on both the individual and societal levels and with the elements described in these two models.

APTA is a membership organization founded in 1921, representing physical therapy, with over 95,000 physical therapists (PT), physical therapist assistants (PTA), and student members.[11] APTA is structured with 51 chapters representing the 50 states and the District of Columbia, and with 18 sections representing special interests in practice.[12] These 18 groups are as follows:

- Acute care.
- Aquatics.
- Cardiovascular and pulmonary.
- Clinical electrophysiology and wound management.
- Education.
- Federal.
- Geriatrics.
- Hand and upper extremity.
- Health policy and administration.
- Home health.
- Neurology.
- Oncology.
- Orthopaedics.
- Pediatrics.
- Private practice.
- Research.
- Sports.
- Women's health.

The history of APTA closely parallels the history of the profession, as the leaders in physical therapy in the early 1900s saw the need to have an organization that would represent the needs of patients by assuring quality and the needs of therapists by providing education and community (see Chapter 1).[13]

APTA as an organization is led by its board of directors, with professional policy direction from its House of Delegates. There are many committees and taskforces involving hundreds of volunteer members that support the work of the Board and House. Also, there is a staff of over 150 employed at APTA's headquarters in Alexandria, Virginia. To learn more about APTA's governance structures, visit APTA.org.[14]

In this chapter, we will explore those resources. As we review the resources, we will identify the elements that can be addressed by using the resource; you will see that many of them help achieve increased competence across more than one of the identified elements. We will begin with those resources designed to help us as individuals meet our obligations to improve practice across our careers and conclude with the resources available to support the profession's role in society.

9.2 Improving Competence in Patient Care

APTA resources that support improving patient care can be found across the APTA website. The resources reviewed in this section can be beneficial in helping to improve clinical expertise, clinical reasoning, access to clinical knowledge, and access to the best available research evidence. Many of these resources have movement as a central focus.

9.2.1 Career Development

APTA resources on career development start with its support of the Commission on Accreditation in Physical Therapy Education (CAPTE). CAPTE makes independent decisions on the status of physical therapist (PT) educational programs using standards developed by CAPTE with stakeholder input. These standards—*PT standards and required elements*—set the baseline for all entry-level education in physical therapy. Graduation from an accredited PT educational program—that is, a program that has met these standards—is required in order to sit for the PT licensure examination. Successful completion of this exam, in turn, is required to enter practice.[15,16]

While a sound preparation at entry-level is essential, it is not sufficient to assure competent practice across a career. APTA has developed several programs to address this issue. They include the following:

- *Specialization:* The specialist certification program was established in 1978 by APTA's House of Delegates to provide recognition of PTs with advanced clinical knowledge, skills and experience in a specialty area of practice. Each specialty area must be approved by the House of Delegates, after a careful assessment of practice in that area. The first specialty area to be approved was cardiopulmonary physical therapy in 1981. Once approved, a standardized examination is prepared, which applicants who meet the experience requirements must pass to become certified. Each certification period is for 10 years. In 2017, there are over 20,000 PTs certified in these areas:
  - Cardiovascular and pulmonary.
  - Clinical electrophysiology.
  - Geriatrics.
  - Neurology.
  - Oncology.
  - Orthopaedics.
  - Pediatrics.
  - Sports.
  - Women's health.

    The American Board of Physical Therapy Specialties (ABPTS), on behalf of APTA's House of Delegates and Board of Directors, manages all of these activities.[17]
- *Residency and fellowship:* APTA has established a program to accredit post-professional educational programs. These programs are designed for PTs to develop clinical reasoning skills in specific areas of practice, through systematic learning experiences that include careful mentoring and feedback in clinical settings to develop clinical reasoning. Residencies are accredited in clinical areas that have been determined to have a valid specialty practice, based on an analysis of practice. Residency programs in areas corresponding to specialist certification are expected to prepare PTs for the specialty examination. As of 2017 there are 253 accredited residency programs in the clinical areas of acute care, cardiovascular and pulmonary care, clinical electrophysiology, geriatrics, neurology, orthopaedics, pediatrics, sports, women's health and wound care management. In addition, there is a residency program in faculty practice. As of 2015, over 2,600 PTs

had completed these residency programs. Fellowship programs are focused on subspecialty areas. As of 2017 there are 42 fellowship programs in critical care, hand therapy, movement system, neonatology, orthopaedic manual physical therapy, spine, sports (Division 1), and upper extremity athlete. As of 2015 over 1,300 PTs had completed fellowships. The American Board of Physical Therapy Residency and Fellowship Education (ABPTRFE) oversees these activities on behalf of the APTA Board of Directors.[18]

These two programs provide excellent opportunities for physical therapists, especially those in the early years of their career, to focus on development of foundational skills in clinical reasoning and specialty knowledge. As stated at the ABPTS website, specialist practice embodies the dimensions identified in the expertise model described earlier. By meeting the requirements for certification, PTs demonstrate that they also embody these dimensions.[17] Competencies that can be achieved by completion of residency education include knowledge, clinical reasoning, clinical skills, and professionalism.[19] Residency education has been shown to bring value to graduates across their careers.[20]

While there is real value in these programs and they should be considered by all therapists as ways to strengthen their clinical practice competency, they also are similar to entry-level education—they generally occur once in a therapist's career.

9.2.2 Continued Competence

APTA has developed several programs that provide continuous opportunities across a therapist's career.

- *Continuing education:* One of the major resources for development across a therapist's career is continuing education (CE). All 50 states and the District of Columbia require continuing education for relicensure, but the true motivation for choosing and completing continuing education should be a careful consideration of one's goals for practice, the gaps in skills and knowledge needed for that practice, and an assessment of how well a particular CE experience will help fill that gap and lead to improved practice. APTA offers many different CE opportunities; every offering must meet rigorous educational standards, including a clear description, learning objectives, teaching methods, and references. These opportunities include the following:
  - Meetings: APTA hosts the largest assembly of physical therapists in the world in its annual Combined Section Meeting, cohosted with APTA's sections. This meeting routinely attracts more than 10,000 PTs and PTAs for over 3 days of concentrated programming in multiple practice areas. NEXT is the other annual APTA meeting. It combines governance activities of APTA's House of Delegates with 3 days of continuing education. Many of the programs at CSM and NEXT also have skills practice components. APTA also hosts several other meetings focused on the interests of specific groups. These include the National Student Conclave and events such as the federal advocacy forum and the state policy and payment forum.[21]
  - Learning center: APTA has developed a comprehensive catalogue of online courses, many of which are free to APTA members. The courses are organized in six categories: patient care, research, prevention and wellness, education and

professional excellence, health care management, and health care leadership. Many courses are organized into themes and progression to allow building of knowledge and skills. There are several packages that are designed to help prepare for the specialization examinations. APTA courses are accepted in all 50 states and the District of Columbia, as allowed by the restrictions in state regulations as to content. Completed courses are stored in online transcripts that can be used to meet CE requirements in the various states.[22]

- APTA also offers several publications that support professional development and increase access to best research evidence. *PT in Motion* features examples of successful practices and highlights important issues in the profession.[23] *Physical Therapy* (PTJ) is one of the premier peer-reviewed journals in rehabilitation.[24] Both of these publications are also free to members. In addition to these publications, many of the APTA Sections produce peer-reviewed journals in their specialty areas.
- The Guide to Physical Therapist Practice is a comprehensive description of physical therapist practice. It has set the language of practice by describing the patient/client management model. The model incorporates the international classification of functioning, disability and health (ICF), and the biopsychosocial model. The guide also describes the many different roles of the physical therapist. Since its first version, published in 1995, the guide has been used as a textbook across physical therapy education. Its current version, Guide 3.0 is available online, free to all APTA members (see ▶ Fig. 9.3).[25]
- *PTNow* is a tremendous resource designed specifically to give practitioners access to the best research evidence from a multitude of sources, both within and outside of physical therapy, relevant to physical therapy care.[26] Its many valuable resources include the following:
  - Article Search: In order to truly assess evidence to see if it is applicable to a particular patient, the evidence needs to be read in full. Reviewing abstracts is not sufficient to make

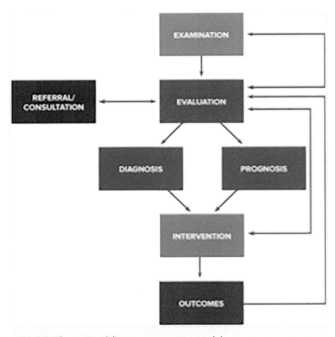

Fig. 9.3 The patient/client management model.

the decision to change practice. Article Search gives APTA members full-text access over 4,500 journals including Cochrane systematic reviews, considered one of the highest levels of evidence.[3] Article Search is an excellent replacement for new graduates for the access they had as students at their academic institutions.

◦ Rehabilitation resource center: This center provides access to many resources across rehabilitation. Content is updated daily to include daily health care news, background data on many conditions treated by PTs, pharmacologic information, materials for patient education, images of exercise for patient education, and full text of several textbooks. As with Article Search, this can replace access to resources lost on graduation.

◦ Clinical summaries synthesize evidence for a particle health problem across the patient/client management model. They integrate evidence across the full range of care from screening and examination through to outcomes measurement. They include links to relevant references and often include case examples.

◦ Tests gives members access to specific tools to use in examination and outcome measurement across the spectrum of patients seen by physical therapists, along with links to references on their psychometric properties and their application in practice. This section of *PTNow* also gives all members access to the work done by the evidence database to guide effectiveness (EDGE) task force. The EDGE task force is a collaborative project between APTA and several of its member sections to identify the best outcome measures currently available.

◦ Clinical practice guidelines (CPG): *PTNow* uses the same criteria as the national guideline clearinghouse.[27] All the CPGs are: based on a systematic review of the evidence, published by APTA sections or by other health care associations, organizations, and societies, not by individuals, and published within the last 5 years. Guidelines are an excellent source of the best research evidence, as they integrate evidence across the entire spectrum of care for a particular patient population.[3] The guidelines created by APTA's sections were developed through an ongoing collaboration among APTA and its sections.

◦ *PTNow* is organized to allow each user to save selected items from each of these areas to a personalized area, My *PTNow*, to make it easier for each therapist to find and use the most relevant clinical resources.

• Specific patient care topics: APTA has identified several specific patient care topics, either through direction from the House of Delegates, or because of environmental scanning on the part of staff. These topics range from specific diseases related issues such as arthritis and concussions, to specific patient populations such as wounded warriors and infants in intensive care, to sites of care such as emergency departments and hospice, to patient centered topics such as cultural competence and behavioral change. For each topic, experts have prepared useful materials, including pertinent websites and references, which provide a rich resource for practice.[28]

One final—and very important—resource available through APTA for improvement in clinical care is membership in any of the 18 sections that are part of APTA (see Info Box 1 (p. 127)). Each

of these sections provides specific resources related to an area of interest. These resources include continuing education programming, publications, access to colleagues through listservs and other online forums, and access to important resources for a particular area of practice.[29]

As can be seen, APTA provides a wide array of valuable resources to help every physical therapist improve competence in clinical care. These resources are all available to APTA members; some, such as meetings, learning center courses, and publications are also available to nonmembers for fees. These resources can help achieve improvement in knowledge, identifying best research evidence, clinical reasoning, and mastery of movement. Using these resources can help a therapist meet a primary obligation to patients—to be a competent practitioner. Competence does not mean doing what was learned at entry-level over and over again. That may result in experience, but it is not experience with the knowledge and skills that may have been shown to be better. That is what competence requires—learning what is better and putting it into practice in order to achieve expertise and excellence.

9.3 Practice Development

While improving knowledge and skills about direct patient care is vital, practice development is also important. Practice development includes three important areas: understanding patient circumstances; practice administration; and advocating for physical therapy patients and profession.

9.3.1 Patient Circumstances

Respecting patient circumstances requires understanding the health care system and its impact on the ability and inclination of patients to seek care. That inclination can include the interest in and motivation to receive care. APTA addresses this through its continuing education programming (meetings and learning center), including courses on topics such as motivation, adherence, cultural competence, and patient centered care.[21,22] The other aspect of patient circumstances is the patient's ability to access and pay for care. APTA has many resources about payment for care and public policy, discussed below.

9.3.2 Practice Administration

Patients cannot receive necessary and valuable physical therapist services if physical therapy practices are not successful. Physical therapists treat a wide variety of patients, in an equally wide variety of facilities, including acute care and rehabilitation hospitals, outpatient facilities, and practices in the community such as schools and home care. The methods of payment for physical therapist services are also varied. This means that there is a great deal of knowledge PTs must have in order to meet regulatory and compliance requirements, to manage practice groups, and to be economically successful. APTA has a great many resources available in this arena:

• Practice administration: Because of the importance of this topic, APTA has a specific portion of its website dedicated to topics related to practice administration.[30] A few of the more important topics include areas around compliance and documentation. APTA has prepared a comprehensive text, defensible documentation for patient/client management that provides descriptions of good documentation, as well as detailing specific requirements from various payment sources. It is used as a text in entry-level programs and for practicing clinicians to improve their documentation skills.[31] Other important areas include information about managing some specific kinds of practice. For example, information is available about the important decision about owning one's own practice.[32] Information on creating and contributing to pro bono care is also available.[33] Materials are also available on details of day-to-day practice management.[34,35] APTA also has a House of Delegates policy that sets the expected standards for practices: standards of practice for physical therapy.[36]

- Practice improvement: APTA has also invested in exciting programs that offer great opportunities to identify ways to improve practices as groups, and therefore improve health care as a whole. One of these is the innovations in practice project. This project debuted with a web-streamed conference viewed live across the country presenting several innovation models of care delivery. Innovations 2.0 continued that effort with a competition to identify additional innovative models of care. Those selected in the competition received APTA funding to continue their work and are participating in activities to mentor more APTA members in adapting these models in their own practices.[37] A second major endeavor is the creation of a registry of physical therapist care. The registry is a repository of data from actual patient care that can be used to analyze patient care by feedback to individual PTs about their decision making, to improve practices by bench marking them against similar ones, and to improve the collective practice of physical therapy. Because of the potential of the range of data, across the entire profession, the registry may well become the largest in health care, with the potential to provide an extraordinary data source for clinicians, researchers, and the profession (see ▶ Fig. 9.4).[38]

- Payment: As with practice administration, APTA has dedicated a specific portion of its website to this topic.[39] There are resources about each of the major entities providing insurance payment for physical therapist services, including Medicare, Medicaid, workers' compensation, VA and Tricare, and private insurances. For each of these, there are materials prepared by experts that explain the insurance coverage, the issues related to physical therapy, ways to ensure compliance with the insurance regulations and to improve the chances of payment by the entities. Also, particular areas where coverage has been questioned are included. One area that crosses over all insurance types is the method of allocating payment. Today, many insurance programs use a common coding system based on the procedures used in care. There is a detailed description of the current coding system, as well as of the plans APTA has in place to improve the coding system to better represent the cognitive effort by PTs in providing care and the complexity of that care.[40,41] While most of this material focuses on those insurance programs that pay physical therapists directly, there are also resources related to those programs that include physical therapy services in consolidated payments, such as those to hospitals, skilled nursing facilities, and home care agencies. There is also a long section on health care reform. Much of this section details the provisions of the current Affordable Care Act as of 2016.[42]

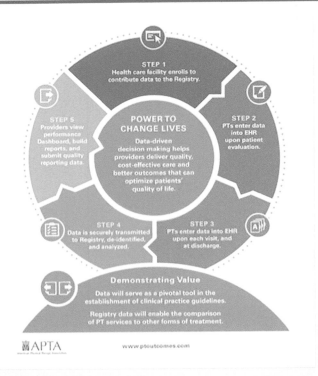

Fig. 9.4 Physical therapy registry.

9.3.3 Advocacy

Advocacy on behalf of the profession is one of APTA's major foci. Advocacy activities are rooted in APTA policies for the profession, which are set by the APTA House of Delegates.[43] These policies can be found at APTA's website, along with many other core documents of the association.[44] The advocacy website also provides several opportunities for people to engage in individual advocacy, including easy to use ways to send direct email to federal and state legislators. The advocacy portion of APTA's website has sections on both federal and state issues.

- Federal advocacy: Federal issues are generally linked to public health topics and the federal level payers, such as Medicare and Medicaid.[45] Transforming health care detailers the current public policy priorities of APTA. They include participating in reducing public health issues such as opioid addiction, concussions, and obesity; increasing access to physical therapist services by reducing barriers to access and the burden of unnecessary regulation and by developing new payment models; improving the supply of PTs in underserved areas; and supporting rehabilitation research and other sources of data that can improve care.[46] There are also many background papers that provide useful information about the reasons for APTA's public policy priorities. APTA also supports the Physical Therapy Political Action Committee, which is the sole fund-raising organization focused on physical therapy issues at the federal level.[47]

- State advocacy: State issues generally focus on topics that arise out of state regulation around licensure and payment.[48] Licensure, in addition to setting entry to practice, also sets the boundaries to access. Scope of practice and direct access to physical therapist services without referral are examples of two important issues governed by licensure.[49] Scope of practice issues include both the types of activities permitted by physical therapists and assuring that others do not impinge on the PT's scope of practice. Both of these issues are founded in the desire to protect patients. Direct access, the ability of patients to seek care from physical therapists without referral from other practitioners, has been a goal of APTA's for over 30 years. In addition, since health insurance companies are also regulated at the state level, many coverage and payment issues need to be addressed within each state. The website has many resources to help with these topics.

Just as the sections can be excellent resources about direct patient care, the chapters can be great resources for practice development. All states and the District of Columbia have a chapter in APTA (see Info Box 1 (p.127)). Each of these chapters has its own website, with resources about issues unique to each state, particularly scope of practice and payment issues. They also have links to individual advocacy opportunities within the chapter.

Many of APTA's resources related to practice development are available to nonmembers. In fact, some are actually designed for specific groups such as legislators and insurers. Taken as a group, these resources can provide the basis for sound practice that can be economically successful, but more importantly can be in the best interests of patients and clients, by giving them access to necessary services, provided with efficiency and effectiveness.

9.4 Responsibility to Society

Professions and members of professions owe an obligation to patients, clients, and society, what Jensen et al describe as exhibiting virtue.[2,5] We turn now to the most important set of resources at APTA, those that support meeting that obligation.

9.4.1 Professional Obligations to Patients and Clients

Some of APTA's most important resources speak to the obligations of the individual therapist to his or her patients and clients.

- Ethics and professionalism: APTA has many resources to assist physical therapists in understanding and choosing appropriate professional behavior.[50] While the code of ethics is primary in providing this guidance, there are also several other resources as well:
  ○ Code of ethics (see ▸ Fig. 9.5): The code of ethics is the principle core document of the profession, adopted by APTA's House of Delegates.[1] As its preamble states, it defines ethical practices for all physical therapists and provides standards that form the basis of accountability to the public. It also serves as guidance and education for PTs and the public in choosing and evaluating behavior. These purposes transcend APTA and apply to all physical therapists. The code also has the purpose to set standards for APTA to determine if a PT has engaged in unethical behavior. The disciplinary action procedural document provides guidance to APTA members about the processes used to respond to unethical or illegal behavior on the part of members.[51] The code is supported by a Guide for Professional Conduct that is developed

and amended by APTA's Ethics and Judicial Committee based on their experience with ethical issues. It serves as a further explanatory guide for the code of ethics. There are also parallel documents for the physical therapist assistant.
  ○ Ethical decision making: Ethical decision making can be a difficult and complex activity, as potential ethical issues can arise in all aspects of a PT's professional life. This section of the APTA website offers assistance in this regard.[52] One especially valuable resource is realm-individual process-situation (RIPS) model of ethical decision making. This model helps physical therapists to identify if a situation represents unethical behavior, and if so, what action to take.[53]
  ○ Professional core values: These are expectations for behavior that describe what society expects of members of a profession in their daily interactions with their patients and clients.[54] APTA has developed a self-assessment to be used to help individual therapists determine how well they are practicing the core values.[55] In addition, APTA has developed a professionalism course series at the learning center. The series has 10 modules that include educational materials, reflection activities, discussion boards, and assessment tools. Professional core values include
    – *Accountability* is active acceptance of the responsibility for the diverse roles, obligations, and actions of the physical therapist including self-regulation and other behaviors that positively influence patient/client outcomes, the profession and the health needs of society.
    – *Altruism* is the primary regard for or devotion to the interest of patients/clients, thus assuming the fiduciary responsibility of placing the needs of the patient/client ahead of the physical therapist's self-interest.
    – *Compassion* is the desire to identify with or sense something of another's experience; a precursor of caring. Caring is the concern, empathy, and consideration for the needs and values of others.
    – *Excellence* is physical therapy practice that consistently uses current knowledge and theory while understanding personal limits, integrates judgment and the patient/client perspective, embraces advancement, challenges mediocrity, and works toward development of new knowledge.
    – *Integrity* is steadfast adherence to high ethical principles or professional standards; truthfulness, fairness, doing what you say you will do, and "speaking forth" about why you do what you do.
    – *Professional duty* is the commitment to meeting one's obligations to provide effective physical therapy services to patients/clients, to serve the profession, and to positively influence the health of society.
    – *Social responsibility* is the promotion of a mutual trust between the profession and the larger public that necessitates responding to societal needs for health and wellness.
  ○ Integrity in practice: APTA has created a major campaign to help physical therapists and the public recognize fraud and abuse in practice.[56] There is a detailed primer that defines fraud and abuse, as well as many suggestions for PTs to avoid any suspicion of either through poor documentation, lack of compliance, or other behaviors that do not have the intent to fraud or abuse, but may give the appearance of doing so. APTA is also one of the first nonphysician groups to join the American Board of Internal Medicine

Preamble

The Code of Ethics for the Physical Therapist (Code of Ethics) delineates the ethical obligations of all physical therapists as determined by the House of Delegates of the American Physical Therapy Association (APTA). The purposes of this Code of Ethics are to:

1. Define the ethical principles that form the foundation of physical therapist practice in patient/client management, consultation, education, research, and administration.
2. Provide standards of behavior and performance that form the basis of professional accountability to the public.
3. Provide guidance for physical therapists facing ethical challenges, regardless of their professional roles and responsibilities.
4. Educate physical therapists, students, other health care professionals, regulators, and the public regarding the core values, ethical principles, and standards that guide the professional conduct of the physical therapist.
5. Establish the standards by which the American Physical Therapy Association can determine if a physical therapist has engaged in unethical conduct.

No code of ethics is exhaustive nor can it address every situation. Physical therapists are encouraged to seek additional advice or consultation in instances where the guidance of the Code of Ethics may not be definitive.

This Code of Ethics is built upon the five roles of the physical therapist (management of patients/clients, consultation, education, research, and administration), the core values of the profession, and the multiple realms of ethical action (individual, organizational, and societal). Physical therapist practice is guided by a set of seven core values: accountability, altruism, compassion/caring, excellence, integrity, professional duty, and social responsibility. Throughout the document the primary core values that support specific principles are indicated in parentheses. Unless a specific role is indicated in the principle, the duties and obligations being delineated pertain to the five roles of the physical therapist. Fundamental to the Code of Ethics is the special obligation of physical therapists to empower, educate, and enable those with impairments, activity limitations, participation restrictions, and disabilities to facilitate greater independence, health, wellness, and enhanced quality of life.

Principles

Principle #1: Physical therapists shall respect the inherent dignity and rights of all individuals. (Core Values: Compassion, Integrity)

1A. Physical therapists shall act in a respectful manner toward each person regardless of age, gender, race, nationality, religion, ethnicity, social or economic status, sexual orientation, health condition, or disability.

1B. Physical therapists shall recognize their personal biases and shall not discriminate against others in physical therapist practice, consultation, education, research, and administration.

Principle #2: Physical therapists shall be trustworthy and compassionate in addressing the rights and needs of patients/clients. (Core Values: Altruism, Compassion, Professional Duty)

2A. Physical therapists shall adhere to the core values of the profession and shall act in the best interests of patients/clients over the interests of the physical therapist.

2B. Physical therapists shall provide physical therapy services with compassionate and caring behaviors that incorporate the individual and cultural differences of patients/clients.

2C. Physical therapists shall provide the information necessary to allow patients or their surrogates to make informed decisions about physical therapy care or participation in clinical research.

Fig. 9.5 Code of ethics for the physical therapist.

2D. Physical therapists shall collaborate with patients/clients to empower them in decisions about their health care.

2E. Physical therapists shall protect confidential patient/ client information and may disclose confidential information to appropriate authorities only when allowed or as required by law.

Principle #3: Physical therapists shall be accountable for making sound professional judgments. (Core Values: Excellence, Integrity)

3A. Physical therapists shall demonstrate independent and objective professional judgment in the patient's/client's best interest in all practice settings.

3B. Physical therapists shall demonstrate professional judgment informed by professional standards, evidence (including current literature and established best practice), practitioner experience, and patient/client values.

3C. Physical therapists shall make judgments within their scope of practice and level of expertise and shall communicate with, collaborate with, or refer to peers or other health care professionals when necessary.

3D. Physical therapists shall not engage in conflicts of interest that interfere with professional judgment.

3E. Physical therapists shall provide appropriate direction of and communication with physical therapist assistants and support personnel.

Principle #4: Physical therapists shall demonstrate integrity in their relationships with patients/clients, families, colleagues, students, research participants, other health care providers, employers, payers, and the public. (Core Value: Integrity)

4A. Physical therapists shall provide truthful, accurate, and relevant information and shall not make misleading representations.

4B. Physical therapists shall not exploit persons over whom they have supervisory, evaluative or other authority (eg, patients/clients, students, supervisees, research participants, or employees).

4C. Physical therapists shall discourage misconduct by health care professionals and report illegal or unethical acts to the relevant authority, when appropriate.

4D. Physical therapists shall report suspected cases of abuse involving children or vulnerable adults to the appropriate authority, subject to law.

4E. Physical therapists shall not engage in any sexual relation- ship with any of their patients/clients, supervisees, or students.

4F. Physical therapists shall not harass anyone verbally, physically, emotionally, or sexually.

Principle #5: Physical therapists shall fulfill their legal and professional obligations. (Core Values: Professional Duty, Accountability)

5A. Physical therapists shall comply with applicable local, state, and federal laws and regulations.

5B. Physical therapists shall have primary responsibility for supervision of physical therapist assistants and support personnel.

5C. Physical therapists involved in research shall abide by accepted standards governing protection of research participants.

5D. Physical therapists shall encourage colleagues with physical, psychological, or substance-related impairments that may adversely impact their professional responsibilities to seek assistance or counsel.

Fig. 9.5 (Continued)

5E. Physical therapists who have knowledge that a colleague is unable to perform their professional responsibilities with reasonable skill and safety shall report this information to the appropriate authority.

5F. Physical therapists shall provide notice and information about alternatives for obtaining care in the event the physical therapist terminates the provider relationship while the patient/client continues to need physical therapy services.

Principle #6: Physical therapists shall enhance their expertise through the lifelong acquisition and refinement of knowledge, skills, abilities, and professional behaviors. (Core Value: Excellence)

6A. Physical therapists shall achieve and maintain professional competence.

6B. Physical therapists shall take responsibility for their profes- sional development based on critical self-assessment and reflection on changes in physical therapist practice, education, health care delivery, and technology.

6C. Physical therapists shall evaluate the strength of evidence and applicability of content presented during professional development activities before integrating the content or techniques into practice.

6D. Physical therapists shall cultivate practice environments that support professional development, lifelong learning, and excellence.

Principle #7: Physical therapists shall promote organizational behaviors and business practices that benefit patients/clients and society. (Core Values: Integrity, Accountability)

7A. Physical therapists shall promote practice environments that support autonomous and accountable professional judgments.

7B. Physical therapists shall seek remuneration as is deserved and reasonable for physical therapist services.

7C. Physical therapists shall not accept gifts or other considerations that influence or give an appearance of influencing their professional judgment.

7D. Physical therapists shall fully disclose any financial interest they have in products or services that they recommend to patients/clients.

7E. Physical therapists shall be aware of charges and shall ensure that documentation and coding for physical therapy services accurately reflect the nature and extent of the services provided.

7F. Physical therapists shall refrain from employment arrangements, or other arrangements, that prevent physical therapists from fulfilling professional obligations to patients/ clients.

Principle #8: Physical therapists shall participate in efforts to meet the health needs of people locally, nationally, or globally. (Core Value: Social Responsibility)

8A. Physical therapists shall provide pro bono physical therapy services or support organizations that meet the health needs of people who are economically disadvantaged, uninsured, and underinsured.

8B. Physical therapists shall advocate to reduce health disparities and health care inequities, improve access to health care services, and address the health, wellness, and preventive health care needs of people.

8C. Physical therapists shall be responsible stewards of health care resources and shall avoid overutilization or under- utilization of physical therapy services.

8D. Physical therapists shall educate members of the public about the benefits of physical therapy and the unique role of the physical therapist.

Fig. 9.5 (Continued)

Foundation's Choosing Wisely campaign.[57] Over 50 specialty societies have created questions that patients and their practitioners should ask about specific areas of care that have been shown to have little efficacy.[58]

These resources provide clear guidance for physical therapists about expectations for their behavior. As they are available to the public, they also serve to alert our patients and clients what they should expect in our behavior.

9.4.2 Professional Obligations to Society

As Colby and Sullivan state, professions need to be aware of and act on their public purpose.[2] This public purpose is part of the implicit contract the profession and society have with each other; society allows a profession a great deal of autonomy; therefore, the profession needs to earn this trust by working to help improve society. There are many APTA resources that speak to this collective professional responsibility, including

- The vision statement for the physical therapy profession: In 2013, APTA's House of Delegates adopted this outward facing vision, "Transforming society by optimizing movement to improve the human experience." This vision is supported by eight guiding principles that describe the goals for society when the profession has met its vision of helping society to see movement as a key element of being a healthy member of society.[59]

This vision has been widely integrated into APTA's activities, as well as the activities of its component chapters and sections.

- Pro bono care: The code of ethics requires that all physical therapists be involved in pro bono care, either directly or supporting the pro bono work of others.[1] To support this obligation APTA has created materials that provide information on how to develop and sustain pro bono clinical services, in the United States and across the world.[60]
- Move forward: APTA has created a consumer portal with a great deal of valuable information for consumers and potential consumers of physical therapist services. The website features APTA's involvement in the campaign to reduce the opioid epidemic. It also has podcasts, videos, and numerous references that can be used in consumer terms to help people better understand their health and movement.[61] Move Forward had nearly 2 million consumer sessions in 2015.[62]

Guiding Principles to Achieve the Vision ⓘ

Movement is a key to optimal living and quality of life for all people that extends beyond health to every person's ability to participate in and contribute to society. The complex needs of society, such as those resulting from a sedentary lifestyle, beckon for the physical therapy profession to engage with consumers to reduce preventable health care costs and overcome barriers to participation in society to ensure the successful existence of society far into the future.

While this is APTA's vision for the physical therapy profession, it is meant also to inspire others throughout society to, together, create systems that optimize movement and function for all people. The following principles of identity, quality, collaboration, value, innovation, consumer centricity, access/

equity, and advocacy demonstrate how the profession and society will look when this vision is achieved.

The principles are described as follows:

- *Identity.* The physical therapy profession will define and promote the movement system as the foundation for optimizing movement to improve the health of society. Recognition and validation of the movement system is essential to understand the structure, function, and potential of the human body. The physical therapist will be responsible for evaluating and managing an individual's movement system across the lifespan to promote optimal development; diagnose impairments, activity limitations, and participation restrictions; and provide interventions targeted at preventing or ameliorating activity limitations and participation restrictions. The movement system is the core of physical therapist practice, education, and research.

- *Quality.* The physical therapy profession will commit to establishing and adopting best practice standards across the domains of practice, education, and research as the individuals in these domains strive to be flexible, prepared, and responsive in a dynamic and ever-changing world. As independent practitioners, doctors of physical therapy in clinical practice will embrace best practice standards in examination, diagnosis/classification, intervention, and outcome measurement. These physical therapists will generate, validate, and disseminate evidence and quality indicators, espousing payment for outcomes and patient/client satisfaction, striving to prevent adverse events related to patient care, and demonstrating continuing competence. Educators will seek to propagate the highest standards of teaching and learning, supporting collaboration and innovation throughout academia. Researchers will collaborate with clinicians to expand available evidence and translate it into practice, conduct comparative effectiveness research, standardize outcome measurement, and participate in interprofessional research teams.

- *Collaboration.* The physical therapy profession will demonstrate the value of collaboration with other health care providers, consumers, community organizations, and other disciplines to solve the health-related challenges that society faces. In clinical practice, doctors of physical therapy, who collaborate across the continuum of care, will ensure that services are coordinated, of value, and consumer centered by referring, comanaging, engaging consultants, and directing and supervising care. Education models will value and foster interprofessional approaches to best meet consumer and population needs and instill team values in physical therapists and physical therapist assistants. Interprofessional research approaches will ensure that evidence translates to practice and is consumer centered.

- *Value.* Value has been defined as "the health outcomes achieved per dollar spent."[63] To ensure the best value, services that the physical therapy profession will provide will be safe, effective, patient/client-centered, timely, efficient, and equitable.[64] Outcomes will be both meaningful to patients/clients and cost-effective. Value will be demonstrated and achieved in all settings in which physical therapist services are delivered. Accountability will be a core characteristic of the profession and will be essential to demonstrating value.

○ *Innovation.* The physical therapy profession will offer creative and proactive solutions to enhance health services delivery and to increase the value of physical therapy to society. Innovation will occur in many settings and dimensions, including health care delivery models, practice patterns, education, research, and the development of patient/client-centered procedures and devices and new technology applications. In clinical practice, collaboration with developers, engineers, and social entrepreneurs will capitalize on the technological savvy of the consumer and extend the reach of the physical therapist beyond traditional patient/client–therapist settings. Innovation in education will enhance interprofessional learning, address workforce needs, respond to declining higher education funding, and, anticipating the changing way adults learn, foster new educational models and delivery methods. In research, innovation will advance knowledge about the profession, apply new knowledge in such areas as genetics and engineering, and lead to new possibilities related to movement and function. New models of research and enhanced approaches to the translation of evidence will more expediently put these discoveries and other new information into the hands and minds of clinicians and educators.

○ *Consumer centricity.* Patient/client/consumer values and goals will be central to all efforts in which the physical therapy profession will engage. The physical therapy profession embraces cultural competence as a necessary skill to ensure best practice in providing physical therapist services by responding to individual and cultural considerations, needs, and values.

○ *Access/Equity.* The physical therapy profession will recognize health inequities and disparities and work to ameliorate them through innovative models of service delivery, advocacy, attention to the influence of the social determinants of health on the consumer, collaboration with community entities to expand the benefit provided by physical therapy, serving as a point of entry to the health care system, and direct outreach to consumers to educate and increase awareness.

○ *Advocacy.* The physical therapy profession will advocate for patients/clients/consumers both as individuals and as a population, in practice, education, and research settings to manage and promote change, adopt best practice standards and approaches, and ensure that systems are built to be consumer centered.

9.5 Conclusion

As stated at the beginning of the chapter, "Becoming a physical therapist means entering a profession and assuming the responsibilities and obligations that members of a profession have to their patients and to society." The resources at APTA make it possible to meet those responsibilities and obligations. APTA's role in developing these resources reflects the priorities of its members as reflected in actions of the APTA House of Delegates, Board of Directors, and staff. As APTA and its component chapters and sections are the primary organization reflecting the profession of physical therapy, it is appropriate that APTA has assumed this role. While membership in APTA is necessary to access many of these resources, many others are available to the public. Physical therapists and the public will be well served by seeking out these resources and using them to guide and define appropriate physical therapy care.

9.6 Review Questions

1. The "therapeutic alliance" associated with evidence-based practice is based on the integration of which criteria?
   a) Clinical expertise, the patient's values, the best research, and the patient's own circumstances.
   b) Clinical expertise, clinical experience, years of practice, reflection.
   c) The therapist's values, the therapist's clinical expertise, the therapist's own circumstances, and the best research.
   d) The therapist's empathy, kindness, emotional maturity, and dedication to task.
2. The patient values referenced in evidence-based practice can refer to which of the following?
   a) The patient's cultural and religious background.
   b) The patient's physical examination.
   c) The patient's ability to pay for care.
   d) The patient's adherence to the therapy program.
3. Clinical expertise in physical is composed of four elements: clinical reasoning, knowledge, virtue, and which of the following?
   a) Empathy.
   b) Dedication to the profession.
   c) Movement.
   d) Customer service.
4. The specialist certification program was established in which year by APTA's House of Delegates to provide recognition to PTs with advanced clinical knowledge?
   a) 1920.
   b) 1955.
   c) 1978.
   d) 2012.
5. The specialist certification program provides certification for how many years?
   a) 1.
   b) 5.
   c) 10.
   d) 20.
6. APTA currently has a program to accredit which postprofessional educational program?
   a) Fellowships.
   b) Residencies.
   c) Continuing education.
   d) Fellowships and residencies.
7. How many U.S. states now require continuing education for licensure?
   a) 20 and the District of Columbia.
   b) 30 and the District of Columbia.
   c) 40 and the District of Columbia.
   d) 50 and the District of Columbia.

8. National and regional meetings are wonderful forums for continuing education. The largest meeting hosted by APTA is which of the following?
   a) Combined sections meeting.
   b) NEXT conference.
   c) National student conclave.
   d) Federal advocacy forum.

9. APTA supports many publications. Which publication listed below can be described as "a comprehensive description of physical therapy practice…. Sets the language of practice by describing the patient/client management model"?
   a) Physical Therapy (PTJ).
   b) Journal of Orthopedic and Sports Physical Therapy.
   c) PT in Motion.
   d) The Guide to Physical Therapist Practice.

10. Which of the following issues is best addressed through federal advocacy?
    a) State licensure requirements.
    b) State practice acts.
    c) Medicare payment issues.
    d) Scope of practice of physical therapy.

9.7 Review Answers

1. The "therapeutic alliance" associated with evidence-based practice is based on the integration of which criteria?
   a. Clinical expertise, the patient's values, the best research, and the patient's own circumstances.

2. The patient values referenced in evidence-based practice can refer to which of the following?
   a. The patient's cultural and religious background.

3. Clinical expertise in physical is composed of four elements: clinical reasoning, knowledge, virtue, and which of the following?
   c. Movement.

4. The specialist certification program was established in which year by APTA's House of delegates to provide recognition to PTs with advanced clinical knowledge?
   c. 1978.

5. The specialist certification program provides certification for how many years?
   c. 10.

6. APTA currently has a program to accredit which postprofessional educational program?
   d. Fellowships and residencies.

7. How many U.S. states now require continuing education for licensure?
   d. 50 and the District of Columbia.

8. National and regional meetings are wonderful forums for continuing education. The largest meeting hosted by APTA is which of the following?
   a. Combined sections meeting.

9. APTA supports many publications. Which publication listed below can be described as "a comprehensive description of physical therapy practice…. Sets the language of practice by describing the patient/client management model"?
   d. **The Guide to Physical Therapist Practice.**

10. Which of the following issues is best addressed through federal advocacy?
    c. **Medicare payment issues.**

References

[1] Code of Ethics. Available at: http://www.apta.org/uploadedFiles/APTAorg/About_Us/Policies/Ethics/CodeofEthics.pdf, Accessed February 2, 2017

[2] Colby A, Sullivan W. Formation of professionalism and purpose: perspectives from the preparation for the professions program. Univ St Thomas Law J. 2008; 5:404–426

[3] Hack LM, Gwyer J. Evidence into Practice: Integrating Judgment, Values, and Research—An Application to Physical Therapist Practice. Philadelphia, PA: F.A. Davis; 2013

[4] Strauss SE, Richardson WS. Glasziou, Haynes RB, Evidence-based Medicine. 3rd ed. Edinburgh, UK: Elsevier Churchill Livingstone; 2005

[5] Jensen G, Gwyer J, Hack L, Shepard K. Expertise in Physical Therapy Practice. 2nd ed. St. Louis, MO: Saunders Elsevier; 2006

[6] Institute of Medicine. Crossing the Quality Chasm: A New Health System for the 21st Century. Washington DC: Institute of Medicine; 2001

[7] Kissick WL. Medicine's Dilemmas. New Haven, CT: Yale University Press; 1994

[8] Law M. Evidence-Based Rehabilitation. Thorofare, NJ: Slack; 2002

[9] Jensen G, Gwyer J, Shepard K, Hack LM. Expertise in clinical practice. Phys Ther. 2000; 80:28–43

[10] Jensen G, Gwyer J, Hack LM, Shepard K. Expertise in Physical Therapy Practice. 2nd ed. St. Louis, CT: Saunders Elsevier; 2006

[11] APTA. Available at: http://www.apta.org/AboutUs/WhoWeAre/. Accessed February 1, 2017

[12] APTA. Chapters and Sections. Available at: http://www.apta.org/apta/components/public/chaptersandsections.aspx?navID=10737421970. Accessed February 5, 2017

[13] Murphy W. Healing the Generations: A History of Physical Therapy and the American Physical Therapy Association. Alexandria, VA: American Physical Therapy Association; 1995

[14] APTA. Available at: http://www.apta.org/AboutUs/

[15] Commission on Accreditation of Physical Therapy Education. Available at: http://www.capteonline.org/AccreditationHandbook/. Accessed February 1, 2017

[16] Federation of State Boards of Physical Therapy. Available at: http://www.fsbpt.org. Accessed February 1, 2017

[17] APTA. American Board of Physical Therapy Specialties. Available at: http://www.abpts.org/home.aspx. Accessed February 1, 2017

[18] APTA. American Board of Physical Therapy Residency and Fellowship Education. Available at: http://www.abptrfe.org/home.aspx. Accessed February 1, 2017

[19] Furze JA, Tichenor CJ, Fisher BE, Jensen GM, Rapport MJ. Physical therapy residency and fellowship education: reflections on the past, present, and future. Phys Ther. 2016; 96(7):949–960

[20] Jones S, Bellah C, Godges J. A comparison of professional development and leadership activities between graduates and non-graduates of physical therapist clinical residency programs. J Phys Ther Educ. 2008; 22:85–88

[21] APTA. Conferences. Available at: http://www.apta.org/Conferences/. Accessed February 1, 2017

[22] APTA. Learning Center. Available at: http://learningcenter.apta.org. Accessed February 12, 2017

[23] APTA. PT in Motion. Available at: http://www.apta.org/PTinMotion/. Accessed February 2, 2017

[24] APTA. Physical Therapy. Available at: https://academic.oup.com/ptj. Accessed February 2, 2017

[25] APTA. Guide to Physical Therapist Practice. Available at: http://guidetoptpractice.apta.org. Accessed February 2, 2017

[26] APTA. PTNow. Available at: http://www.ptnow.org/Default.aspx. Accessed February 2, 2017

[27] National Guideline Clearinghouse. Available at:https://www.guideline.gov. Accessed February 2, 2017

[28] APTA. Patient Care. Available at: http://www.apta.org/PatientCare/. Accessed February 4, 2017

[29] APTA. Sections. Available at: http://www.apta.org/apta/components/public/chaptersandsections.aspx?navID=10737421970. Accessed February 2, 2017

[30] APTA. Practice Administration. Available at: http://www.apta.org/PracticeAdministration/. Accessed February 4, 2017

[31] APTA. Defensible Documentation. Available at: http://www.apta.org/Documentation/DefensibleDocumentation/. Accessed February 4, 2017

[32] APTA. Practice Ownership. Available at: http://www.apta.org/PracticeOwnership/. Accessed February 4, 2017

[33] APTA. Pro Bono Care. Available at: http://www.apta.org/ProBono/. Accessed February 4, 2017

[34] APTA. Tools for Practice Managers. Available at: http://www.apta.org/ToolsforPracticeManagers/. Accessed February 4, 2017

[35] APTA. Supervision and Teamwork. Available at: http://www.apta.org/SupervisionTeamwork/. Accessed February 4, 2017

[36] APTA. Standards of Practice. Available at: http://www.apta.org/uploadedFiles/APTAorg/About_Us/Policies/Practice/StandardsPractice.pdf#search=%22standards%20of%20practice%22. Accessed February 5, 2017

[37] APTA. Innovations in Practice. Available at: http://www.apta.org/InnovationsinPractice/. Accessed February 4, 2017

[38] APTA. Physical Therapy Outcomes Registry. Available at: http://www.ptoutcomes.com/Home.aspx. Accessed February 4, 2017

[39] APTA. Payment. Available at: http://www.apta.org/Payment/. Accessed February 4, 2017

[40] APTA. Coding and Billing. Available at: http://www.apta.org/Payment/CodingBilling/. Accessed February 5, 2017

[41] APTA. Payment Reform. Available at: http://www.apta.org/PaymentReform/. Accessed February 5, 2017

[42] APTA. Health Care Reform. Available at: http://www.apta.org/HealthCareReform/. Accessed February 5, 2017

[43] APTA. Advocacy. Available at: http://www.apta.org/Advocacy/. Accessed February 5, 2017

[44] APTA. Policies and Bylaws. Available at: http://www.apta.org/Policies/. Accessed February 5, 2017

[45] APTA. Federal Advocacy, http://www.apta.org/FederalAdvocacy/. Accessed February 5, 2017

[46] APTA. Transforming Health Care. Available at: http://www.apta.org/FederalIssues/PublicPolicyPriorities/Document/. Accessed February 5, 2017

[47] PTPAC. Available at: http://www.ptpac.org. Accessed February 5, 2017

[48] APTA. State Advocacy. Available at: http://www.apta.org/StateAdvocacy/. Accessed February 5, 2017

[49] APTA. State Issues. Available at: http://www.apta.org/StateIssues/. Accessed February 5, 2017

[50] APTA. Ethics and Professionalism. Available at: http://www.apta.org/EthicsProfessionalism/. Accessed February 5, 2017

[51] APTA. Disciplinary Action Procedural Document. Available at: http://www.apta.org/uploadedFiles/APTAorg/About_Us/Policies/Judicial_Legal/DisciplinaryActionProceduralDocument.pdf#search=%22disciplinary%20action%22. Accessed February 5, 2017

[52] APTA. Decision Making Tools. Available at: http://www.apta.org/Ethics/Tools/. Accessed February 5, 2017

[53] APTA. Realm-Individual Process-Situation (RIPS) Model of Ethical Decision Making. Available at: http://www.apta.org/uploadedFiles/APTAorg/Practice_and_Patient_Care/Ethics/Tools/RIPS_DecisionMaking.pdf. Accessed February 5, 2017

[54] APTA. Professionalism. Available at: http://www.apta.org/Professionalism/. Accessed February 5, 2017

[55] APTA. Core Values Self-Assessment. Available at: http://www.apta.org/CoreValuesSelfAssessment/. Accessed February 5, 2017

[56] APTA. Integrity in Practice. Available at: http://integrity.apta.org/. Accessed February 5, 2017

[57] ABIM. Choosing Wisely. Available at: http://www.choosingwisely.org. Accessed February 5, 2017

[58] ABIM. Five Things Physical Therapists and Patients Should Question. Available at: http://www.choosingwisely.org/societies/american-physical-therapy-association/. Accessed February 5, 2017

[59] APTA. Vision. Available at: http://www.apta.org/Vision/. Accessed February 5, 2017

[60] APTA. Pro Bono. Available at: http://www.apta.org/ProBono/. Accessed February 5, 2017

[61] APTA. Move Forward. Available at: http://www.moveforwardpt.com/Default.aspx. Accessed February 5, 2017

[62] APTA, Consumer Information Available on the APTA Website. (RC 30–05), Annual Report to the 2016 House of Delegates. Available at: http://communities.apta.org/p/do/sd/sid=2721&fid=11720&req=direct. Accessed February 5, 2017

[63] Porter ME, Teisberg EO. Redefining health care: creating value-based competition on results. Boston, MA: Harvard Business School Press; 2006

[64] Crossing the Quality Chasm. A New Health System for the 21st Century. Washington, DC: Institute of Medicine of the National Academies; 2001. 66

10 Professionalism in Society

Sean F. Griech

Keywords: American Physical Therapy Association, American Physical Therapy Association Code of Ethics, autonomous practice, autonomy, direct access, doctor of physical therapy, evidence-based practice, leadership, practitioner of choice, professional behavior, professional behaviors assessment tool, professional identity, professionalism, Vision 2020

Chapter Outline

1. Introduction
   a) What is Professionalism?
   b) History of Professionalism in Physical Therapy
2. Role of Professionalism in Health Care and Physical Therapy
3. Developing a Professional Identity
4. Professional Behaviors
5. Professionalism and Leadership
6. American Physical Therapy Association's Code of Ethics

"From my earliest days, I loved words. My mom once told me that when I was five and sitting on Santa's lap and asked by the great man himself what I wanted for Christmas, I said 'typewriter.' Santa tried to convince me to ask for a baseball or a football. I stood firm and later that month, under our Christmas tree, he delivered a Remington typewriter. That typewriter still sits in my attic.

"Words can be spoken or written. Words can rhyme. Words can hurt and they can heal. Words can tell a coherent or confusing story. Words can define our relationships. Words explain. Words can be trusted or they can lie. Words can have one meaning or they can have many meanings.

"On my first day in my entry-level physical therapy program 35 years ago, the first words out of my chairperson's mouth as he greeted us were 'from today forward you are a professional.' He spoke it with such assuredness and finality! From that moment forward the word 'professional' became a holy grail to me: how do I define it? How do I become it? How do I protect it? How do I teach it?

"The root of the word 'professional' comes from old French noun 'profession' and refers to the vows taken upon entering a religious order. The original word has evolved into many now commonly used words in today's lexicon: profess, professor, profession, professional, professing, professed, and professorial. The roots can now be found in nouns, adjectives, adverbs, and verbs.

"One of the commonalities of most of the definitions of professional is the word 'character.' I find this interesting because I once believed that the standards of being a professional were defined by an administrative practice act or code of ethics. However, the word character, to me, seems to imply that the behavior defined as being professional is derived from within each of us. This seems to make sense to me. When faced with a difficult decision—especially a behavioral decision—our innate character, our professionalism can be expressed if we give it time through reflection, asking for counsel with mentors, and learning how great men and women handled similar difficult issues.

"I have also learned that crossing the professional line is tantamount to crossing the Rubicon; one can never go back. Once professionalism is lost, we too, are lost. As physical therapists we need to seek the highest of moral grounds in all administrative, behavioral, and clinical activities. Our professionalism, our character, must be protected at all costs.

"As I sit on my back porch typing this reflection on my laptop I cannot help think of the words that old Remington typewriter—still in my attic—typed over the past 50 years. I doubt I will ever type on that old friend again. However, when I am gone and someone is tasked with cleaning my attic, I hope they find that Remington and think of me. I hope they say, 'He was a professional. He was a professional who loved words.'"

—George A., Pipersville, Pennsylvania

10.1 Introduction

10.1.1 What is Professionalism?

Professionalism has many lay definitions. Definitions often change based on the aim of the use or context of the word in writing or speech. Is the word used as an explanation, rationalization, expectation, excuse, description, approbation, punishment? A generic definition of professionalism we may wish to consider for this chapter is *the conduct, aims, or qualities that characterize or mark a profession or a professional person.*[1] As an actual or aspiring doctor of physical therapy student it is important to have a clear understanding of what professionalism entails and the behavioral and clinical expectations the word brings to clinical life.

Catherine Worthingham, PT, PhD, FAPTA, was a giant in the long history of physical therapy, a change agent who was effective, respectful, and honest in her efforts to move the profession forward. Dr. Worthingham was a visionary who demonstrated professionalism and leadership across the domains of physical therapy: movement, advocacy, education, clinical practice, and research.

The highest professional honor which can be bestowed on a physical therapist is the designation of Catherine Worthingham Fellow of the American Physical Therapy Association (FAPTA), which honors Dr. Worthingham and inspires all physical therapists to attain through the highest levels of professional excellence and impact to advance the profession she continuously exemplified. Her prescient statement made in 1965, "As much as we would like to think so, physical therapy is not yet completely recognized as a profession,"[2] challenged the profession to make advancements across all domains to earn the title among health care peers and the public of "profession."

It has been long debated how an occupation becomes a profession, and in fact the term profession is often viewed as a virtual nonconcept due to the ambiguity and nonagreement on its definition.[3] Despite the disagreement on a universal definition, the term profession historically consists of at least four traits[4]:

1. A body of theoretical knowledge.
2. Some degree of professional autonomy.
3. An ethic that the members enforce.
4. Accountability to society.

These four traits are present in physical therapy and we will explore each in this chapter. The chapter will also contain a discussion about the desire for autonomy and autonomous practice and how that desire led the American Physical Therapy Association's (APTA) leadership to develop its current mission and our vision statements. Additionally, there will be a discussion of the APTA code of ethics for the physical therapist, as well as the professionalism in physical therapy: core values and the professional behaviors assessment tool. The content of each document will be explored through the lens of professionalism to assist the reader with his or her continued behavioral and clinical growth and development as a future physical therapist, as well as advancing the profession of physical therapy.

10.1.2 History of Professionalism in Physical Therapy

Autonomy, one of the four traits of a profession, is discussed frequently in the physical therapy literature. Autonomy has received a significant amount of attention beginning in the 1980s with a shift toward managed care.[4] Autonomy has been defined as: "The feeling that the practitioner ought to be allowed to make decisions without external pressures from clients, from others who are not members of his profession, or from his employing organization."[3] Managed care, in a dual-pronged effort to reduce costs and move toward a preventive model of health care management, placed most of the clinical decision making in the hands of the primary care practitioner (PCP)—the gate keeper. The PCP "managed care" through the referral system. The patient could not visit a specialist—such as the physical therapist—without a referral from the PCP without considerable financial penalties. Managed care significantly limited autonomy of health care providers, including physical therapists. Managed care's hard evidence of administrative restriction to the services of the physical therapy profession prompted leadership within APTA to take action to advance the *profession* of physical therapy. This initiative to advance physical therapy led the House of Delegates (HOD) of APTA to adopt Vision 2020.[5] This strategic plan, introduced in 2000, was inclusive of transitioning to a doctoring profession and consisted of six elements: doctor of physical therapy, evidence-based practice, autonomous practice, direct access, practitioner of choice, and professionalism.

In 2003, 3 years after the approval of Vision 2020, APTA's board of directors adopted professionalism in physical therapy: core values (see: http://www.apta.org/ Professionalism/).[6] This document lists seven attributes of professionalism for physical therapists as well as definitions and sample indicators for each. Professionalism is expected by those who are trained to do a job well and is demonstrated when that professional uses skill, good judgment, and polite behavior expected

from a professional. Professionalism is the continual and judicious use of service, advocacy, communication, knowledge, technical skills, self-directed learning and improvement, clinical reasoning, emotions, values, and reflection in daily practice for the benefit of the individual and community being served. The APTA core values delineate the professional obligations of a physical therapist and physical therapist assistant (see ► Table 10.1).

APTA leadership believed that in order to move Vision 2020 forward, "professionalism" needed to be explicitly defined and described. APTA's official position on professionalism begins with clearly stating the expectations that graduate physical therapist educational program should demonstrate in regard to professionalism and professional education. It was APTA's hope that physical therapist professional behaviors could be expressed in a way that would describe the expectations of the individual practitioner in daily practice.[6] In this way, APTA leadership felt that the definition could be universal and applicable

Table 10.1 Professionalism in physical therapy: core values[5]

Core value	Definition
Accountability	Accountability is active acceptance of the responsibility for the diverse roles, obligations, and actions of the physical therapist including self-regulation and other behaviors that positively influence patient/client outcomes, the profession and the health needs of society
Altruism	Altruism is the primary regard for or devotion to the interest of patients/clients, thus assuming the fiduciary responsibility of placing the needs of the patient/client ahead of the physical therapist's self-interest
Compassion/Caring	Compassion is the desire to identify with or sense something of another's experience; a precursor of caring Caring is the concern, empathy, and consideration for the needs and values of others
Excellence	Excellence is physical therapy practice that consistently uses current knowledge and theory while understanding personal limits, integrates judgment and the patient/client perspective, embraces advancement, challenges mediocrity, and works toward development of new knowledge
Integrity	Integrity is steadfast adherence to high ethical principles or professional standards; truthfulness, fairness, doing what you say you will do, and "speaking forth" about why you do what you do
Professional duty	Professional duty is the commitment to meeting one's obligations to provide effective physical therapy services to patients/clients, to serve the profession, and to positively influence the health of society
Social responsibility	Social responsibility is the promotion of a mutual trust between the profession and the larger public that necessitates responding to societal needs for health and wellness

Source: http://www.apta.org/uploadedFiles/APTAorg/About_Us/Policies/Judicial_Legal/ProfessionalismCoreValues.pdf.

to all physical therapists. In an effort to achieve Vision 2020, a task force was developed in 2007 which concisely operationalized the definition of professionalism. The following statement was the result of that charge: "Physical therapists and physical therapist assistants demonstrate core values by aspiring to and wisely applying principles of altruism, excellence, caring, ethics, respect, communication, and accountability, and by working together with other professionals to achieve optimal health and wellness in individuals and communities."[7,8] This document is intended to be used as a tool to help assess and determine areas that student and practicing physical therapists may need to identify, reflect on, expand, and use in clinical practice to facilitate the growth of physical therapy into a profession. Box 10.1 (p.141) provides an opportunity for the reader to explore this effort.

Professionalism in Physical Therapy: Core Values–Self Assessment Activity

Download the self-assessment tool from http://www.apta.org/CoreValuesSelfAssessment/, and follow the directions for completing the document. Once completed, reflect as an individual or group on the following questions:
- On what sample indicators did you or the group consistently score yourself/themselves on the scale at the 4 or 5 levels?
- Why did you or the group rate yourself/themselves higher in frequency for demonstrating these sample behaviors?
- On what sample indicators did you or the group score yourself/themselves on the scale at level 3 or below?
- Why did you or the group rate yourself/themselves lower in frequency for demonstrating these sample behaviors?
- Identify, develop, and implement approaches to strengthening the integration of the core values within your practice environment.
- Establish personal goals for increasing the frequency with which you demonstrate specific sample behaviors with specific core value(s).

Conduct periodic reassessment of your core value behaviors to determine the degree to which your performance has changed in your professionalism maturation.

(Adapted from APTA: http://www.apta.org/CoreValuesSelfAssessment/.)

As a continuation of efforts begun with Vision 2020, APTA (HOD) adopted the vision statement for the Physical therapy profession in 2013. APTA acknowledged that although elements of Vision 2020 are not explicitly mentioned in the current vision or its guiding principles, the values of Vision 2020 remain significant to the successful fulfillment of the new vision.[9] This new vision statement refocused physical therapists to their core clinical function, improving movement: "Transforming society by optimizing movement to improve the human experience."[9] APTA has developed a strategic plan to achieve this vision (see ▶ Fig. 10.1) as well as guiding principles to achieve the vision which demonstrate what the profession and society will look like once this vision is achieved. (All of these documents can be accessed from APTA's website: http://www.apta.org/Vision/.)

Vision 2020

Physical therapy, by 2020, will be provided by physical therapists who are doctors of physical therapy and who may be board-certified specialists. Consumers will have direct access to physical therapists in all environments for patient/client management, prevention, and wellness services. Physical therapists will be practitioners of choice in patients'/clients' health networks and will hold all privileges of autonomous practice. Physical therapists may be assisted by physical therapist assistants who are educated and licensed to provide physical therapist directed and supervised components of interventions.

Guided by integrity, lifelong learning, and a commitment to comprehensive and accessible health programs for all people, physical therapists and physical therapist assistants will render evidence-based services throughout the continuum of care and improve quality of life for society. They will provide culturally sensitive care distinguished by trust, respect, and an appreciation for individual differences.

While fully availing themselves of new technologies, as well as basic and clinical research, physical therapists will continue to provide direct patient/client care. They will maintain active responsibility for the growth of the physical therapy profession and the health of the people it serves.

(Adapted from APTA: APTA Vision Statement for Physical Therapy 2020, HOD P06–00–24–35, House of Delegates Standards, Policies, Positions, and Guidelines, Alexandria, VA, 2009, APTA.)

10.2 Role of Professionalism in Health Care and Physical Therapy

Historically, the study of professionalism until recently was limited to the sociology literature. As the field of health care continues to change and adapt to internal and external variables so has the practice of health care providers. Although payment and reimbursement of services has played an integral role in the formation of more modern health care delivery, other variables have played significant roles. Patients expect a certain "experience" when they seek the advice and care of a health care professional, and physical therapy is no exception. Consider for a moment a recent experience with a health care provider. Was it positive? Was it negative? What factors were considered to determine the quality of this encounter? Was the quality of the encounter defined by outcome, or did the personal experience with the provider impact perceptions of the effectiveness of the encounter? There is a phrase for this type of "soft skill": bedside manner. Student physical therapists and novice physical therapists soon learn that the patient's perception of the quality of services rendered is based on soft skills rather than clinical decision making and outcome. Everyone has an opinion about customer service; not many patients can accurately judge clinical decision making and outcomes. Soft skills are personal attributes or characteristics that allows someone to effectively navigate their environment, interact well with others, and perform well.[10,11] Soft skills, depending on their employment in the clinical setting, may not have an impact on

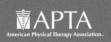

20 18 AMERICAN PHYSICAL THERAPY ASSOCIATION
StrategicPlan

In Pursuit of APTA's Vision for the Profession:
Transforming Society by Optimizing Movement to Improve the Human Experience

The Strategic Plan is the association's roadmap to decisions and actions over the next 3 to 5 years that will move us toward realizing APTA's Vision Statement for the Physical Therapy Profession. It is guided by the vision, the Association Purpose, and the Association Organizational Values and builds on our past successes while *preparing* the association and the profession to thrive in the future.

The Strategic Plan is never "done." APTA reviews the plan regularly and updates as needed through an active, mindful process that looks at environmental changes and member input. By keeping the plan contemporary and relevant, the association better provides representation, services, and community to APTA members.

In 2015, APTA's Board of Directors updated the Strategic Plan to address 3 areas of transformation, in line with the vision: transforming society, transforming the profession, and transforming the association. The plan correlates closely with the 8 guiding principles of the vision: Identity, Quality, Collaboration, Value, Innovation, Consumer-Centricity, Accessibility, and Advocacy.

Keep in mind that the Strategic Plan addresses much of what APTA does, but not everything. Some operational activities aren't mentioned in the plan, yet they do some heavy lifting toward the mission of the association, enabling the activities of the Strategic Plan to continue.

The following objectives and sub-objectives outlined below build upon the 2017 Strategic Plan for work to be completed or. for significant progress to be made in 2018.

TRANSFORM SOCIETY
Barriers to movement will be reduced at population, community, workplace, home, and individual levels.

1	Reform payment policy to allow individuals access to high-quality physical therapist services.
2	Establish mutually beneficial partnerships.
3	Improve society's recognition and understanding of physical therapy and physical therapists.
4	Leverage technology to advance physical therapists' role in enhancing movement.

Fig. 10.1 APTA 2017 strategic plan. (Adapted from: http://www.apta.org/StrategicPlan/Plan/.)

clinical decision making and outcomes; they may camouflage poor clinical decision making and outcomes; or, they can camouflage good clinical decision making and outcomes. In the best of scenarios, soft skills are complementary to clinical skills. Soft skills can include several characteristics such as communication, social skills, and professionalism. The lay public often defines soft skills as "professionalism." The variability in the definition of professionalism between lay persons and clinical persons may lead to unmet customer service expectations. How often do we hear a friend or family member express frustration over a negative experience with a health care provider by saying, "They weren't professional." And how often do we hear from a clinical peer citing a customer service complaint, "I don't understand why my patients are not happy; my outcomes are first rate!"

TRANSFORM THE PROFESSION

Best practices in education will lead to physical therapist practice marked by value and associated with use of evidence, best practice principles, and outcomes research.

1	Further develop and implement strategies to address unwarranted variations in clinical practice, so that physical therapists demonstrate consistency in practice based on outcomes, evidence, and cultural competence.
2	Integrate the movement system as a concept into practice, education, and research.
3	Engage with the Education Leadership Partnership to reduce unwarranted variations in student qualifications, readiness, and performance across the continuum of physical therapist professional education.
4	Provide academic and clinical faculty with quality professional development opportunities and provide PT/PTA programs with updated resources and student assessment tools.
5	Advance diversity and inclusion within the physical therapy profession.
6	Identify roles and promote physical therapist participation in primary care delivery models.
7	Assess current strategies established to advance physical therapy health services and outcomes research.

TRANSFORM THE ASSOCIATION

APTA will be a relevant organization that is entrepreneurial, employing disciplined agility to achieve its priorities.

1	Develop and refine data sources to drive business intelligence in the areas of public affairs, professional affairs, finance, business affairs, and member affairs.
2	Identify the sources and users of physical therapy information in an effort to make APTA the definitive source of such information.
3	Achieve a greater market share of membership.
4	Demonstrate leadership in establishing and adopting best practices in association management.

Fig. 10.1 (Continued)

Developing professional behaviors should be a goal of every student and practicing physical therapist. In 2004, Lopopolo et al conducted a Delphi study to determine knowledge and skills needed by physical therapists entering practice in the areas of leadership, administration, management, and professionalism (LAMP).[12] One of the overwhelming findings of the LAMP study determined professional involvement and ethical practice were highly rated for both areas of needed knowledge and skill. The authors concluded that the student physical therapist and novice graduate (physical therapists) need to appreciate, define, and be able to incorporate into clinical practice information related to being fully involved in the profession of physical therapy to utilize professional behaviors in the practice arena. The authors also recommended the need for focal and targeted guidance for the student and novice therapist to meet expected professional norms.[11]

The questions thus emerge: how does a student or novice therapist develop the skills expected of a professional and how are the quantity and quality of these behaviors assessed? For years, health care professional education programs have been trying to answer these questions. In 1985 Jefferson Medical College developed three instruments to measure professionalism in its medical students, specifically in the area of empathy, collaboration and teamwork (interprofessional health care), and lifelong learning.[13] These instruments continue to be used today in multiple health care disciplines. In fact, the antecedents used in studying these measures by Stern[13] (altruism, attitudes, compassion, empathy, humanism, integrity, lifelong learning, noncognitive attributes, patient–physician relationships, personality, respect for others, and relationships with other members of the health care team) were considered in APTA's 2007 definition of professionalism, which can be found at http://www.apta.org/Professionalism/. The importance of incorporating professionalism in physical therapy education was described by Richardson in 1999. The author counseled on the importance of ensuring physical therapists are equipped with a clear understanding of professional behavior expectations to assist in making intelligent, independent, professional actions.[14] Richardson used the term "professionalize" to describe the action of acting with professionalism.

Novice physical therapists tend to narrow their focus to the clinical intrigues of the patient presentation they are treating and only tangentially consider the behavior aspects of their clinical persona.[14] With the growing complexity of health care today, this narrow view will limit success as a physical therapist. A directed effort is required to assist the novice therapist to realize the impact of professionalism in interacting with patients and to the ultimate clinical outcome.[15,16] According to Richardson: "Taking responsibility for professionalization must be perceived as integral to being a physical therapist and the spur to continual professional development over the professional lifespan."[14]

One way to grow professionalism, previously discussed in this chapter, is the APTA core values checklist. This document can assist the student and/or practicing clinician in developing the skills of professionalism. Utilizing this document in physical therapy education as well as by individual students as part of a reflective practice can help ensure that these behaviors become second engrained in clinical practice. Significant time and focus should be spent during physical therapy education to develop the hard skills of patient examination and treatment and to the soft skills such as professionalism. A survey of physical therapy educators revealed that 98% viewed professionalism as an important component of physical therapy curriculum.[17] Besides using the core values checklist, Box 10.3 (p.144) provides some additional activities that you can do to help promote professional behavior development.

Activities to Help Promote Professional Development   ℹ

- Formal continuing education courses.
- Educational opportunities such as in-services by employers.
- Participation in mentorship opportunities.
- Participation in formal residency/fellowship.
- Accepting additional or new challenges in work positions.
- Research in topics of interest.
- Reading professional journals/participation in journal clubs.
- Exploring additional opportunities as part of the interdisciplinary health care team.
- Involvement in professional association activities and events.
- Clinical specialization.
- Career advancement opportunities.
- Peer-review processes.
- Self-assessment and reflection.
- Post-professional education.
- Study groups.
- Leadership in professional associations.
- Development of a professional portfolio.
- Participation in association-sponsored advocacy.

(Adapted from: Swisher and Page[4])

10.3 Developing A Professional Identity

An assumption exists among professionals that every professional must have a professional identity.[18] Although this may seem intuitive, it is possible that professionals cannot list or thus self-reflect on their professional values and commitments. Professionals are taught to daily reflect on their day's actions: "What did I do well today and what could I improve on?" Areas of success should be dissected to identify and categorize the reason for the success; which decisions and actions led to the success? Areas noted for requiring improvement should also be reflected on and an action plan for remediation should be developed. Though the author of this chapter has not been able to find studies related to frequency of clinical versus behavioral self-reflection one can assume that most practicing therapists tend to reflect more on clinical outcomes rather than professional behaviors. In other words, many professionals either choose not to or cannot purposefully draw on the core of their identity within their profession to identify strengths and weaknesses and thus develop a self-improvement plan.[18] In 2012, Trede et al performed a review of literature regarding professional identity development.[19] The authors concluded that there was little consensus on the definition of professional identity but were able to synthesize three descriptions from the literature. First, professional identity can be defined as the sense of being a professional.[19,20] The authors noted several elements of professionalism that are present during development of an individual's professional identity. Technical skills and interpersonal skills alone are not sufficient to becoming an expert clinical therapist; the professional also needs to embrace the use of professional judgment and reasoning, critical self-evaluation, and self-directed learning in order to fully realize their professional identity.[20] Second, professional identity can be described as a "self-image which permits feelings of adequacy and satisfaction in the performance of an expected role."[21] Adequacy and satisfaction can both be achieved when the professional also includes in his professional role the behaviors that society expects of that individual.[19] For example, most patients expect their physical therapists to be compassionate. When the PT is able to self-realize and develop this trait, the patient therapist collaborative alliance will be facilitated because the therapist is meeting one of the behavioral expectations of the patient. Finally, professional identity is discussed specifically in context of the health professional. It is described as occurring when a member of a profession develops the "attitudes, beliefs, and standards which support the practitioner role and a clear understanding of the responsibilities of being a health professional."[22]

One important requirement for all novice physical therapists is the development of the professional identity. Discourse of the role of the professional identify should begin early in the professional curriculum and continue as a thematic curricular track.[23] Doctor of physical therapy students should be required to formally reflect either in directed discussion by university or the clinical instructor or in journaling as to the professional identity when on clinical internship. The clinical internship permits the student to continue the development of the professional identity, to practice skills related to professional identity, to observe physical therapists modeling professional identity, and to reflect on his professional identity. Reflective practice will facilitate the student therapist's transition from a novice to expert clinician and will be instrumental in continuously developing the professional identity. Without having a clear understanding of self and social image students will not be able to truly develop this professional identity.[23] The activity in Box 10.4 (p. 145) will assist you in starting this personal journey.

Professional Identity

Developing a professional identity is a personal journey that will require a great deal of self-reflection and having a clear understanding of self and your social image.[23] It may be beneficial to begin a professional portfolio or journal that will help you progress as a professional. To assist you in this, take a minute to:

- Create a list of characteristics that you think characterizes the skills and behaviors of a *professional* physical therapist.
- Consider the characteristics (traits) that you observed in a *successful* physical therapist during your clinical observations or internships.
- Reflect on what a *successful* and *effective* physical therapist looks like.

These considerations should act as a launching pad for future reflection along your professional journey as a future physical therapist. Conduct periodic reassessment of your core value behaviors to determine the degree to which your performance has changed in your professionalism maturation.

(Adapter from APTA: http://www.apta.org/CoreValuesSelfAssessment/.)

Professional development is a transformative process. Socialization is a transformative professional development process, which involves clinical instructors, family/friends, nonacademic mentors, and colleagues. Socialization will play a significant role in one's development as a professional.[24,25] This model highlights the importance of personal communities—those individuals beyond the academic program—who will help to shape the professional identity. Take a moment to complete the following exercise: consider individuals who have been extremely strong influences your life up to this point. The influences can be positive or negative. The only requirement is that these influences be sentinel; they stand out for their impact on your development. Socialization is the ability to reflect on these individuals' impact on your life—to dissect and eventually understand why these individuals brought you to the path you are currently journeying. Positive experiences can teach us through role modeling and the reinforcement of proper professional ethics, morals, and ideals. However, negative experiences often have an even more powerful impact if we are able to successfully dissect them and develop corrective or preventive behaviors. When asking students in my entry-level courses what has helped to shape the career path they have chosen, most describe a personal experience with an injury or a family member who required physical therapy care as influential in their decision to become a PT. A number of students also describe a Christian humanism calling to service through concrete works with the poor, sick, and impaired. Some students have observed a therapist working with a patient and noticed the professional way in which he/she dealt with their patient. Individual contacts, relationships, observations, and exemplars all play an important role in the student and novice physical therapist developing a professional identity as a physical therapist. Learning—especially in the development of the professional identity—does not only occur in the formal classroom. Socialization occurs everywhere. We need to keep our eyes and ears open for these experiences, identify them, reflect on them, and use the experience to enrich our professional identity.

10.4 Professional Behaviors

Students in preparation to enter the profession of physical therapy are strongly immersed in coursework with the objective of developing the requisite didactic and psychomotor skills of an expert physical therapist. Courses such as human anatomy, neuroanatomy, neuroscience, clinical skills, modalities, and therapeutic exercise are precisely directed to develop the background scientific knowledge the clinical skills used by therapists. Perhaps not as overt to the student is the curricular content related to the professional identity. Some programs contain courses such as "professionalism," "professional identity," and "professional development" as well as other programs have aspects of the development of the professional identity as in all courses as a continuous theme. As previously discussed in this chapter, APTA strongly supports and encourages the development of the professional identity and while in the professional program your curriculum will provide to you many of the basic concepts of building the identity. However, as the professional program tapers in the third year, all physical therapists must transition from spoon-fed to lifelong learners. Upon graduation, there will no longer be faculty directing your education clinically or professionally; at that point the novice therapist must self-direct the development of his/her professional identity. Novice therapist's attention often is directed toward the first professional position, the licensing examination, payment of student loans, finding new housing and other such practical demands. Oftentimes the requirement to transition to a lifelong learning outlook is forgotten. We must remember that our profession is a science and science never rests. Novel basic science and clinical science research emerges almost daily and changes our practice patterns—and just as frequently, social research, social opportunities, exemplars, and experiences—reshape our professional identity.

Several tools exist to assist the student and novice physical therapist with professional development. "Physical therapy–specific generic abilities" was originally developed in 1991 by the faculty of the University of Wisconsin–Madison physical therapy program. In response to the changing landscape of physical therapy—which has been influenced by economics, enlargement of the scope of practice of physical therapists, Vision 2020, and evidence-based practice—the research team of Warren May, PT, MPH, Laurie Kontney PT, DPT, MS, and Z. Annette Iglarsh, PT, PhD, MBA, updated the PT-Specific Generic Abilities.[26] The updates included data related to the current health policy and on generational differences of the "Millennial" —or "Y" —Generation (born 1980–2000). These are the graduates of the classes of 2004 and beyond who will shape clinical practice in the 21st century.[26] The team initially worked to identify and rank in order professional behaviors expected of the newly licensed physical therapist. Next, they wrote/revised behavior definitions, behavioral criteria and placement within developmental levels (beginning, intermediate, entry level, and postentry level) for the 10 statistically identified behaviors.[26] The updated document, professional behaviors assessment tool (see **Appendix**), was the result. The 10 behaviors identified were actually identical to the original generic abilities; however, the rank orders changed.[26] Another change was in the title of the document itself. It is now referred to as "professional behaviors," not only to differentiate it from the generic abilities but to better reflect the objective of assessing professional behaviors determined to be critical for professional growth and development in physical therapy education and practice.[26]

10.5 Professionalism and Leadership

Leadership has been the topic of many discussions, books, and a significant body of research. Leadership a highly sought and valued commodity.[27] Leadership, despite the broad nature of this topic, belongs in any discussion of professionalism—including physical therapy. Despite the instinctive inclination to promote the importance of leadership skills, a universally accepted definition does not exist. Leadership has been compared to words such as democracy, love, and peace—although we may intuitively know the definition of each word, they can all have different meanings to different people.[27] Many theoretical frameworks exist to help define and characterize leadership and its traits or characteristics. Some popular examples in health care include transformational leadership[28] and servant leadership.[29,30,31] Explanations of the many existing leadership theories is beyond the scope of this text; however, it is recommended that novice professionals become aware of the different traits and characteristics of these leadership styles. Often different leadership styles are required depending on the situation the leader is presented with. Leadership in the profession of physical therapy may take on several appearances. Physical therapists have opportunities to lead, whether it be in the clinic, community, or within the association. APTA's Leadership Development Committee has developed resources to assist physical therapists in improving and developing their leadership skills. One such resource is the core competencies of leadership development.[32] This document has identified four competencies—vision, self, people, and function (see ▶ Fig. 10.2) to assist those who wish to develop their leadership skills. APTA offers a variety of resources grouped according to each of these four competencies to assist therapists to "embrace the responsibilities of leadership to influence growth of the profession of physical therapy" (see http://www.apta.org/LeadershipDevelopment/Recommended Resources/). Additionally, APTA supports and provides many opportunities to develop and advance leadership abilities. For example,

Fig. 10.2 APTA leadership core competencies. (Adapted from: http://www.apta.org/Leadership-Development/.)

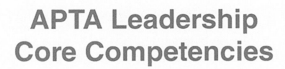

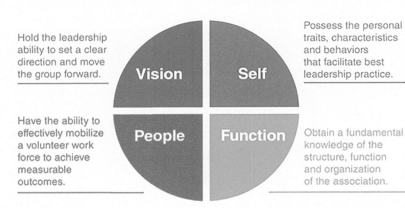

the Health Policy and Administration (HPA) section of the APTA website offers a program entitled the LAMP Institute for leadership in physical therapy (see: http://www.aptahpa.org/?page=57). This program focuses on "leadership development through structured self-assessments of strengths and weaknesses, identification of tools needed to lead successfully, empowerment, and mentoring through applied leadership development projects. These offerings are valuable for all PT professionals (PTs and PTAs) practice owners, clinicians, educators, researchers, and students who want to develop their leadership effectiveness."[33]

10.6 American Physical Therapy Association's Code of Ethics

We have discussed in some detail and provided resources to the student and novice physical therapists in developing the professional identity and to describe the behaviors expected of a professional physical therapist. All health care professions, including physical therapy, govern themselves through a code of ethics that helps to guide and measure professional behaviors.[34] The first code of ethics for our profession was introduced in 1936, 15 years after the first organizational meeting of the American Woman's Physiotherapeutic Association, APTA's precursor.[35] This document has undergone significant changes, modifications, and updates over the years. The most recent version of the code of ethics for the physical therapist (see http://www.apta.org/ uploadedFiles/ APTAorg/About_Us/Policies/Ethics/CodeofEthics.pdf) was adopted in 2009 by the HOD, and went into effect on July 1, 2010. According to this document, its purpose is to[36]

1. Define the ethical principles that form the foundation of physical therapist practice in patient/client management, consultation, education, research, and administration.
2. Provide standards of behavior and performance that form the basis of professional accountability to the public.
3. Provide guidance for physical therapists facing ethical challenges, regardless of their professional roles and responsibilities.
4. Educate physical therapists, students, other health care professionals, regulators, and the public regarding the core values, ethical principles, and standards that guide the professional conduct of the physical therapist.
5. Establish the standards by which APTA can determine if a physical therapist has engaged in unethical conduct.

The code of ethics is comprehensive, but is not exhaustive. The preamble of the document is transparent to this fact stating that not every situation can be addressed and recommends advice or consultation on matters not discussed. Within the Code of ethics document, there are eight "principles" along with very specific and comprehensive definitions for each. APTA offers many resources to help clarify the interpretation and use of this document (see http://www.apta.org/Ethics/Core/). ▶ Table 10.2 provides a brief summary.

Table 10.2 Brief description of the APTA code of ethics for the physical therapist[36]

Principle	Core value	Take home message
Physical therapists shall respect the inherent dignity and rights of patients/clients	Compassion, integrity	PTs respect each patient or client without bias, recognizing their own personal biases and doing their best to prevent those biases from affecting patient/client care
Physical therapists shall be trustworthy and compassionate in addressing the rights and needs of patients/clients	Altruism, compassion, professional duty	PTs respect patients' and clients' autonomy by giving them the information they need to make informed decisions. Furthermore, the PT helps patients and clients with their decision making, and both the PT and the PTA—the latter in collaboration with the PT—protect the patient's or client's confidentiality
Physical therapists shall be accountable for making sound professional judgments	Excellence, integrity	PTs exercise autonomous professional judgment, based on evidence and in collaboration with other health care professionals as necessary
Physical therapists shall demonstrate integrity in their relationships with patients/clients, families, colleagues, students, research participants, other health care providers, employers, payers, and the public	Integrity	PTs are expected to act with integrity in relationships with patients, coworkers, students, and any other vulnerable individuals. PTs are responsible for protecting vulnerable populations from harmful or potentially harmful behaviors
Physical therapists shall fulfill their legal and professional obligations	Professional duty, accountability	PTs recognize that their legal and professional or ethical responsibilities may extend beyond what is required by practice acts and into the moral realm to protect patients, colleagues, and society
Physical therapists shall enhance their expertise through the lifelong acquisition and refinement of knowledge, skills, abilities, and professional behaviors	Excellence	PTs must stay current in enhancing their knowledge and skills. Furthermore, PTs must support patient care with evidence-based interventions
Physical therapists shall promote organizational behaviors and business practices that benefit patients/clients and society	Integrity, accountability	PTs accept responsibility for their actions, support full disclosure, and avoid employment relationships that prevent them from fulfilling their responsibilities to patients
Physical therapists shall participate in efforts to meet the health needs of people locally, nationally, or globally	Social responsibility	PTs help provide services to people whose access to physical therapy is limited. PTs and PTAs also accept use services responsibly and help people understand the benefits of physical therapy

Source: Kirsch NR. New and Improved. PT—Magazine of Physical Therapy. Available at: http://www.apta.org/PTinMotion/2009/10/EthicsinPractice/. November, 2009. Accessed January 16, 2017.

10.7 Review Questions

1. A profession typically includes which of the following traits?
   a) A body of theoretical knowledge.
   b) Some degree of professional autonomy.
   c) An ethic that members enforce.
   d) All of the above.
2. "Autonomy" in the professional research is best defined by which statement?
   a) That members of the organization are permitted to make decisions without external pressure from clients, from nonprofessional members, and from the employing organization.
   b) Freedom to bill insurance companies directly.
   c) Freedom to treat clients without a referral.
   d) The ability to operate one's business independently.
3. The new vision statement for physical therapy reads?
   a) Transforming society by optimizing movement to improve the human experience.
   b) Direct access for all.
   c) Equal pay for equal work.
   d) Professionalism in health care.
4. Most research related to professionalism is published in which type of literature?
   a) Psychology.
   b) Sociology.
   c) Physical therapy.
   d) Computer science.
5. With regard to clinical care, which of the following characteristics is considered a "soft skill"?
   a) Range of motion measurements.
   b) Manual muscle testing.
   c) Communication.
   d) Wound debridement.

10.8 Review Answers

1. A profession typically includes which of the following traits?
   d. All of the above.
2. "Autonomy" in the professional research is best defined by which statement?
   a. That members of the organization are permitted to make decisions without external pressure from clients, from nonprofessional members, and from the employing organization.
3. The new vision statement for physical therapy reads?
   a. Transforming society by optimizing movement to improve the human experience.
4. Most research related to professionalism is published in which type of literature?
   b. Sociology.
5. With regard to clinical care, which of the following characteristics is considered a "soft skill"?
   c. Communication.

References

[1] Professionalism. Merriam-Webster website. Available at: https://www.merriam-webster.com/dictionary/professionalism. Accessed December 21, 2016

[2] Worthingham CA. Complementary functions and responsibilities in an emerging profession. Phys Ther. 1965; 45(10):935–939

[3] Forsyth PB, Danisiewicz TJ. Toward a theory of professionalization. Work Occup. 1985; 12(1):59–76

[4] Swisher LL, Page CG. Professionalism in Physical Therapy: History, practice, & development. Philadelphia, PA: Elsevier Health Sciences; 2005

[5] APTA. Available at: http://www.apta.org/vision2020/. Accessed July 30, 2017

[6] Professionalism in Physical Therapy. Core Values. Available at: http://www.apta.org/uploadedFiles/APTAorg/About_Us/Policies/Judicial_Legal/ProfessionalismCoreValues.pdf. Updated July 27, 2012. Accessed December 16, 2016

[7] Professionalism for the Physical Therapist. Available at: https://www.apta.org/Professionalism/. Updated November 22, 2015. Accessed December 15, 2016

[8] Ries E. The Power of Professionalism: What's in a Word? A term with profound implications for patients, PTs, the profession, and society. Available at: http://www.apta.org/PTinMotion/2013/9/Feature/PowerofProfessionalism/. September, 2013. Accessed December 15, 2016

[9] Vision Statement for the Physical Therapy Profession and Guiding Principles to Achieve the Vision. Available at: http://www.apta.org/Vision/. September 9, 2016. Accessed December 29, 2016

[10] Cruess SR, Johnston S, Cruess RL. Professionalism for medicine: opportunities and obligations. Med J Aust. 2002; 177(4):208–211

[11] Lippman LH, Ryberg R, Carney R, Moore KA. Workforce connections key "soft skills" that foster youth workforce success: toward a consensus across fields. Child Trends.. 2015; 24:1–56

[12] Lopopolo RB, Schafer DS, Nosse LJ. Leadership, administration, management, and professionalism (LAMP) in physical therapy: a Delphi study. Phys Ther. 2004; 84(2):137–150

[13] Stern DT. Measuring Medical Professionalism. New York, NY: Oxford University Press; 2006:19

[14] Richardson B. Professional development: professional socialisation and professionalisation. Physiotherapy. 1999; 85(9):461–467

[15] Olsen SL. Teaching treatment planning. A problem-solving model. Phys Ther. 1983; 63(4):526–529

[16] Schon DA. The Reflective Practitioner. London. Maurice Temple Smith; 1991

[17] Davis DS. Teaching professionalism: a survey of physical therapy educators. J Allied Health. 2009; 38(2):74–80

[18] Trede F. Role of work-integrated learning in developing professionalism and professional identity. Asia-Pac J Coop Educ. 2012; 13(3):159–167

[19] Trede F, Macklin R, Bridges D. Professional identity development: a review of the higher education literature. Stud High Educ. 2012; 37(3):365–384

[20] Paterson M, Higgs J, Wilcox S, Villeneuve M. Clinical reasoning and self-directed learning: key dimensions in professional education and professional socialisation. Focus Health Prof Educ. 2002; 4(2):5–21

[21] Ewan C. Becoming a doctor. In: Cox K, Ewan C, eds. The Medical Teacher. Edinburgh: Churchill Livingstone. 1988: 83–7

[22] Higgs J. Physiotherapy, professionalism and self-directed learning. Journal of the Singapore Physiotherapy Association.. 1993; 14:8–11

[23] Davis J. The importance of the community of practice in identity development. Internet J Allied Health Sci Pract. 2006; 4(3):1–8

[24] Sweitzer VB. Towards a theory of doctoral student professional identity development: a developmental networks approach. J Higher Educ. 2009; 80 (1):1–33

[25] Weidman JC, Twale DJ, Stein EL. Socialization of graduate and professional students in higher education: a perilous passage. ASHE-ERIC High Educ Rep. 2001; 28(3)

[26] May W, Kontney L, Iglarsh Z. Professional Behaviors for the 21st Century. Available at: http://www.marquette.edu/physical-therapy/documents/ProfessionalBehaviors.pdf. Published 2010. Accessed January 15, 2017

[27] Northouse PG. Leadership: Theory and Practice. 6th ed. Thousand Oaks, CA: Sage Publications; 2013

[28] Burns JM. Leadership. New York, NY: Harper & Rowe; 1978

[29] Greenleaf RK. The Servant as Leader. Westfield, IN: The Greenleaf Center for Servant Leadership; 1970

[30] Greenleaf RK. The Institution as a Servant. Westfield, IN: The Greenleaf Center for Servant Leadership; 1972

[31] Greenleaf RK. Servant Leadership: A Journey Into the Nature of Legitimate Power and Greatness. Westfield, IN: The Greenleaf Center for Servant Leadership; 1977

[32] Leadership Development. Available at: http://www.apta.org/LeadershipDevelopment/. Accessed January 15, 2017

[33] LAMP Leadership Development Certificate Program. HPA section of the APTA website. Available at: http://www.aptahpa.org/?page=57. Accessed January 16, 2017

[34] Greenfield B, Jensen GM. Beyond a code of ethics: phenomenological ethics for everyday practice. Physiother Res Int. 2010; 15(2):88–95

[35] Kirsch NR. Bringing Us Up To Code. PT—Magazine of Physical Therapy. Available at: http://www.apta.org/PTinMotion/2009/10/EthicsinPractice/. October, 2009. Accessed January 16, 2017

[36] Code of Ethics for the Physical Therapist. American Physical Therapy Association website. Available at: http://www.apta.org/uploadedFiles/APTAorg/About_Us/Policies/Ethics/ CodeofEthics.pdf. Updated July 1, 2010. Accessed January 16, 2017

Appendix

Professional Behaviors Assessment

DeSales University Physical Therapy Program

Student Name _____ Semester _____

Advisor _____

Directions: 1. Read the description of each Professional Behavior.

2. Become familiar with the behavioral criteria described in each of the levels.

3. Self assess your performance continually, relative to the Professional Behaviors, using the behavioral criteria.

4. To complete this form:

a) Using a Highlighter Pen, highlight all criteria that describes behaviors you demonstrate in Beginning (column 1), Intermediate (column 2), Entry Level (column 3) or Post-Entry Level Professional Behaviors.

b) Identify the level within which you predominately function.

c) Document specific examples of when you demonstrated behaviors from the highest level highlighted.

d) For each Professional Behavior, list the areas in which you wish to improve.

5. Schedule a meeting with your faculty advisor to review your professional behaviors and complete your professional development plan.

**Professional Behaviors were developed by Warren May, Laurie Kontney, and Annette Iglarsh (2010) as an update to the Generic Abilities.

Fig. 10.3

1. Critical Thinking: The ability to question logically; identify, generate and evaluate elements of logical argument; recognize and differentiate facts, appropriate or faulty inferences, and assumptions; and distinguish relevant from irrelevant information. The ability to appropriately utilize, analyze, and critically evaluate scientific evidence to develop a logical argument, and to identify and determine the impact of bias on the decision making process.

Beginning Level:	*Intermediate Level:*	*Entry Level:*	*Post-Entry Level:*
Raises relevant questions Considers all available information Articulates ideas Understands the scientific method States the results of scientific literature but has not developed the consistent ability to critically appraise findings (i.e. methodology and conclusion)	Feels challenged to examine ideas Critically analyzes the literature and applies it to patient management Utilizes didactic knowledge, research evidence, and clinical experience to formulate new ideas Seeks alternative ideas Formulates alternative hypotheses	Distinguishes relevant from irrelevant patient data Readily formulates and critiques alternative hypotheses and ideas Infers applicability of information across populations Exhibits openness to contradictory ideas Identifies appropriate measures and determines	Develops new knowledge through research, professional writing and/or professional presentations Thoroughly critiques hypotheses and ideas often crossing disciplines in thought process Weighs information value based on source and level of evidence

Fig. 10.3 (*Continued*)

Recognizes holes in knowledge base Demonstrates acceptance of limited knowledge and experience in knowledge base	Critiques hypotheses and ideas at a level consistent with knowledge base Acknowledges presence of contradictions	effectiveness of applied solutions efficiently Justifies solutions selected	Identifies complex patterns of associations Distinguishes when to think intuitively vs. analytically Recognizes own biases and suspends judgmental thinking Challenges others to think critically

I function predominantly in the **beginning/intermediate/entry/post entry** *level*

Examples of behaviors to support my self-assessment:

Fig. 10.3 (*Continued*)

Regarding this Professional Behavior, I would like to improve in the following ways:

2. Communication: The ability to communicate effectively (i.e. verbal, non-verbal, reading, writing, and listening) for varied audiences and purposes.

Beginning Level:	*Intermediate Level:*	*Entry Level*	*Post-Entry Level:*
Demonstrates understanding of the English language (verbal and written): uses correct grammar, accurate spelling and	Utilizes and modifies communication (verbal, non-verbal, written and electronic) to meet the	Demonstrates the ability to maintain appropriate control of the communication exchange with	Adapts messages to address needs, expectations, and prior knowledge of the audience to maximize learning

Fig. 10.3 (*Continued*)

expression, legible handwriting	needs of different audiences	individuals and groups	Effectively delivers messages capable of influencing patients, the community and society
Recognizes impact of non-verbal communication in self and others	Restates, reflects and clarifies message(s)	Presents persuasive and explanatory verbal, written or electronic messages with logical organization and sequencing	Provides education locally, regionally and/or nationally
Recognizes the verbal and non-verbal characteristics that portray confidence	Communicates collaboratively with both individuals and groups	Maintains open and constructive communication	Mediates conflict
Utilizes electronic communication appropriately	Collects necessary information from all pertinent individuals in the patient/client management process	Utilizes communication technology effectively and efficiently	
	Provides effective education (verbal, non-verbal, written and electronic)		

*I function predominantly in the **beginning/intermediate/entry/post entry** level*

Fig. 10.3 (*Continued*)

Examples of behaviors to support my self assessment:

Regarding this Professional Behavior, I would like to improve in the following ways:

Fig. 10.3 *(Continued)*

3. Problem Solving: The ability to recognize and define problems, analyze data, develop and implement solutions, and evaluate outcomes.

Beginning Level:	Intermediate Level:	Entry Level	Post-Entry Level:
Recognizes problems	Prioritizes problems	Independently locates, prioritizes and uses	Weighs advantages and disadvantages of
States problems clearly	Identifies contributors to problems	resources to solve problems	a solution to a problem
Describes known solutions to problems	Consults with others to clarify problems	Accepts responsibility for implementing solutions	Participates in outcome studies
Identifies resources needed to develop solutions	Appropriately seeks input or guidance	Implements solutions	Participates in formal quality assessment in
Uses technology to search for and relocate resources	Prioritizes resources (analysis and critique of resources)	Reassesses solutions	work environment
Identifies possible solutions and probable outcomes	Considers consequences of possible solutions	Evaluates outcomes	Seeks solutions to community health-related problems
		Modifies solutions based on the outcome and current evidence	Considers second and third order effects of solutions chosen
		Evaluates generalizability of current evidence to a particular problem	

Fig. 10.3 (Continued)

*I function predominantly in the **beginning/intermediate/entry/post entry** level*

Examples of behaviors to support my self assessment:

Regarding this Professional Behavior, I would like to improve in the following ways:

Fig. 10.3 *(Continued)*

4. Interpersonal Skills: The ability to interact effectively with patients, families, colleagues, other health care professionals, and the community in a culturally aware manner.

Beginning Level:	Intermediate Level:	Entry Level:	Post-Entry Level:
Maintains professional demeanor in all interactions	Recognizes the non-verbal communication and emotions that others bring to professional interactions	Demonstrates active listening skills and reflects back to original concern to determine course of action	Establishes mentor relationships
Demonstrates interest in patients as individuals	Establishes trust	Responds effectively to unexpected situations	Recognizes the impact that non-verbal communication and the emotions of self and others have during interactions and demonstrates the ability to modify the behaviors of self and others during the interaction
Communicates with others in a respectful and confident manner	Seeks to gain input from others	Demonstrates ability to build partnerships	
Respects differences in personality, lifestyle and learning styles during interactions with all persons	Respects role of others	Applies conflict management strategies when dealing with challenging interactions	
	Accommodates differences in learning styles as appropriate		

Fig. 10.3 (*Continued*)

Maintains confidentiality in all interactions Recognizes the emotions and bias that one brings to all professional interactions		Recognizes the impact of non-verbal communication and emotional responses during interactions and modifies own behaviors based on them	

I function predominantly in the **beginning/intermediate/entry/post entry** *level*

Examples of behaviors to support my self assessment:

Fig. 10.3 *(Continued)*

Regarding this Professional Behavior, I would like to improve in the following ways:

---

5. Responsibility: The ability to be accountable for the outcomes of personal and professional actions and to follow through on commitments that encompass the profession within the scope of work, community and social responsibilities.

Beginning Level:	Intermediate Level:	Entry Level:	Post-Entry Level:
Demonstrates punctuality Provides a safe and secure environment for patients Assumes responsibility for actions	Displays awareness of and sensitivity to diverse populations Completes projects without prompting Delegates tasks as needed	Educates patients as consumers of health care services Encourages patient accountability Directs patients to other health care	Recognizes role as a leader Encourages and displays leadership Facilitates program development and modification

Fig. 10.3 (Continued)

| Follows through on commitments Articulates limitations and readiness to learn Abides by all policies of academic program and clinical facility | Collaborates with team members, patients and families Provides evidence-based patient care | professionals as needed Acts as a patient advocate Promotes evidence-based practice in health care settings Accepts responsibility for implementing solutions Demonstrates accountability for all decisions and behaviors in academic and clinical settings | Promotes clinical training for students and coworkers Monitors and adapts to changes in the health care system Promotes service to the community |

I function predominantly in the **beginning/intermediate/entry/post entry** *level*

Fig. 10.3 (*Continued*)

Examples of behaviors to support my self assessment:

Regarding this Professional Behavior, I would like to improve in the following ways:

Fig. 10.3 *(Continued)*

6. Professionalism: The ability to exhibit appropriate professional conduct and to represent the profession effectively while promoting the growth/development of the Physical Therapy profession.

Beginning Level:	*Intermediate Level:*	*Entry Level:*	*Post-Entry Level:*
Abides by all aspects of the academic program honor code and the APTA Code of Ethics Demonstrates awareness of state licensure regulations Projects professional image Attends professional meetings Demonstrates cultural/generational awareness, ethical values, respect, and continuous regard for all classmates,	Identifies positive professional role models within the academic and clinical settings Acts on moral commitment during all academic and clinical activities Identifies when the input of classmates, co-workers and other healthcare professionals will result in optimal	Demonstrates understanding of scope of practice as evidenced by treatment of patients within scope of practice, referring to other healthcare professionals as necessary Provides patient/family centered care at all times as evidenced by provision of patient/family education, seeking patient input and informed consent for all aspects of care and	Actively promotes and advocates for the profession Pursues leadership roles Supports research Participates in program development Participates in education of the community Demonstrates the ability to practice effectively in multiple settings

Fig. 10.3 (*Continued*)

162

| academic and clinical faculty/staff, patients, families, and other healthcare providers | outcome and acts accordingly to attain such input and share decision making Discusses societal expectations of the profession | maintenance of patient dignity Seeks excellence in professional practice by participation in professional organizations and attendance at sessions or participation in activities that further education/professional development Utilizes evidence to guide clinical decision making and the provision of patient care, following guidelines for best practices Discusses role of physical therapy within the healthcare system and in population health | Acts as a clinical instructor Advocates for the patient, the community and society |

Fig. 10.3 (*Continued*)

		Demonstrates leadership in collaboration with both individuals and groups	

I function predominantly in the **beginning/intermediate/entry/post entry** *level*

Examples of behaviors to support my self assessment:

Regarding this Professional Behavior, I would like to improve in the following ways:

Fig. 10.3 *(Continued)*

7. Use of Constructive Feedback: The ability to seek out and identify quality sources of feedback, reflect on and integrate the feedback, and provide meaningful feedback to others.

Beginning Level:	Intermediate Level:	Entry Level:	Post-Entry Level:
Demonstrates active listening skills Assesses own performance Actively seeks feedback from appropriate sources Demonstrates receptive behavior and positive attitude toward feedback Incorporates specific feedback into behaviors Maintains two-way communication without defensiveness	Critiques own performance accurately Responds effectively to constructive feedback Utilizes feedback when establishing professional and patient related goals Develops and implements a plan of action in response to feedback	Independently engages in a continual process of self-evaluation of skills, knowledge and abilities Seeks feedback from patients/clients and peers/mentors Readily integrates feedback provided from a variety of sources to improve skills, knowledge and abilities Uses multiple approaches when	Engages in non-judgmental, constructive problem-solving discussions Acts as conduit for feedback between multiple sources Seeks feedback from a variety of sources to include students/supervisees/ peers/supervisors/patients Utilizes feedback when analyzing and updating professional goals

Fig. 10.3 (*Continued*)

	Provides constructive and timely feedback	responding to feedback Reconciles differences with sensitivity Modifies feedback given to patients/clients according to their learning styles	

I function predominantly in the **beginning/intermediate/entry/post entry** *level*

Examples of behaviors to support my self assessment:

Fig. 10.3 *(Continued)*

Regarding this Professional Behavior, I would like to improve in the following ways:

8. Effective Use of Time and Resources: The ability to manage time and resources effectively to obtain the maximum possible benefit

Beginning Level:	*Intermediate Level:*	*Entry Level:*	*Post-Entry Level:*
Comes prepared for the day's activities/responsibilities Identifies resource limitations (i.e.	Utilizes effective methods of searching for evidence for practice decisions	Uses current best evidence Collaborates with members of the team to maximize	Advances profession by contributing to the body of knowledge

Fig. 10.3 (*Continued*)

information, time, experience)	Recognizes own resource contributions	the impact of treatment available	(outcomes, case studies, etc)
Determines when and how much help/assistance is needed	Shares knowledge and collaborates with staff to utilize best current evidence	Has the ability to set boundaries, negotiate, compromise, and set realistic expectations	Applies best evidence considering available resources and constraints
Accesses current evidence in a timely manner	Discusses and implements strategies for meeting productivity standards	Gathers data and effectively interprets and assimilates the data to determine plan of care	Organizes and prioritizes effectively
Verbalizes productivity standards and identifies barriers to meeting productivity standards	Identifies need for and seeks referrals to other disciplines	Utilizes community resources in discharge planning	Prioritizes multiple demands and situations that arise on a given day
Self-identifies and initiates learning opportunities during unscheduled time		Adjusts plans, schedule etc. as patient needs and circumstances dictate	Mentors peers and supervisees in increasing productivity and/or effectiveness without decrement in quality of care

Fig. 10.3 (Continued)

		Meets productivity standards of facility while providing quality care and completing non-productive work activities	

*I function predominantly in the **beginning/intermediate/entry/post entry** level*

Examples of behaviors to support my self assessment:

Regarding this Professional Behavior, I would like to improve in the following ways:

Fig. 10.3 (*Continued*)

9. Stress Management: The ability to identify sources of stress and to develop and implement effective coping behaviors; this applies for interactions for: self, patient/clients and their families, members of the health care team and in work/life scenarios.

Beginning Level:	Intermediate Level:	Entry Level:	Post-Entry Level:
Recognizes own stressors	Actively employs stress management techniques	Demonstrates appropriate affective responses in all situations	Recognizes when problems are unsolvable
Recognizes distress or problems in others	Reconciles inconsistencies in the educational process	Responds calmly to urgent situations with reflection and debriefing as needed	Assists others in recognizing and managing stressors
Seeks assistance as needed	Maintains balance between professional and personal life	Prioritizes multiple commitments	Demonstrates preventative approach to stress management
Maintains professional demeanor in all situations	Accepts constructive feedback and clarifies expectations	Reconciles inconsistencies within professional, personal and work/life environments	Establishes support networks for self and others
	Establishes outlets to cope with stressors	Demonstrates ability to defuse potential	Offers solutions to the reduction of stress
			Models work/life balance through health/wellness

Fig. 10.3 (*Continued*)

		stressors with self and others	behaviors in professional and personal life

I function predominantly in the **beginning/intermediate/entry/post entry** *level*

Examples of behaviors to support my self assessment:

Regarding this Professional Behavior, I would like to improve in the following ways:

Fig. 10.3 *(Continued)*

10. Commitment to Learning : The ability to self-direct learning to include the identification of needs and sources of learning; and to continually seek and apply new knowledge, behaviors, and skills.

Beginning Level:	Intermediate Level:	Entry Level:	Post-Entry Level:
Prioritizes information needs Analyzes and subdivides large questions into components Identifies own learning needs based on previous experiences Welcomes and/or seeks new learning opportunities Seeks out professional literature	Researches and studies areas where own knowledge base is lacking in order to augment learning and practice Applies new information and re-evaluates performance Accepts that there may be more than one answer to a problem Recognizes the need to and is able to verify solutions to problems	Respectfully questions conventional wisdom Formulates and re-evaluates position based on available evidence Demonstrates confidence in sharing new knowledge with all staff levels Modifies programs and treatments based on newly-learned skills and considerations	Acts as a mentor not only to other PT's, but to other health professionals Utilizes mentors who have knowledge available to them Continues to seek and review relevant literature Works towards clinical specialty certifications Seeks specialty training Is committed to understanding the

Fig. 10.3 *(Continued)*

Plans and presents an in-service, research or cases studies	Reads articles critically and understands limits of application to professional practice	Consults with other health professionals and physical therapists for treatment ideas	PT's role in the health care environment today (i.e. wellness clinics, massage therapy, holistic medicine) Pursues participation in clinical education as an educational opportunity

*I function predominantly in the **beginning/intermediate/entry/post entry** level*

Examples of behaviors to support my self-assessment:

Fig. 10.3 (*Continued*)

Regarding this Professional Behavior, I would like to improve in the following ways:

Professional Development Plan:

Based on my self-assessment of my progress toward these Professional Behaviors, I have

identified the following areas for improvement and I am setting the following goals:

Fig. 10.3 *(Continued)*

To accomplish these goals, I will take the following specific actions:

By my signature below, I indicate that I have completed this self-assessment and sought

feedback from my faculty advisor.

Student Signature: _____

Date: _____

Advisor feedback/suggestions:

Advisor signature: _____

Date: _____

Fig. 10.3 (Continued)

11 Acquisition of a First Job

Julie M. Skrzat

Keywords: Licensure, interview, first professional position, organizational culture, salary, benefits, mentorship, orientation

Chapter Outline

1. Overview
2. Licensure
   a) Licensure Exam Preparation
3. First Job
   a) Where to Start
   b) Other Considerations
   c) Job Search
   d) Application Process
   e) Scheduling the Interview
   f) Preparing for the Interview
   g) Day of Interview
      1. What to Wear
      2. What to Bring to the Interview
      3. Potential Employer Questions
      4. Potential Applicant Questions for the Interviewer
      5. After the Interview
      6. Acceptance
4. Conclusion

"I am a professor in a large Doctor of Physical Therapy (DPT) educational program in the midwest. I have been asked to write this first-person account for this chapter. After much deliberation, I decided to write about the National Physical Therapy Examination (NPTE). Perhaps no other aspect of the entire entry level DPT educational process produces as much anxiety among students. I believe, after preparing hundreds of students for the licensure examination, I have come up with a bit of conventional wisdom that I wish to share with the reader.

"Even after thirty years of practice I still cringe a bit when the NPTE is mentioned. I remember my anxiety as I entered the test-taking arena as if it were yesterday. A typical examination within the professional program provokes some anxiety but nothing as profound as the NPTE. Perhaps this is because most DPT courses have multiple assessment tools; performing poorly in one can be remediated by a good performance in the next. However, the NPTE is dichotomous: pass or fail. There is no method of remediating the grade. Plus, everyone—friends, family, fellow students, and faculty—knows you are taking the exam and are intimately interested in your outcome. Passing leads to much joy and celebration. Failing... well, let's not go there.

"With common curricula, common accreditation standards, numerous ongoing didactic and clinical assessments, and numerous clinical internships—each student who successfully completes one of these challenging programs has the tools to excel on the NPTE. The question must be asked: why do students fail the NPTE? The numbers of failures are not insignificant. Students do fail.

"I believe students fail for two reasons. The first is the obvious reason: lack of preparation. The NPTE is a comprehensive examination. There is no way a student can remember all the esoteric facts learned over three years without restudying. In preparation for the NPTE students need to develop a systematic, encompassing study algorithm which touches all content taught in the professional program—and the plan must be carried out. I have never met a new graduate from my program who didn't have the goal of months of studying for the NPTE. However, I have met many students who failed to carry out their plan of study. Freedom from the rigors of the classroom, part-time jobs, relationships, vacations, unread novels and unseen movies, and binge television watching can all derail the best study plan.

"The second—and often more overlooked—reason why students fail to pass the NPTE is test-taking anxiety. Today, we are all well aware that anxiety can negatively impact decision making and cognitive recall. The sympathetic nervous system outflow—the sweating, cold hands, rapid heart rate—can all impact test taking. Avoiding anxiety is easier said than done. Taking practice tests in environments similar to the testing center surely helps. Knowledge of a strong preparation plan also helps. However, the biggest enemy of anxiety is confidence. Know you are well-prepared! Believe you will do well! Have faith in your academic preparation!

"Get in there and pass!"

—Arnold Z., Chicago, Illinois

11.1 Overview

As a new graduate, finding the correct position in the correct location and with the correct salary and the correct benefits may seem daunting. Rather than feeling overwhelmed, the new graduate should feel a sense of opportunity and excitement as the realization that the years of formal, spoon-fed education are nearing an end and a new and exciting professional life chapter is dawning. The first job search provides the new graduate with an opportunity to formally reflect on the challenges and successes of the past and to consider, often with the aid of mentors, the professional future.[1] Rarely does life provide such an impressive jumping-off point as it does between the end of formalized education and the first professional position. Graduation from the professional program is a period of changes: from a customer of the educational system to a provider of health care services; from a spoon-fed learner to a self-directed learner; from following to leading; from little responsibility and decision making to an ability to charter one's future; with personal accountability transitioning from the doctor of physical therapy (DPT) program to the clinical patient; and, from the role of "student" where expenses greatly exceed income to "wage earner" where, hopefully, income exceeds expenses. During periods of great social and professional upheaval, as exampled by the transition from student to licensed therapist, the new graduate, to maintain proper perspective, should focus on his mission—to serve the poor, sick, impaired, disabled and disenfranchised by the performance of physical therapy services. Remember that the mission is more important than the arena in which it is delivered, the salary earned, the benefits awarded, and professional companionship found. To solidify and reinforce one's mission, the period of graduation is an excellent time to rewrite the personal mission statement and keep it nearby as the transition unfolds. The mission statement is the compass which will assist in keeping the professional aims and goals in view and prevent dilution from life's many confounding variables.

11.2 Licensure

Prior to practicing physical therapy, the graduated DPT is required to obtain a temporary or permanent state license to practice physical therapy in the jurisdiction of practice. The purpose of becoming a licensed clinician is to "meet and maintain prescribed standards" established by the jurisdiction's (state's) regulatory board of physical therapy.[2] Licensure assists to ensure the public that the therapist providing evaluation, assessment and intervention is qualified at the entry level criteria determined by the Commission on Accreditation in Physical Therapy Educational to serve the public via the provision of physical therapy services.[2] General guidelines for licensure can be found at http://www.apta.org/Licensure/.

One of the main tools used by a state's regulatory entity to determine if a physical therapist (PT) or physical therapist assistant (PTA) meets the entry-level criteria is the national physical therapy exam (NPTE) of the Federation of State Boards of Physical Therapy (FSBPT).[2] The NPTE is "competency specific" and covers the entire scope of physical therapy practice. The PT exam and the PTA exam contain questions about theory, examination and evaluation, diagnosis, prognosis, treatment intervention, prevention, and consultation. An exam blueprint is developed yearly by the FSBPT to determine the percentage of questions on the NPTE pertaining to each aspect of physical therapy practice.[2] Every graduate of a physical therapy or physical therapist assistant education program must receive a passing score on the NPTE to become a licensed PT or licensed/certified PTA (or to regain licensure/certification if lapsed) in the United States.[3] Licensure is state specific with each state having a unique practice act detailing the scope of physical therapy practice in that state. Therapists may be licensed in more than one state.

As of 2017, the NPTE is a computer-administered examination. The PT licensure examination has five sections each with 50 questions. Of the 250 multiple-choice questions, only 200 are scored. The other 50 questions are being pre-tested to determine validity and reliability for possible inclusion in future examinations. The PTA licensure examination has four sections with a total of 200 multiple-choice questions. As in the PT examination, 50 of these questions are being pre-tested and are not scored. The scoring ranges from 200 to 800. The minimum passing score is 600 for both the PT and PTA exam. Further information can be found at http://www.apta.org/Licensure/NPTE/ and https://www.fsbpt.org.

Licensure is managed by the individual state boards.[2] Depending on which state a new graduate plans to practice, temporary licensing may not be available; therefore, passing the national licensing exam is necessary in order to practice. Practice Acts for all 50 states, the District of Columbia, Puerto Rico, and the Virgin Islands can be found at http://www.apta.org/Licensure/StatePracticeActs/.

"As a graduate from a moderately sized DPT program in a major eastern city I feel I was fortunate in that our Department Chairperson and her Administrative Assistant actively supported and guided the entire licensure process for our class. Our Program graduates every May and we targeted the July date for our licensure examination. During a meeting the previous January our chairperson provided the students with a very specific timeline of events leading up to the NPTE including what needed to be done, the date it needed to be done, and who needed to do it. Our chairperson met with us weekly from January to May to help us with the process.

"To help us prepare for the actual NPTE our program contracted with an outside study group to assist in our preparation. Three full days were scheduled where the outside group prepped us for the exam. We were told about the test, reviewed major content areas, learned test-taking techniques, were given a practice textbook, and all took a practice exam. The exam was graded the day we took it and we were given feedback about our scores in each content area. The practice test was probably the most beneficial for me. I thought my strongest clinical area was cardiopulmonary but the teste results indicated that I needed to improve my knowledge in this key content area.

"I took the test in July and passed!"

—Jackie C., Philadelphia, Pennsylvania

11.2.1 Licensure Exam Preparation

Preparation for the licensure exam is a relatively complex process. The school conferring the DPT degree to the new graduate will notify the FSBPT of each individual student's planned graduation. The DPT student will then receive an email from the FSBPT with instruction to create an account. Once the DPT degree has been officially conferred by the university or college, the university or college will notify the FSBPT of the successful conferral. The FSBPT will then notify the graduate that he or she may register for the NPTE. Once registered for the NPTE through the FSBPT, the new graduate must also notify the jurisdiction (state) in which he or she plans to practice. Appropriate vetting is performed by the jurisdiction prior to granting approval to sit for the examination. Once the FSBPT *and* jurisdiction have approved the request to sit for the NPTE, the new graduate will receive an Authorization to Test (ATT) communication from the FSBPT and the jurisdiction. The new graduate is then permitted to schedule a test date. The FSBPT grades the examination and reports the grade to the jurisdiction. If the new graduate's score meets the minimum passing grade, a license to practice in the jurisdiction is issued. Testing occurs four times per year—January, April, July, and October.[4] FSBPT and the state boards of physical therapy have strict criteria regarding when retakes can occur and how often they can be taken.

Once this process has been understood, the new graduate should work backward to determine a timeline for a plan of study. A number of study aids, including practice tests, study guides, and tutorials, are available through the FSBPT and commercial vendors to assist in preparation for the NPTE. DPT program directors often counsel the program's students on which materials are most valid and helpful in preparation for the NPTE. Many programs sponsor review sessions prior to the examination.

11.3 First Job

Acceptance of the first professional position initiates a career trajectory that the new graduate will most likely follow for some time. In the best of all worlds, the first professional position should provide a strong orientation to professional life, skilled and compassionate mentorship, a challenging but not overwhelming work environment, time for reflection, opportunities for ongoing professional education, and assistance in learning and practicing behavioral skills which will compliment clinical expertise.[1] The first job allows the new graduate to self-examine and reflect on his preparedness and capacity as a professional and to determine which behavioral and clinical skills require further develop to permit maximal contribution to society and to one's career goals.[1]

> "Upon graduation I decided to postpone my job search until I passed the NPTE. Graduation was in early June and the NPTE was scheduled for late July so I only had eight weeks for full-time studying. Fortunately, I passed the boards on my first try.
>
> "Unlike many of my classmates I was unsure of where I wanted to work. I was unsure of the arena of physical therapy (outpatient, inpatient, pediatrics, geriatrics). There were so many choices and I loved them all. I was sure that I wanted to stay in the Baltimore area, which would allow me to move back home to save on rent and thus facilitate the repayment of my loans.
>
> "A faculty member gave me some advice which I remember. He said if we were unsure of the arena of physical therapy in which we wished to practice to identify three or four mentors from the field of PT and meet individually with each one to discuss our future. I chose two faculty members and two previous clinical instructors. We met individually over a period of a week over coffee and I was amazed at not only the cogent advice they offered, but how, with their experience, they 'saw' things differently than I and gave me a terrific perspective on my future. They all helped me realize that employment in an acute care tertiary care hospital is what would benefit me the most."
>
> —Paul V., Baltimore, Maryland

We reside in a free society. In the majority of cases—save for those with contractual or legal obligations—we are free to leave a position and organization for one which may better benefit us professionally, geographically, academically, financially, and from a quality-of-life viewpoint. Few physical therapists remain at their first professional position for their entire professional career. Therefore, the question often arises: How long should I stay at my first job if it does not meet my expectations? There is no easy answer. Certainly, if a new employee finds his new organization acting unethically or illegally, there is every reason

for a quick resignation. One should never risk one's reputation or license for a sense of loyalty to an employer. Because all work histories should be included on a resume, potential future employers may question the short time frame of employment at a specific site. This should be explained by a narrative describing that the short duration of employment was due to a "value issue" with the employer. There is no need (and potential legal danger in) detailing the specific reasons for the resignation. This act will not be held against the applicant.

A less clear situation is when the first position, for subtler reasons, does not meet the needs of the new graduate and an offer of employment at another organization is suddenly available. What is the correct time frame to stay with the first organization: 3 months, 6 months, a year, or more? Traditionally, employment at the first job should be maintained for at least a year. From the employer's perspective, the organization spent a good deal of time and capital in recruiting, hiring, and training the new employee and does deserve the respect of the new employee providing the organization with every opportunity to improve conditions. The first job is often the first professional position one may take, and therefore the new graduate may have an incorrect or blurred perspective of what professional work is really like. Time is often required to assimilate perspective into reality. In addition, resigning from a position after a few months of employment because "I was offered a better position (or money, or hours, or location)" is not something the hiring entity wishes to hear.[5]

> "As a physical therapy director in a large acute medical rehabilitation hospital, one of the scenarios that really upsets me is when new graduates accept a position in my department (or any physical therapy department department) and after a few months resign to take a similar position with a competitor. Some graduates do not realize that accepting a position is an agreement between both parties: the employer and the therapist. As the employer I agree to pay the therapist, provide benefits, pay for his compliance checks, orient him, provide mentorship, develop a professional plan of advancement, and slowly—through training and supervision—bring his work load up to full productivity. This may take three to six months. The hired therapist agrees to work hard, follow policies, be trained, and utilize good customer service skills with his clients.
>
> "Last month, a new hire—she hadn't been with us for more than two months—tendered her resignation. When asked why she was resigning she told me that a hospital across town was offering a higher salary. She loved working for me but 'could not turn down the extra money—you know, with school loans and stuff.' I can fully appreciate when new graduates resign new positions based upon personal problems or social issues, ethical or legal concerns, or simply unhappiness with the work environment. Things happen. But to leave to make a few extra dollars, after the employer spent so much time and money to train the new employee without the employee reciprocating by staying with us for at least a year... well, I personally find that unprofessional."
>
> —M. Wilding, Raleigh, North Carolina

11.3.1 Where to Start

There are a multitude of job options available to the physical therapist. These options include part-time, full-time, or per diem employment; the geographic location of practice; the arena of physical therapy in which to practice such as acute care, orthopedic outpatient, school-based physical therapy, and home care; and the professional pathway in which one wishes to travel: clinical, academia, or administration. The most traditional route is for the new graduate to take a clinical position where classroom knowledge can be transitioned to direct patient care. This clinical pathway can lead to further opportunities such as clinical specialization and residency. Clinical practice can assist the new graduate with identifying a patient population for future specialization. The clinical pathway also provides an immediate revenue stream to assist with student loan payments.

The academia pathway is a strong calling for many physical therapists. The term "academia" relates to obtaining a faculty position at a college or university. Along with teaching, most academicians also perform some level of research. Though there are academics with the DPT degree, most academics have returned to the university to obtain a nonclinical doctorate degree, such as the PhD. The PhD offers additional benefits in academia as compared with the DPT including, for many universities, the ability to obtain tenure, promotion, and funding for research projects.

With health care being a hierarchical industry there are ample opportunities for administrative positions especially in larger clinical facilities. These positions may be in physical therapy such as ownership of a private practice, managing a physical therapy site in a large hospital system, and managing a particular program within a larger setting such as lymphedema services or wheelchair clinic, or they may be in health care management, such as a hospital vice president, nursing home administrator, or CEO. Administrators in health care may have a clinical degree such as the DPT, an administrative/ management degree such as the master's in business administration (MBA), or both degrees. Often the dual degree is most beneficial. The MBA prepares the applicant for the rigors of management such as human resources, finance, and accounting, and the clinical degree provides the applicant with a broad understanding of clinical medicine. If the new graduate believes an administrative position is of future interest perhaps obtaining a first position with the possibility of upward mobility should be a consideration.

With the many professional options afforded the new physical therapy graduate consideration should be directed to developing, along with a personal mission statement, a 5-year professional action plan (see ▶ Fig. 11.1). The 5-year professional action plan consists of the step-by-step actions with a timeline in order to facilitate reaching one's ultimate professional goals.

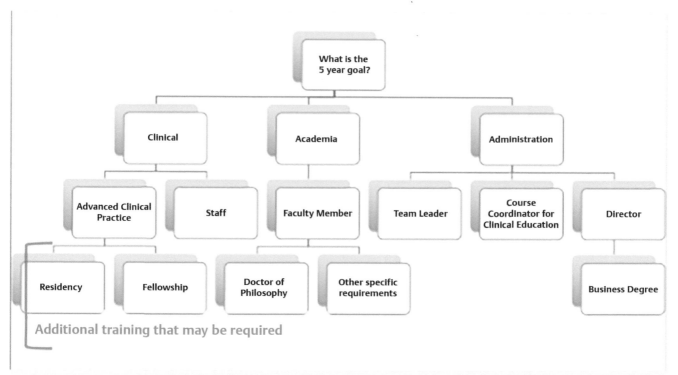

Fig. 11.1 The development of a 5-year professional plan. At graduation from the professional program and perhaps every 2 years thereafter during the course of a professional career, physical therapists, with the assistance of reflection, self-directed learning, and mentorship, develop a 5-year professional plan. The 5-year professional plan provides a mechanism for the development of a concrete map of professional growth.

"At the urging of one of my faculty members back in DPT school I developed a 5-year professional plan at graduation. I wrote it myself but asked a number of mentors to review it and discuss it with me. This is what we produced:

1. Year 1
   a) Pass licensure board examination in New Jersey.
   b) Obtain a staff physical therapist position at a large outpatient facility where I could concentrate my clinical practice in women's health.
   c) Join the APTA and the Women's Health Section.
   d) Attend the Combined Sections Meeting (CSM).
2. Year 2
   a) Continue to gain experience in women's health.
   b) Join a Women's Health Special Interest Group.
   c) Attend CSM.
   d) Decide whether to continue to pursue women's health as my area of concentration.
3. Year 3
   a) If I decide to pursue a career in women's health apply for a position in a Women's Health residency.
   b) Continue to gain clinical experience.
   c) Offer myself as a lab assistant in a local DPT program to investigate my enjoyment of teaching.
4. Year 4
   a) Begin my Women's Health residency.
   b) Continue clinical work through the residency under the supervision and mentorship of my residency faculty.
5. Year 5
   a) Complete the Residency.
   b) Pass the specialization examination.
   c) Obtain a full time clinical position in women's health.
   d) If I enjoy teaching, begin to investigate PhD programs."

—Candace B., New York, New York

When selecting a career pathway consider the following questions listed in ▶ Table 11.1 to aid in the decision. To assist with developing the 5-year professional plan, therapists should utilize the clinical decision-making tree for career pathway to facilitate reflection on professional growth. APTA has also developed a resource entitled "Considerations for Practice Opportunities and Professional Development" and is available at http://www.apta.org/CareerManagement/ConsiderationsforOpportunities/?navID=10737421106. In addition, when beginning the first job search, identify and meet with three to four trusted mentors who are well-acquainted with the new graduate's strengths and weaknesses and who also have a broad understanding of the profession of physical therapy. Mentors can provide advice on choosing the professional pathway, offer insight about job prospects in specific geographic locations, and offer cogent counsel on working in the various arenas of physical therapy practice. In addition,

Table 11.1 Clinical decision-making tree for career pathway

Clinical	Academic	Administration
What type of setting do I want to practice in?	What am I interested in studying?	Why do I want to be a leader?
Am I interested in a particular patient population?	Why am I interested in studying this?	What skills do I have to be a leader?
Are resources, including equipment, available to meet my practice needs?	What institutions provide such a program?	Do I have any leadership experience? If so, what did I do well? What are areas to improve on?
What mentorship is offered through the position?	Which faculty are involved in the program?	Based on past experiences, what are good and bad characteristics of an administrator?
What, if any, other team members will I be working with?	Is the faculty member of interest recently published or productive in the field?	
What are the professional growth opportunities?		
What is required to advance up the clinical ladder?		

meeting with trusted mentors external to the profession of physical therapy may provide an opportunity for the new graduate to listen to unique and unbiased viewpoints.

11.3.2 Other Considerations

Once the career pathway is confirmed, there are additional considerations which may impact the first job search. These include the following:

- Geographic location.
- Arena of practice.
- Organization culture and reputation.
- Workplace environment (fast vs. slow placed, etc.).
- Orientation program.
- Mentorship availability.
- Professional growth opportunities such as specialization, promotion, and continuing education.
- Human resource benefits, including medical/dental insurance, retirement plans, disability insurance, life insurance, and other associated things.
- Family, friends, and personal beliefs.

This list is not inclusive, and must be modified on an individual basis.

"When looking at possible first jobs do not exclude culture from the decision-making equation. Like most small community hospitals my workplace is struggling financially, but I applaud leadership for its openness and willingness to work with the employees. From my first day here, I have been amazed at the altruism and empathy of the staff. Everyone works hard. People help each other. The patient definitely comes first. My supervisor works harder than everyone and she keeps telling us that her job is to make our job easier. She leads and supports the staff. We may not have the coolest equipment. Our continuing education budget is small. The carpet in our waiting room needs replacement. But I am proud of what we are doing and I love my coworkers. I have been here five years and have no intention of leaving. How wonderful to go home each evening feeling I am doing good work and supported by administration and my coworkers in my efforts. I will never forget when my mom died unexpectedly two years ago the chief of the medical staff stopped by the funeral and hugged me."

—Jenny M., Philadelphia, Pennsylvania

Geographic location relates to the location in the United States (or world) that the new graduate prefers to work. Fortunately, unlike many industries, health care services can be accessed with minimal commute from just about everywhere in the United States' large cities, small cities, rural areas, north, south, east, west, coastal, mountains—all have health care services. Therefore, choosing a geographic area in which to reside is not based on the availability of work but rather one's preference of where one wishes to live. In addition, with the current need for physical therapists in practically all geographic locations, jobs are relatively plentiful.[6]

There are an amazing number of arenas of health care where physical therapy is practiced. While enrolled in a DPT educational program, the clinical internships provide the student with a number of opportunities to experience physical therapy services in multiple arenas. Broadly, arenas of physical therapy practice are divided into inpatient and outpatient services (though some arenas provide both). Examples of inpatient arenas of practice include acute care, acute medical rehabilitation, skilled nursing facility, subacute facility, nursing home, long-term acute care hospital, specialty hospital such as children's or maternity hospital, hospice, and critical access hospital. Outpatient arenas include general outpatient practice, specialty practice such as lymphedema, wound care, and pediatrics, home care, school-based therapy, and multidisciplinary clinic practice such as wheelchair clinic and prosthetic/orthotic clinic. Some arenas of physical therapy practice are nonclinical such as academia, research, consultant, or insurance company case reviewer.

Organizational culture and organizational reputation deal with the implicit and explicit "curriculum" of organization. Organization culture deals with the written and unwritten rules of the organization. Written rules begin with the mission and vision statements and extend to specific organizational policies and procedures. Unwritten rules include those esoteric but important items, such as: do employees take long lunches, do employees gossip about the boss, do employees come in on weekends, do employees socialize together, and do managers manage with a centralized or decentralized style? Organizational reputation is how the public perceives the organization. Is it a good place to work or bad? Are the quality of the organization's products and services well respected in the community? Organizational reputation is easily gauged by talking with customers of the company. Organizational culture, especially for the applicant, is very difficult to measure unless the applicant has friends in the organization or the applicant performed an internship at the organization. Potential applicants often ask permission to observe for a day in order to better understand an organization's culture.

Though the services and products offered in rehabilitation departments are relatively consistent, there are obvious differences in the pace of services offered from arena to arena and clinic to clinic. Pace is often measured through a productivity index. Productivity index is the volume of work, measured in patients seen or interventions performed, required by each practicing therapist per day. Some therapists enjoy working in a high-volume clinic while other therapists prefer a slower-paced environment. Failure to meet the organization-specific productivity index may lead to punitive measures. Applicants should always inquire about productivity indexes during the interview process.

"As a new graduate I had heard of 'productivity indexes' but I guess I did not appreciate the magnitude of the impact of these numbers on my daily work life. On graduation I accepted a position in a national chain outpatient physical therapy organization. We are in 33 states and have well over 100 sites. We are for-profit. Our productivity index is a relatively complex model. A specific number of 'points' is given for initial evaluation and a lesser number of points is given for treatment. Certain treatments such as lymphedema and wound care are given a higher percentage of points than other treatments such as modalities and therapeutic exercise. Each morning in my email I receive notification from my supervisor of my productivity numbers from the day before, week to-date, month to-date, and year to-date. Also included are my variances from the expected norms. In our office is a banner with the entire department's year-to-date productivity score. (You can see that productivity is a big thing here!) If I exceed the expected productivity over the year I receive a bonus; if I am below the expected productivity the effect may be no bonus or raise or even being placed on probation. On clinical internship I was only concerned about making the correct clinical decisions; now, along with the clinical side of things I need to constantly think of how busy I am. I guess I understand the aim of a productivity index but I am not sure I think it is the best way to measure the quality of an employee. One of my coworkers is not the best PT; her outcomes are not very good but she works hard and she always exceeds her productivity. For this reason, she is well respected by our administration and is paid much better than me."

—Robert K., Nashville, Tennessee

Orientation and mentorship programs are formal, facility-developed educational programs designed for the new graduate to assist with easing the new employee's transition to the organization. Orientation programs are typically one to four weeks in duration and include a thorough review of organizational policies and procedures, a facility tour, review of the mission and vision statements and scope of care, introduction to all staff members, education related to computer software and hardware, and the performance of mandatory competency learning activities required by accreditation standards. A mentorship program is the assignation of an experienced staff member to partner with the new employee to guide the employee through the first 6 months of employment. The mentor formally meets with the new employee weekly to answer any arisen questions and to provide counsel with problematic issues. A strong orientation and mentorship program are highly valued concepts among most new employees.

Professional growth as exampled by promotion availability, ongoing educational opportunities, and additional responsibilities is highly valued by physical therapists. Larger organizations tend to offer more promotional opportunities as compared with smaller organizations. Most jurisdictions of practice require a specific number of continuing education credits in order to maintain licensure. Will the potential work environment offer support for continuing education? Will the environment offer paid time off for employees to attend these courses? These activities can be very expensive. Will the organization support an employee's attempt at gaining specialization?

Lastly, personal beliefs and the opinions of friends and family will influence work decisions. Examples of work place variables which may impact personal beliefs include such items as not for profit versus for profit organization, religious versus secular ownership, and the willingness of the organization to provide free medical care for those uninsured or underinsured. Friends and family influences are important especially if the job offer requires relocation, weekend and holiday work, and limited vacation or sick benefits.[1]

To assist with prioritization of these variables, a worksheet shown in ▶ Table 11.2 has been created to assist the new graduate in rank-ordering these variables based on importance to the new graduate. As the therapist nears graduation and begins to consider arenas and locations of the first professional position, this worksheet is helpful to rank order a number of variables. Rank ordering of these variables will assist in narrowing the position search. Rank ordering provides two opportunities for the new graduate searching for the first professional position. First, it is a method to assist the new graduate with reflection on one's personal goals related to the work environment, and second, the table can be used to compare and contrast various organizations in meeting the applicant's personal goals.

11.3.3 Job Search

When the new graduate has selected a pathway, geographical area, and arena of practice, the next step is to search for a position that meets those criteria. New graduates should search opportunities offered through current and past clinical instructors, faculty mentors, colleagues, and professional and job websites. Specific websites include, but are not limited to

- APTA red hot jobs (http://www.apta.org/apta/hotjobs): This website allows searches based on job category (i.e., director,

Table 11.2 Rank ordering of important job variables for the new graduate

Criteria	Things I must have[1]	Things I would like to have[2]	Things to which I am indifferent[3]
Geographic location			
Arena of practice			
Organization culture and reputation			
Workplace environment (fast vs. slow placed, etc.)			
Orientation program			
Mentorship availability			
Productivity standards			
Professional growth opportunities such as specialization, promotion, and continuing education			
Human resource benefits, including medical/dental insurance, retirement plans, disability insurance, life insurance, and other associated things			
Family, friends, and personal beliefs			

faculty, academic, PT, etc.), practice setting (i.e., acute care hospital, inpatient rehab, private practice, etc.), practice area (i.e., cardiopulmonary, neurology, pediatrics, etc.), job type (i.e., full time, part time, etc.), and/or state.
- APTA virtual career fair for PTs and PTAs (http://www.apta.org/VirtualCareerFair/).
- Specific organizations' websites: Once pathway, geographic location, and practice setting are identified, specific institutions and organizations within the area can be located. Search the organization's website to identify if there are job openings. Many organizations, due to the costliness of advertising online, in journals, and in newspapers, only advertise job openings on their websites.
- Indeed (www.indeed.com).
- Monster (www.monster.com).

When searching, map each organization's characteristics on the Rank Ordering of Important Job Variables Form to permit comparison.

11.3.4 Application Process

Most cover letters and resumes are submitted to organizations electronically. The actual "application" is often completed at the interview. Most DPT and PTA professional programs include education related to cover letter and resume content and formatting. If additional guidance is needed, the APTA's *Career Resources for Current Students*—http://www.apta.org/Current-Students/Employment/—has a curriculum vitae (CV) template.

Always have mentors review the cover letter and resume for content, grammar, spelling, formatting, and syntax prior to submission. Do not rely on spell-check programs to identify all errors. A cover letter and resume submitted with errors always reflects poorly on the applicant.

11.3.5 Scheduling the Interview

The timeframe for a submitted cover letter and resume to be reviewed by an organization is variable—often based on the imperative of the need of the organization to fill the position. Applicants should not become discouraged if weeks or even a month passes between submission and notification of an interview decision. Larger companies tend to require longer times to review cover letters and resumes than smaller companies due to the complex hierarchy.

Applicants benefit by the knowledge that organizations spend much time and capital to review resumes, schedule interviews, research references, and interview candidates.[7] If granted an interview, the organization perceives a benefit to taking the time and spending the money to interview the candidate. Therefore, the candidate should take advantage of this opportunity by preparing for the interview.

11.3.6 Preparing for the Interview

Preparation prior to the actual interview enhances the possibility of a job offer.[8] The applicant should realize that his or her resume impressed human resources sufficiently to facilitate the offer of the interview but simply because an offer to interview was made does not indicate that an offer of employment is forthcoming. Organizations often choose three to five applicants to interview meaning that each applicant has, at best, a 33% chance of an offer for employment. The percentage chance of an offer of employment can increase significantly with a strong interview preparation plan.

The first preparatory act is simply to confirm as quickly as possible the plan to attend the interview. Rapidity of response is the first "behavioral metric" about the applicant the organization will collect. Organizations value promptness as an employee's attribute. Ensure that the organization will only witness in person, via e-mail, by telephone, or by written communication, the highest ethical and moral professional behavior. The second preparatory act is for the applicant to familiarize himself or herself with the mission, vision, scope of care, and history of the organization. A standard question asked by interviewers to applicants is why the applicant chose this company as part of the job search. Quoting the mission and vision of the organization and how it relates to one's personal goals is an excellent way of answering this question. Verbally quoting the mission and vision of the organization is a wonderful exemplar of the applicant's interest in the organization.

Preparation for the actual interview is difficult because, in most cases, the applicant is not aware of the type of interview which is planned. There are a variety of interview techniques available to an organization. Currently, the most commonly utilized technique is the behavioral interview. A behavioral interview is where the organization asks for responses related to applicant potential or past experiences. Potential behavioral interview questions may include the following:

- How would you handle a situation where a coworker had alcohol in his breath?
- Provide an example of an occasion when you used logic to solve a problem.
- Give an example of a goal you set for yourself and the plan you used to achieve it.
- Give an example of a goal you did not meet and how you handled the frustration of not achieving it.
- Describe a stressful situation which occurred within the past month and how you handled it.
- Tell me about how you worked effectively under pressure.
- How do you handle a challenge?
- Have you been in an employment situation where you didn't have enough work to do?
- In school if you performed unexpectedly below what you expected on an examination, what actions did you take?
- Describe a decision you made that was unpopular and how you handled implementing it.
- Have you ever dealt with company or classroom policy you weren't in agreement with? How did you handle this?
- If a coworker was doing something unethical how would you handle it?
- Have you gone above and beyond the call of duty? If so, then how? When you worked on multiple projects how you did prioritize?
- How do you handle a situation in which you are given an aggressive timeline for accomplishment?
- Give an example of how you set goals and achieve them.
- What do you do when your schedule is interrupted? Give an example of how you handle it.
- Have you had to convince a team to work on a project they weren't thrilled about? How did you do it?
- In school I am sure you were on many teams. Discuss a situation where the team was floundering and how you helped the team meet its goals.
- Have you handled a difficult situation with a coworker? Describe the situation and tell me how you resolved the issue.
- Share an example of how you were able to motivate employees or coworkers.
- Give an example of when you did or when you did not listen.
- Provide an example of how you handled a difficult situation with a supervisor? How?
- What do you do if you disagree with your boss?
- How would you react if a clerk at a local supermarket insulted you?

The behavioral method of interviewing assumes that the physical therapy candidate either possesses or can learn the necessary clinical skill set to practice based on the organization's mission. By using a behavioral interview technique, the organization is attempting to learn if the candidate has the necessary behavioral skills to be successful. Situational interviewing, another common interview technique is where the physical therapy applicant may be provided a simulated patient and asked to perform a segment of the evaluation or intervention process. Often the situational "role play" is recorded for future dissection by the search committee. A free-form interview is where there is no set agenda and the interviewer asks questions based on the applicant's responses. Group interviews are where an applicant may simultaneously meet with three to four representatives of the organization. A serial interview is when an applicant will meet with a number of organizational representatives one after another. Regardless of the interview type always formulate an answer mentally prior to speaking. Respond only to the question asked; do not add unrelated information. Be honest with responses. Lying or withholding integral information from an interview (or on the resume), if discovered, may be cause for later termination. Keep all responses positive. Avoid criticisms of any kind but especially of previous work and educational experiences. It is not necessary to lead off with negative things about your past experiences but timely truthfulness will go a long way in demonstrating solid character to future employers.

11.3.7 Day of the Interview

What to Wear

Proper applicant interview attire is an expectation of an organization. Wearing the correct clothes will not add to the value of an applicant but not wearing the correct clothes may diminish the applicant's value. Wearing the correct attire reinforces the belief that the applicant is professional, is knowledgeable about professional mores, and is taking the interview opportunity seriously. Not only are the correct clothes a marketing tool for the candidate, correct clothes can also boost the interviewee's confidence.

- There is much difference between causal dress, smart casual dress, and professional dress. Search the web for examples of professional dress to reinforce the appropriate attire to wear to the interview.
- When in doubt, err on the side of slightly overdressed.
- Conservative is the key. Do not opt for an outfit which will "stand out" or "make others take notice of me." Avoid the plaid sports coat and floor-length floral print skirts. For men and women, a dark (black, gray, or navy blue) suit, white shirt, and shined shoes are always appropriate. Men's ties should be conservative. Women's shoes should have low to medium heels. If wearing a dress or skirt, the hem length should not be above the knee.
- Ensure clothes are cleaned and pressed.
- Minimize cologne/perfume, do not wear artificial nails (these are banned due to being an infection hazard in most health care arenas), and keep makeup to a minimum. Many persons today use a variety of body art including tattoos, piercings, hair dyes, and asymmetrical haircuts as a message of individuality. This is certainly fine for most occasions but the applicant should remind himself or herself that he or she is interviewing for essentially a customer contact position and, in addition, the supervisors performing the interview may have a different perspective than the applicant as to the definition of professional appearance.
- Fingernails should be clean and well-trimmed. Hair should be styled conservatively. Men's facial hair should be worn neatly and kept trimmed. An import consideration is that the organization is hiring someone to be its face with the public. The applicant should always consider: "If I owned this organization, what type of image would I like my physical therapists

to present to our customers and their families?" and even better: "What type of image do the organization's customers want me, as a prospective employee, to project?"
- Take the sit-down test. Sit in a chair in front of a mirror and ensure that there are no problem areas. If problems are identified, adjust accordingly.

What to Bring to the Interview

The well-prepared applicant will bring a number of items to the interview. The first item is identification. In this post-9/11 world applicants must present a number of forms of identification to potential hirers. Bring originals of the passport, driver's license, and one other form of picture identification. Bring the social security number. Bring a leather-bound agenda, three copies of the resume, three copies of reference contacts, and two pens. Bring the name, address, and contact information of an emergency contact. Lastly, bring a list of potential questions for you, as the applicant, to ask the organization's reputation. Every interviewer, at one point, will ask the interviewee: "Do you have questions for me?" It is best to be prepared with a list of questions.

"I was on clinical internship two states away when I received an email asking me to schedule an employment interview. This was the hospital in my home town—the hospital I had targeted for employment for years. After discussing this opportunity with my clinical instructor, she kindly offered to allow me to miss one day of internship the next week to travel home for the interview. I scheduled the interview for Friday and drove home Thursday evening. I awoke Friday to six inches of fresh snow. The roads were terrible. I called the hospital and asked for human resources and asked if my interview was cancelled. The representative said it was not. I changed into my suit and went out to my car for the ride to the hospital. As I walked onto my driveway I slipped and fell, drenching my suit in snow, slush, and salt. Being a poor college student, I only had one suit so I changed into corduroys and a sweater. I cleaned off my car and drove to the hospital arriving just in time for my interview. The interview with the human resources director went well as did my interview with the Director of Rehabilitation Services. Even though my I felt my interview answers were good and I showed proper deference and interest, I could not help but feel that for want of a clean suit I lost the job. As the Director of Rehabilitation Services walked me to my car we looked at the door and saw the heavy snow still falling. She turned to me and said: 'We interviewed three persons today for the PT spot. You will receive an offer of employment early next week. You were the only interviewee who dressed for the occasion.' As I looked at her I noticed she was wearing corduroys and a sweater."

—Anita B., Rochester, New York

Potential Employer Questions

Regardless of the interview type: behavioral, situational et al, most potential employers will ask a few standard questions.

Formulate and memorize your answers to these simple questions prior to the interview:

- Basic interview
  - Tell me about yourself.
  - What are your strengths?
  - What are your weaknesses?
  - What do you offer that other candidates do not?
- Career development
  - Why are you interested in this position?
  - Why are you interested in working at this company?
  - How do your professional goals align with the company's mission?
  - Where do you see yourself professionally in 5 years?
- Behavioral interview
  - Describe a situation of conflict and how it was resolved.
  - What is your greatest failure and what did you learn from it?
  - Have you ever been on a team where someone was not pulling their own weight? How did you handle it?
  - If I were your supervisor and asked you to do something that you disagreed with, what would you do?
- Other
  - How would you describe your work style?
  - Tell me about your proudest moment.
  - Was there a person in your career who made a difference? If so, why or why not?

Potential Applicant Questions for the Interviewer

Come prepared with questions. Remember, a new graduate is interviewing the organization as much as the organization is interviewing the new graduate. The new graduate needs to ensure this is also a good match for his or her professional goals and growth. Additionally, asking questions shows interest in the company.

- Does the organization offer an orientation and mentorship program to new employees?
- What are the opportunities for professional growth?
- What are the options for advancement within the company? Are the advancements in the clinical or administrative arena?
- What are productivity standards? How are they calculated? What are the implications for therapists meeting the standards and not meeting the standards?
- Will I be required to work weekends and holidays?
- If offered the position would I be a salaried or hourly employee?

There are a number of questions to avoid asking potential employers during the interview. These typically involve salary and benefits. Conventionally, these are not mentioned at the interview. If an offer of employment is at a later date to the applicant, the salary and benefits package will be included in the offer. The time between the offer of employment and the decision deadline is the time for the applicant to ask question of the potential employer about salary and benefits.

After the Interview

Write down everything recalled, such as details about patient care, how scheduling is done, clinic dynamics, information about support staff, etc. Additionally, write down personal feelings and impressions. Can you imagine working at such a place? What was the culture? Did the employees appear happy?

Acceptance

Employment decisions usually occur anywhere from a week to 3 weeks after the interview; rarely, if ever, is a decision made and forwarded to the applicant at the interview. If an offer is forwarded, read the offer thoroughly. It may be advised to have an additional person, who you trust, to review as well. Further guidance on employment agreements is found at http://www.apta.org/uploadedFiles/APTAorg/About_Us/Policies/HOD/Employment/studentNewGrad.pdf.

11.4 Conclusion

This chapter provides guidance for the first physical therapist job search once the academic tenure ends. The first job search can easily be overwhelming, but by taking the process one step at a time, the applicant may find it to be professionally enriching and exciting.

Physical therapy is a dynamic profession that truly combines the science of healing and the art of caring. Realize that every job, patient encounter, educational experience, and conference attendance is a stepping stone to your ultimate goal. Take advantage of what is provided to you. Be open minded. Also remember that the job as a physical therapist is a job. And the job, no matter how extrinsically or intrinsically rewarding it is, should never assume the number one spot on the list of important items in one's life. Family, religion or personal philosophy, friends, relationships and the like should occupy the top positions as items of import in one's life. A particular job in a particular location, and to a lesser extent, a career, can always be replaced. These other items cannot.

Lastly, the following are quotes from my colleagues, all of whom have different career trajectories, reflecting on their first job search. Hopefully, their comments will provide counsel, comfort, and opportunity for reflection.

- "Find a setting that supports learning. Find a setting which makes you excited. Find a setting where you feel comfortable. Find a setting with strong mentorship. The first professional position will forever color your professional life."
- "I would suggest new graduates to take their time with the interview and job application process and to maximally ensure that the position is the right one. I would encourage new graduates to ask questions regarding the mentorship opportunities available for both experienced and newer staff members and what types of other opportunities are available (research, committees, community outreach, teaching, etc.). I would also encourage new graduates to ask about the company's clinical ladder and how their specific organization fosters achievement of those tasks as outline within the clinical ladder."
- "Finding a position where the new graduate will be able to grow and receive mentorship is one of the most important attributes of a first professional position. I also believe it important not to expect too much from the first professional position. The academic years often provide a skewed perspective of the first position. Experience teaches us that every position has its benefits and difficulties."

- "The best advice I can provide to the new graduate approaching the first professional position is to work with mentors to determine the arena of physical therapy in which to practice prior to any other actions. Too many new graduates apply to positions via a shotgun approach—apply to every opening. Choose an arena such as home care, acute care, acute medical rehabilitation, outpatient orthopedics and such and only apply those facilities which meet the arena requirement. Comparing like to like is much easier than comparing different arenas."

- "My first position was a bit different from the norm but it worked for me. I took a position as a traveling therapist. I specifically requested acute care placements. Every 13 weeks for my first year and a half as a professional I worked at a different hospital. I was placed in four different states—California, Alaska, Florida, and Georgia—and enjoyed seeing the country. I learned adaptation techniques and learned to be very flexible. I had some great and not-so-great mentors but when I finally returned home for a 'permanent job' I felt extremely well prepared."

Best of luck.

11.5 Review Questions

1. Tools to assist jurisdictions to ensure that new doctor of physical therapy graduates meet the prescribed entry-level criteria include all of the following, except
   a) The national physical therapy examination.
   b) Graduation from an accredited doctor of physical therapy program.
   c) Criminal background check.
   d) All of the above.
2. The national physical therapy exam includes how many "official" questions?
   a) 100.
   b) 150.
   c) 200.
   d) 250.
3. Physical therapist licensure is regulated at which government level?
   a) Federal.
   b) State.
   c) County.
   d) Township.
4. A multitude of employment options are available to physical therapists. Which option includes a typical 40-hour work week and a full benefits package?
   a) Full time.
   b) Part time.
   c) Per diem.
   d) Flex time.
5. For therapists wishing to eventually enter into an administrative/management position, which degree, along with the doctor of physical therapy degree, is most beneficial?
   a) Doctor of philosophy.
   b) Doctor of education.
   c) Masters of business administration.
   d) Bachelors in accounting.

6. A respected and wise person with specialized knowledge in the field of physical therapy, who provides career and professional advice to a physical therapist, is known by which professional term?
   a) Advisor.
   b) Counselor.
   c) Mentor.
   d) Guru.
7. Organizational culture is an important criterion which requires consideration by any potential employee. Organizational culture is defined as which of the following?
   a) The public's perception of the organization.
   b) The sum total of the written and unwritten rules of an organization.
   c) The benefits package offered to new employees.
   d) The willingness of an organization to hire underrepresented minorities.
8. For physical therapists, productivity index can be defined as which of the following?
   a) The typical workload expected to be performed by a clinical therapist.
   b) The therapist's dollar value of salary plus benefits.
   c) The average number of hours worked per week per therapist.
   d) The number of professional publications per therapist per year.
9. Most jurisdictions require licensed physical therapists to accrue a specific number of which item listed below?
   a) Publications.
   b) Paid time off to rejuvenate.
   c) Continuing education credits.
   d) College credits.
10. Which term best expresses the clothing style to wear to a formal employment interview?
    a) Conservative and dark.
    b) Formal wear.
    c) Comfortable.
    d) Bright and modern.

11.6 Review Answers

1. Tools to assist jurisdictions to ensure that new doctor of physical therapy graduates meet the prescribed entry-level criteria include all of the following, except
   d. All of the above.
2. The national physical therapy exam includes how many "official" questions?
   c. 200.
3. Physical therapist licensure is regulated at which government level?
   b. State.
4. A multitude of employment options are available to physical therapists. Which option includes a typical 40-hour work week and a full benefits package?
   a. Full time.
5. For therapists wishing to eventually enter into an administrative/management position, which degree, along with the doctor of physical therapy degree, is most beneficial?
   c. Masters of business administration.

6. A respected and wise person with specialized knowledge in the field of physical therapy, who provides career and professional advice to a physical therapist, is known by which professional term?

   c. Mentor.

7. Organizational culture is an important criterion which requires consideration by any potential employee. Organizational culture is defined as which of the following?

   b. The sum total of the written and unwritten rules of an organization.

8. For physical therapists, productivity index can be defined as which of the following?

   a. The typical workload expected to be performed by a clinical therapist.

9. Most jurisdictions require licensed physical therapists to accrue a specific number of which item listed below?

   c. Continuing education credits.

10. Which term best expresses the clothing style to wear to a formal employment interview?

    a. Conservative and dark.

References

[1] Ree EJ, Weber RJ. What to look for in your first job. Hosp Pharm. 2014; 49(8):773–779

[2] American Physical Therapy Association. Licensure. Available at: www.apta.org/licensure. Accessed December 27, 2016

[3] American Physical Therapy Association. About the National Physical Therapy Examination. Available at: www.apta.org/licensure/NPTE. Accessed December 27, 2016

[4] The Federation of State Boards of Physical Therapy. Exam Candidates. Available at: http://www.fsbpt.org/ExamCandidates.aspx. Accessed December 27, 2016

[5] Forbes. Job Seekers: How to Gracefully Quit Your Job. Available at: http://www.forbes.com/sites/lisaquast/2014/04/14/job-seekers-how-to-gracefully-quit-your-job/#6825df61644c. Accessed January 2, 2017

[6] American Physical Therapy Association. Working Outside the United States. Available at: www.apta.org/careermanagement/workingoutsideus/. Accessed December 27, 2016

[7] Lundy DW. The view from the other side of the desk: what an employer looks for during an interview. J Orthop Trauma. 2013; 27 Suppl 1:S5–S7

[8] Siegel J. Finding your first job in academics: interviewing strategies. J Orthop Trauma. 2011; 25 Suppl 3:S104–S107

12 Evaluating the Job Offer

Deborah Smith Brown

Keywords: Benefits, business expenses, dental insurance, disability insurance, health insurance, hourly versus salary employee, interview, life insurance, pretax benefits, retirement, salary, tax benefits, tax bracket, vacation

Chapter Outline

1. Overview
2. Salary
3. Benefits
   a) Paid Time Off
   b) Health Insurance
   c) Short- and Long-Term Disability
   d) Retirement Plans
   e) Life Insurance
   f) Business Expenses
   g) Continuing Education
   h) Performance Reviews
   i) Job Location
4. Student Loan Repayment
5. Salary and Benefits Review Form

"As a director of human resources at a large Pittsburgh hospital, I have had the opportunity to interview many candidates for physical therapy positions within our hospital. Overall, I have found the candidates well-prepared, professional, and engaging. This aim of this 'First Person' is to provide the reader with a few dos and don'ts of hiring as seen from the human resource director's perspective.

"First, research the company you are applying to. So many of our therapy applicants only have a tangential appreciation of the mission, vision, and scope of care of our hospital. Many do not know that we are a full-service hospital treating persons of all ages. Many applicants believe we are a pediatric hospital. I am amazed that candidates consider a specific place for employment without knowing much about the facility. Look at the website. Talk to employees. Search us in the internet. I always ask our applicants to tell me about this hospital. Too often I receive a blank stare.

"Dress appropriately for the interview. This means business attire: dark suits, white shirts, and polished shoes for men and conservative dark clothes for women. Just last week a candidate arrived for his interview in jeans and a flannel shirt. Next applicant, please!

"Everyone has a resume these days but not everyone has it reviewed by competent friends for spelling, grammatical, and syntax errors. Nothing spoils a good resume more than these types of errors.

"Be on time for the interview. On time is defined as arriving five to ten minutes prior to the scheduled interview time. Arriving too early is almost as bad as arriving late.

"Practice the interview. There are specific questions that all interviewers ask. For instance: Tell me about yourself? Tell me about your strengths? Tell me about your weaknesses? Why do you want to work here? Prepare your answers and practice

orating these answers to friends, classmates, or family prior to your interview.

"Leave your cell phone in the car.

"Bring to the interview an agenda with blank paper, a pen, and extra copies of your resume and references.

"When providing references provide a number of contact methods to reach these persons such as cell phone, email, address, employment address. This makes life much easier for the reference checkers.

"Monitor your body language during the interview. Avoid slouching which may indicate disinterest. Force yourself to make eye contact. Speak slowly and clearly. Do not fidget. Lean forward. Offer a strong but not forceful handshake. Do not cross your legs.

"After the interview thank the interviewer for taking time from his or her busy day to meet with you. Shake hands. As soon as you arrive home write a personal (not email) thank you card to each person who interviewed you. Thank them for their time and consideration and reiterate your strong interest in the position.

"Hopefully, these thoughts will permit the reader to view the interview process from the perspective of the interviewer."

—Rita P., Pittsburgh, Pennsylvania

12.1 Overview

The applicant's goal following application and interview is the offer of a job. The job offer is accompanied by an offer of salary and a benefits package. The salary is the amount of reimbursement the employee will receive either hourly or yearly for the work provided to the organization. The benefits package consists of items either provided to the employee free of charge by the organization or in which the organization assumes partial financial responsibility for the provision of these items. Examples of items within the benefits package include vacation time, sick time, bereavement time, continuing education allowances, retirement benefits, health benefits, and dental benefits. The savvy applicant must be skilled at weighting these extrinsic rewards (salary and benefits package) with the intrinsic rewards (joy of a particular job, self-satisfaction, challenging environment, ability to make decisions) to make the correct job choice. There is much more to evaluating a job offer than simply the comparisons of salary and benefits package. The aim of this chapter is to provide the prospective employee with an outline of methods to evaluate the salary and benefits package offered. Evaluating the intrinsic rewards of one position over another is an individual decision and will not be discussed here.

Following the review of this chapter, the student will be able to

- Outline and define the components of the salary and benefits package.
- Estimate the valued and financial worth of the entire benefits package to facilitate comparison with other offers.
- Discuss methods of the facilitation of reducing educational debt.

12.2 Salary

Employees may be hired as full time, part time, or per diem. Full-time employees work what is considered a "full week," which may be either 36, 37.5, or 40 hours per week. Full-time employees typically receive a full benefits package. A part-time employee is hired to work less than full-time and often the benefits package is prorated based on the number of hours worked per week. Most prorated systems of benefits end with fewer than 20 hours of scheduled work per week; if an employee averages fewer than 20 hours per week there are either no benefits or a very limited array. A part-time employee is typically scheduled a fixed number of hours to work per week. A per diem employee has no scheduled hours but may be "called in" if needed. Per diem employees in physical therapy are often paid more per hour worked than full-time or part-time employees. This small salary bump is in consideration for the lack of benefits offered and lack of guaranteed hours. Often during times of difficulty finding employment, such as in economic downturns or industry changes, employees will accept a part-time or per diem position with hopes of eventually transitioning to a full-time position.

Gross salary does not equal take-home pay. Take-home pay is the gross salary plus additions such as bonuses and awards less deductions for federal, state and local taxes, as well as deductions for benefits provided by your employer that require an employee contribution such as health insurance, dependent care, specific retirement benefits, and so forth. The federal tax brackets as of this writing are shown in ▶ Table 12.1.

Social security tax (6.2%) and Medicare tax (1.45%) along with federal tax will reduce the paycheck by 17.65% before state and local taxes are calculated. The federal withholding tax is not a fixed percentage of income as are Social Security and the Medicare tax. The federal income tax rate depends on each wage earner's tax situation. Individuals with high deductions, such as mortgage interest and real estate taxes, could be in a lower tax bracket even though their gross pay is the same as another individual without those deductions.

Some states and localities collect taxes through a fixed percentage of gross pay while other states and localities use an incremental rate similar to the federal tax system. There are also local services tax and occupational privilege taxes that may be assessed depending on your locality.

Because an employer is not aware of an employee's personal tax situation, the salary portion of the reimbursement package presented at hiring will be as gross salary. True take-home pay will need to be calculated based on the individual tax situation. In some situations, signing bonuses are offered as an incentive to accept an offer of employment. Applicants must realize that this is a one-time payment and will not be included in future year's salary adjustments. For instance, if the organization grants an across-the-board salary increase the following year of 2%, only the employee's prior year salary—and not the additional bonus dollars—will be included in the salary increase calculation. The employee will benefit by beginning employment with a higher salary as compared with a lower salary and a hiring bonus. Over a number of years this accrual of raises based on a higher initial salary may be substantial. Bonuses may be paid at hire, incrementally over the course of the first year, or at the end of the first year of employment. Prior to accepting a signing bonus, understand the terms of the bonus. Check to see if there is a repayment clause if resigning by a specific date.

Potential hires should also be made aware whether they are being hired as a salaried or hourly employee. A salaried employee, also called an "exempt" employee, receives a salary package based on gross salary per year. The gross salary is then disbursed to the employee in equal amounts determined by the number of pay periods per year. For instance, for ease of calculation, if the salary offered is $52,000 per year and the paychecks are disbursed by the organization on a weekly basis, the employee will receive a paycheck with the gross being $1,000 per week. If paychecks are disbursed biweekly, each paycheck's gross will be $2,000. An hourly employee, also called a "nonexempt" employee, is reimbursed for working at an hourly rate. For ease of calculation, if the employee is hired at $20 per hour, if the employee works 40 hours per week, the gross pay per week would be $800 per week. There are additional advantages to each hiring status. Salaried, unlike hourly employees, are not typically required to punch a timeclock. Hourly employees eligible for overtime, shift pay differentials, and holiday pay while salaried employees are not. Salaried employees typically have more freedom than hourly employees in developing their work schedules. Salaried employees are often able to work from home.

Also, inquire about the frequency of the disbursement of paychecks. Companies may pay employees weekly, biweekly, or monthly. The frequency of paycheck disbursement is an important variable in household budgeting. For instance, if only one paycheck is received per month, the employee must be adept at budgeting the income to last for an entire month. In addition, if the paycheck disbursement is monthly, there may, depending on date of hire, be a full month of employment prior to receiving the first paycheck.

12.3 Benefits

The second major component of the reimbursement package is the benefits package. During the past decade, the importance of

Table 12.1 2018 tax brackets (for taxes due April 16, 2019) (IRS.gov)

Tax rate	Single filers	Married filing jointly or qualifying widow/ widower	Married filing separately	Head of household
10%	Up to $9,525	Up to $19,050	Up to $9,525	Up to $13,600
12%	$9,526 to $38,700	$19,051 to $77,400	$9,526 to $38,700	$13,601 to $51,800
22%	$38,701 to $82,500	$77,401 to $165,000	$38,701 to $82,500	$51,801 to $82,500
24%	$82,501 to $157,500	$165,001 to $315,000	$82,501 to $157,500	$82,501 to $157,500
32%	$157,501 to $200,00	$315,001 to $400,000	$157,501 to $200,000	$157,501 to $200,000
35%	$200,001 to $500,000	$400,001 to $600,000	$200,001 to $300,000	$200,000 to $500,000
37%	Over $500,000	Over $600,000	Over $300,000	Over $500,000

the careful evaluation of the benefits package offered has gained significant importance. Historically, the post-World War II employment benefits packages were fairly equal, with the primary variable being vacation hours. However, this practice has changed dramatically in recent years due to the rising cost of health care copays, deductibles, and prescription medicine coverage. A very common mistake among new members of the workforce is to believe that all benefits packages are created equally.

12.3.1 Paid Time Off

An employer is not required by law to offer paid vacation, personal, or sick time. This is a benefit that is offered as a quid pro quo to encourage the retaining of qualified employees. On average, an employee who has been with an organization for 1 year will receive 1 to 2 weeks paid vacation time. Regardless of whether the employee is hired as a salaried or hourly employee, vacation accrual tends to increase with years duration of employment. Personal and sick time offered in the benefits package will be less than the vacation offered. Extended sick time (2–3 or more consecutive days) may require a doctor's note. Vacation, personal, and sick time off may not be given in total on the first day of work, but accrued in increments each week worked over the course of the year. Some employers will permit employees to remain home when sick even without accrued sick days. These days are considered unpaid days. There are often organization rules regarding the use of unpaid days.

Unfortunately, some employees view the benefit of sick days as additional vacation days. For this reason, some employees will "use" all their accrued sick days by the end of the calendar year as vacation days—the once ubiquitous practice of taking "mental health days." To counter this practice, some employers are transitioning to a system of paid time off (PTO). Under the PTO system, employees receive a set number of days to use for vacation, sick, and personal rather than the individual classifications.

In addition to paid vacation, personal, and sick time, an employer may offer paid holidays. If required to work on a holiday, the holiday benefit may be replaced by a day that the employee chooses either during the calendar year or, depending on organization policy, within the same pay-period as the holiday falls. Salaried employees do not receive additional pay for working holiday; oftentimes full-time hourly employees receive additional pay for working the holiday.

When voluntarily leaving employment, unused vacation pay—equivalent to the hours of vacation accrued but unused—must be paid. In most but not all organizations the monetary value of unused sick and personal time is not reimbursable.

There is a law governing unpaid leave, the federal Family and Medical Leave Act (FMLA).[1] This allows qualified employees to take up to 12 weeks of unpaid leave under certain circumstances. FMLA applies to employers with at least 50 employees. A qualified employee is an employee who has worked for the employer for at least a year and has worked for 1,250 hours during the previous 12 months. The employee can take unpaid leave:

- To care for a newborn, an adopted child, or a child placed in the employee's home by the foster care system during the first year of arrival.

- To care for an immediate family member (spouse, child, parent) with a serious mental or physical health condition.
- Because the employee suffers from a serious mental or physical condition that prevents the employee from working.

In addition, many states provide additional benefits through their own family leave programs. As an example, New York governor Andrew Cuomo executed sweeping legislation on April 4, 2016, the New York Paid Family Leave Benefits Law (PFLBL), that raised the minimum wage in New York to $15 an hour *and* provides a phased-in system of paid family leave benefits providing covered employees up to 12 weeks of paid family leave—currently the most comprehensive paid family leave program in the nation. The PFLBL is a series of amendments to the New York State Workers' Compensation Law.[2] When the amendments are fully phased in, covered employees will be eligible for up to 12 weeks of paid family leave annually to care for an infant or a family member with a serious health condition, or to assist with family obligations when a family member is called into active military service. Eligible employees will be paid by a state fund—not their employers—financed by deductions taken directly from employees' wages, not from tax contributions paid by employers. Notably, the paid family leave is not available for an employee's *own* serious health condition, although an employee may be eligible for income protection benefits under New York's existing short-term disability insurance program.[3]

Many organizations provide for bereavement days. Bereavement days may be used in lieu of vacation days. Bereavement days are used in the event of a close family member: to prepare for the funeral, to comfort loved ones, and to grieve. Most organizations offer three bereavement days per year.

12.3.2 Health Insurance

Health insurance is a benefit offered to attract and retain qualified employees. Employer sponsored health insurance, as a standard full-time employment benefit, began in the 1940s as a method of recruiting and retaining skilled employees and by the 1960s became *de rigueur* with full-time employment. In this decade, there has been an emerging paradigm shift where employers are no longer providing full-time employees with a health insurance benefit. The reason for this is the escalating costs of providing health care coverage. Even if the benefit is not withdrawn altogether, many employers are shifting the insurance premiums burden to the employee via limiting plan coverage, increasing deductibles, and increasing copays. If the employer does not offer health insurance to employees the employee is then responsible for obtaining coverage independently of the employer. Purchased individually, health care coverage is extremely expensive due to the lack of purchase discounts available to large purchasers such as major organizations.

Even if the employer offers health insurance as part of the benefits package the premiums the employee is responsible for, even with large buyer discounts, is significant. Therefore, this aspect of the benefits package is not inconsequential. If offered, coverage may vary widely. Of all aspects of the offered benefits package, health insurance coverage requires the most careful review because of the hidden costs to the employee. In an attempt to lower premium costs, employers may require employees to be responsible for a portion of the monthly premiums. This is known as the employee insurance copay and typically ranges from 10 to 50% of the monthly insurance premium and is automatically withheld from the paycheck. The IRS has established Section 125 of the Internal Revenue Code[4] to allow the employee to deduct the payment of insurance premiums and other employee benefits, we will discuss later, on a "pretax" basis. If your employer has established this plan, often called a "cafeteria plan," the employee's federal taxable income will be reduced by the health insurance premiums paid, thus saving on the federal income tax burden.

Insurance companies are also attempting to reduce costs by either limiting benefits or, like the employer, cost shifting to the employee. One method of cost shifting is called the practitioner copay. A practitioner copay is a dollar amount the employee must pay directly to the health practitioner (doctor, specialist, physical therapist, laboratory) prior to the intervention. Copays typically range from $10 to $100. Copays are not additional earnings by the practitioner; rather they are subtracted from the reimbursement to the practitioner typically provided by the insurer. Another common method of cost shifting employed by the insurance companies is the technique of a deductible. A deductible is the dollar amount which must be paid by the employee for health care services before health insurance benefits are available to offset the cost of medical interventions. Oftentimes there are individual deductibles for outpatient care and inpatient care. Deductibles can range into the thousands of dollars. The deductible amount must be paid by the employee directly to the practitioner prior to the use of the insurance coverage to cover interventions. Health care policies should be carefully reviewed by the employee for the amount of practitioner copays, coverage, the deductibles, and the insurance copays.

As of January 1, 2015, employers with 50 or more full-time employees are required to provide health coverage that meets the Affordable Care Act (ACA) standards to full-time employees and their dependents. The ACA mandates the benefits package offered provide specific coverages. However, all health care items and services are not required to be covered. Examples of nonmandated services include dental coverage, long-term hospital coverage, durable medical equipment purchases and rental, optometry/optician services, and prescription benefits. Therefore, the out-of-pocket costs for these specific health care benefits (and any other required by the employee or expected to be required by the employee) should be investigated during the review of the benefits package.

Typically, the larger the organization, the more variety of types of health care plans offered to employees. Below is a brief overview of the more commonly offered plans:

- *Health maintenance organizations (HMOs):* This plan requires the employee choose a primary care physician (PCP) who acts as the "gatekeeper" for services provided. These plans restrict which health care professionals and which services can be utilized by the employee by requiring preapproval via referral from the PCP and, if approved, referral only to those health care professionals and services within network of the HMO. HMOs cover expenses related to illness and offers preventive care services.

- *Preferred provider organizations (PPOs):* These plans are similar to an HMO but offer wider access to doctors. Permission to see a specialist does not require preauthorization.
- *Point of service plan:* This plan is the most flexible of all. It encompasses the HMO and PPO elements in addition to being able to see physicians not associated with the plan. No preauthorization is required. Employee copay for out of network physicians is higher than in network physicians.
- *Health savings accounts (HSAs):* HSAs were established as part of the Medicare Prescription Drug, Improvement, and Modernization Act,[5] which included the enactment of Internal Revenue Code Section 223, signed into law by President George W. Bush on December 8, 2003. HSAs were developed to replace the medical savings account system. An HSA is a tax-advantaged medical savings account available to taxpayers in the United States who are enrolled in a high-deductible health plan (HDHP). The funds contributed to an account are not subject to federal income tax at the time of deposit. Unlike a flexible spending account (FSA, discussed later), HSA funds roll over and accumulate year to year if they are not spent. HSAs are owned by the individual, which differentiates them from FSAs. This is a savings account that assists with offsetting the costs of HDHP through the savings of the employee not being responsible for the federal income tax on income deposited. The funds in the savings account are used to pay the medical expenses not covered by insurance. Both the employer and the employee can contribute to the HSA. Contributions made by the employee to the HSA are tax free and money not spent at the end of the year may be rolled over to pay for future medical expenses. Money from the HSA can be withdrawn for any reason, but if not used for qualified medical expenses the withdrawal is subject to a penalty and is included in gross income for tax purposes. The contribution limit and penalty is set each year by tax law.
- *Flexible spending account (FSA):* This is similar to an HSA but with slightly different rules. As with the HSA, contributions are made to an account by the employee, with the employee not being responsible for the federal tax burden on money deposited. Employers cannot contribute to the employee FSA. The dollars in the FSA are used to offset copays, medical expenses, deductibles, and other medical debts. Any balance in the FSA that is not utilized by the end of the year is forfeited.
- *Health reimbursement arrangements (HRA):* An HRA, commonly referred to as a health reimbursement account, is an IRS-approved, employer-funded, tax-advantaged employer health benefit plan that reimburses employees for out-of-pocket medical expenses and individual health insurance premiums. An HRA is not health insurance. An HRA allows the employer to make contributions to an employee's account and provide reimbursement for eligible expenses. An HRA plan is an excellent way to provide health insurance benefits and allow employees to pay for a wide range of medical expenses not covered by insurance.

12.3.3 Short- and Long-Term Disability

Short-term disability insurance is an insurance policy that protects an employee from loss of income in the case that he or she is temporarily unable to work due to illness, injury, or accident.

Short-term disability insurance does not protect against work-related accidents or injuries, as these would be covered by workers' compensation insurance.

Short-term disability insurance is usually provided by employers, and there are a variety of differing plans available for employers to offer their employees. Employees can provide group insurance packages as part of a benefits package.

If an organization doesn't offer short-term disability insurance or if an employee wants additional coverage, the employee has the option of purchasing an individual plan from an insurance agent. Most commonly, though, the insurance is available through the employer.

Most short-term disability insurance plans include certain specifications regarding the employee's eligibility to receive benefits. For example, some plans indicate a minimum service requirement or the minimum length of time that a worker must have been employed for, and may require that the employee works full-time or has worked consecutively for a certain period of time.

In addition to these requirements, some employers specify that an employee must use all of their sick days before becoming eligible for short-term disability benefits. Employers may also require a doctor's note to verify an employee's affliction, commonly including illnesses such as arthritis or back pain, cancer, diabetes, or other nonwork-related injuries.

Short-term disability insurance benefits vary by plan. Typically, a package offers about 64% (usual range: 50 to 70%) of an employee's pre-disability salary. Short-term disability insurance plans may provide benefits for as few as 10 weeks, but most commonly provide benefits for 26 weeks.

Following the expiration of insurance benefits, many employers offer their employees access to the benefits available from a long-term disability insurance provision.

Long-term disability insurance is an insurance policy that protects an employee from loss of income in the event that he or she is unable to work due to illness, injury, or accident for a long period of time.

Long-term disability insurance is usually provided by employers, and there are a variety of differing plans available for employers to offer as part of a comprehensive employee benefits package. If a company doesn't offer long-term disability insurance or if an employee wants additional coverage, he or she has the option of purchasing an individual long-term disability plan from an insurance agent. Most frequently, though, long-term disability insurance is available through the employer; it is expensive to purchase as an individual. Some employers, if they do not provide long-term disability insurance will develop a relationship with a long-term disability insurance company to create an employee discount for their staff who choose to purchase it.

Long-term disability insurance is also often available through an employee's professional associations at a discounted rate.

Long-term disability insurance, provided by an employer, may be inadequate to meet a disabled employee's needs. This is the second reason employees might want to consider purchasing supplemental long-term disability insurance. Additionally, payments to the employee from their employer's long-term disability insurance are taxable income whereas payments from an employee purchased plan are usually not.

Long-term disability insurance begins to assist the employee when short-term disability insurance benefits end. Once the employee's short-term disability insurance benefits expire (generally after 3–6 months), the long-term disability insurance pays an employee a percentage of their salary, typically 50 to 70%. Long-term disability payments to the employee, in some policies, have a defined period of time (e.g., 2–10 years). Others pay an employee until he or she is 65 years old; this is the preferred policy.

Each long-term disability insurance policy has different conditions for payout, diseases or preexisting conditions that may be excluded, and various other conditions that make the policy more or less useful to an employee. Some policies, for example, will pay disability benefits if the employee is unable to work in his or her current profession; others expect that the employee will take any job that the employee is capable of doing—that is a big difference and consequential.

12.3.4 Retirement Plans

As an employee, there are a number of retirement options that may be offered. Your employer is not required to offer a retirement plan or required to fund a retirement plan. There are a number of qualified plans: pension plans, profit-sharing plans, 401(k) and 403(b) plans, and stock bonus plans. All plans are required to be provided to the employee in writing. Normally there is an age and years of service level that must be met for the employee to participate in the plan.

Employer-sponsored pension plans were once widely offered by most organizations as a recruitment and retention tool but are slowly falling out of favor with employers due to their high cost. In employer-sponsored pension plans the employer pays into a pension fund. When an employee retires after a specified number of years of service, the employee receives a regular check from the pension fund for the remainder of his or her life. Employers are required to fund the pension fund with sufficient dollars to ensure the meeting of the future expenses of providing checks to retired employees.

In the United States, a 401(k) plan is the tax-qualified, defined-contribution pension account defined by the Internal Revenue Code. Under the plan, retirement savings contributions are provided (and sometimes proportionately matched) by an employer, deducted from the employee's paycheck before taxation (therefore tax-deferred until withdrawn after retirement or as otherwise permitted by applicable law), and limited to a maximum pretax annual contribution of $18,500 (as of 2018). Other employer-provided defined-contribution plans include 403(b) plans for nonprofit institutions and 457(b) plans for governmental employers. These plans are all established under section 401(a) of the Internal Revenue Code. Also, 401(a) plans may provide total annual addition of $55,000 (as of 2018) per plan participant, including both employee and employer contributions.

Stock bonus plans are a hybrid version of profit-sharing plans. In profit-sharing plans, employers grant employees deposits into retirement accounts based on the profits that the company has made during the year. Stock bonus plans are similar but employers give shares to employees instead of direct dollars. Stock bonus plans are not guarantees for money, and can vary greatly from year to year. Employers have a choice whether or not to place any money in stock bonus plans, and in a bad year they might choose to not grant any stock. However, there are typically limits as to how much stock an employer can grant in 1 year to employees. Sometimes 401(k) plans are also part of stock bonus plans, depending on the company's benefit arrangements. There are a number of requirements that a stock bonus plan must meet. Participants must have to pass through voting rights on the stock held by the plan, and must have the ability to demand that the employer buy back the securities if the stock is not publicly traded. Employers must distribute the stock within 1 year of retirement, death, or disability or within 5 years if the employee is terminated but still eligible. When there is an employer match or employer contribution to the fund, ask the details of vesting policy on the employer contribution. Vesting is a time table when the employer contribution becomes fully the employee's. Some plans are immediate vesting, meaning all employers' contributions are 100% the employee's. Others use a 5-year cliff vesting, where from 1 to 4 years of service the contributions are forfeited if the employee leaves the company. During year 5 and beyond the employers' contributions are 100% the employee's. Other plans use a gradual vesting from 2 to 7 years to reach 100% vesting. The details of the vesting will be in the plan description.

12.3.5 Life Insurance

Most large employers offer the equivalent of 1-year's salary of life insurances as a benefit to their employees without additional copay required. Coverage in excess of the 1-year equivalency is usually at the employee's expense. This additional expense can be passed through to the employee on their W2 as additional taxable income. Employer-sponsored life insurance plans are typically "term" plans meaning that the benefit ends at the termination of employment.

12.3.6 Business Expenses

Beginning in 2018, employee business expenses are no longer a federal tax deduction. Depending on your state of residency, a deduction for employee business expenses my still be available on your state and local income tax return.

From an employee's standpoint, an "accountable reimbursement" plan provided by the employer is the most beneficial. The requirements of an "accountable" plan are outlined by the IRS. These plans provide reimbursement directly to the employee for qualified work-related expenses. The reimbursement would not be included in taxable income. If the reimbursement is not included in wages, then there is no deduction taken on a state or local tax return. Employees will be reimbursed dollar for dollar with no reduction for itemized tax limitations.

If the employer's reimbursement plan does not meet the requirements of an "accountable" plan, then the reimbursement will be included in taxable wages and the employee is eligible to deduct the expenses on his or her state and/or local tax return. Depending on the employee's tax situation the employee may not receive a dollar for dollar write-off of the expense and therefore will be paying tax on some or all of the reimbursement.

Commuting costs are not deductible expenses. However, transportation from one work location to another is deductible. Some general business deductions include travel, licenses, continuing education, uniforms, dues, insurances, and supplies. This is not an exhaustive list and based on the profession the list will contain items specific to that profession.

12.3.7 Continuing Education

A requirement of physical therapy licensure, by the state issuing the license, is for the holder of the license to sit for a specific number of continuing education credits per year to maintain the license. Attendance at these events must be documented and available if the state licensing board requests proof of attendance. Continuing education content may be mandated by the state, the state board of practice, by the clinical specialization organization, or may be self-determined by the practitioner based on work environment and career goals. As part of the benefits package, employers often offer a fixed dollar amount per year which may be used by the employee to offset the cost of mandated continuing education. If the employer does not reimburse the employee for continuing education credits, the employee is responsible for this cost. If the employee is not reimbursed for this expense it is deductible as a business expense; if the employer pays for the continuing education courses the employee may not deduct the cost as a business expense.

12.3.8 Performance Reviews

An important question to ask during the interviews or during review of the benefits package is regarding performance reviews. Most companies perform reviews yearly and some even more frequently. These may be a stressful meeting for the employee. An employee should try to change his mindset concerning reviews from a potentially punitive discussion to more of a coaching strategy durig which the employee is open to instruction, mentorship, and constructive criticism. Be prepared for the review. Know the job description and the specific duties of the position. If there is no written description of the position, begin to clarify with the supervisor the duties the employer expects. Spend time prior to the performance review to reflect on the past year and to develop a list of behavioral and job-specific goals for the coming year. Document the progress toward these goals, especially if they are discussed in prior meetings. An example would be citing the courses completed toward an advanced degree or certificate. Have a positive attitude. Do not be defensive when receiving criticism. Take notes. Take time to think about the comments in light of the business and other factors in the environment. On reflection of the performance review discussion, the employee can schedule a follow-up appointment if further clarification is needed. Supervisors greatly respect employees who are motivated to perform well and who are able to develop a list of performance goals. These discussions need not only occur during the yearly performance review. Maintain an open dialog with the supervisor on a daily or weekly basis. Be aware that reviews are often as uncomfortable for the reviewer as for the employee. The supervisor wants the employee to perform well to improve company performance. The employee wants to do well for self-improvement, advancement, and perhaps a salary increase. If an employee approaches the performance review with the goal of obtaining information and direction that will facilitate professional growth this positive attitude will be noted and appreciated by the supervisor. The common goal is to progress as an employee, a department and a business. The employee and supervisor are on the same side.

12.3.9 Job Location

There are many intangible benefits and drawbacks to a job. One of the largest is the location. Before selecting a position consider the commuting time and cost. If the work schedule requires traveling on nonrush hour times, the commuting time may not be as much a factor as commuting during rush hour. The commuting costs—such as gas, wear and tear on the vehicle, parking—and commuter expenses—such as public transportation—should be calculated before accepting a position. Employees in large cities are often amazed at the cost of parking; most urban employers do not offer free parking. In some major cities, the cost of parking per month may be as high as $200. Some companies will offer transportation benefits under Section 132 of the Internal Revenue Code.[4] This is for qualified transportation benefits associated with mass transportation. Mass transportation includes all public transportation services, vanpool, and carpool. This benefit will reduce the tax burden if commuting is done using one of the qualified methods. Getting to and from the job can add an hour or more to the work day. Careful consideration of the process of commuting can ease much downstream work stress and costs.

12.4 Student Loan Repayment

While receiving a professional degree is a celebratory accomplishment, accepting the first position in one's chosen field truly marks the passage from student to professional. Sadly, this period of one's life is typically the time to begin the process of repaying college loans. Though the repayment burden of loan principal and accrued interest can be challenging and daunting, a strong, preplanned repayment strategy may save the borrower tens of thousands of dollars. The following pages will outline a variety of plans that are currently available for the repayment of student loans.

The borrowing student should maintain excellent records of all student loan original documentation. A file of these papers and forms, organized by lender, should be maintained during and after the college experience. Along with original forms, a list of lenders, access passwords, and usernames should be saved. Additionally, a spread sheet of lenders, loan durations, interest rates, contact information, balances, and terms should be maintained and routinely updated. Borrowers should be aware of "grace periods" for each loan. A grace period is the time between graduation and the due date for the first payment of interest and principal. Monthly payments should never be missed. Missed payments may result in financial penalties and may also impact the borrower's credit rating. A low credit rating may require years to remediate and will most assuredly negatively impact the borrower's future ability to obtain loans for a home or car. If a hardship arises and payments cannot be made, contact the lender immediately. Let the lender know as soon as possible of any difficulties making payments. Always make the lender aware of any change in address, e-mail, or telephone number.

The best strategy for repayment is to pay the minimum due payment for those loans with the lowest interest rate and pay the minimum payment *plus* as much toward the principal as the borrower's budget permits. Make sure to include instructions that the additional payment amount be applied to the principal of the loan. The borrower does not want the additional payment applied to next month's bill.

In most cases, a direct withdrawal of the loan payment from the borrower's checking account will offer a slight reduction in interest rate. This small reduction may not seem like much, but over the life of the loan the small discount may save much in the way of interest.

If the borrower has many high-interest loans, there may be an advantage to consolidating high-interest rate loans into one lower-interest rate loan. Interest rates, especially in the past few decades, have been widely fluctuating. The optimum time to refinance would be when interest rates are at or near all-time lows. However, refinancing should be investigated if current loan rates are less than the rates of the loan. Loan consolidation into one loan also lessens the payment burden of multiple monthly payments. Private loans cannot be consolidated into a federal loan but federal loans can be repaid early using private loans.

Savvy borrowers use bonuses, tax refunds, and other one-time cash receipts for principal payment of loans. Because this type of payment is not incorporated in the borrower's budget, this type of payment is especially useful in paying down principal.

There is a student loan interest tax deduction on the federal tax return. Borrowers may be able to deduct up to $2,500 per year of student loan interest on the federal return. This deduction is available for all years paying interest. Consider consulting a tax advisor to assist with using tuition credits which are available if in school and paying tuition.

Most loans will be serviced through a provider associated with the Department of Education's Federal Student Aid Division. The lending institution that services the loan may be different than another student's or even a different provider than a loan taken for tuition at an earlier date. Federal student aid provides the following options for repayment of student loans.[6] Payment plans are selected when beginning to pay back student loans but may be changed at any time without a fee:

- Standard repayment plan.
- Graduated repayment plan.
- Extended repayment plan.
- Income-driven repayment plans.

Standard repayment plan: If no repayment plan is selected, the standard repayment plan is the default option. The standard plan will result in higher monthly payments and lower interest over the life of the loan, thereby saving money. The length of the repayment period depends on the amount of student loan debt and can vary from 10 to 30 years. There is no prepayment penalty on this or any student loan administered with the Federal Student Aid Department.

- *Graduated repayment plan:* In this plan the payments are low in the first few years and gradually rise on average every 2 years. This plan is designed for wage earners who will have lower income after graduation and then expect gradual increases in their salary. The graduated repayment plan is from 10 to 30 years depending on the amount of student debt. There is no prepayment penalty. This plan is generally more expensive in the long term than the standard repayment plan due to the length of the repayment terms, the very low first few years' required payment, and the gradual increase in repayment.

- *Extended repayment plan:* This plan is for loans greater than $30,000. Borrowers will have a fixed or graduated monthly payment that will be lower than the standard or graduated repayment plans. Payments will be made for up to 25 years. Usually this plan will have more interest paid than the two other plans and therefore may be a more expensive option.
- *Income-driven repayment plans:* This is not a single repayment plan but a group of plans. There are four options under this plan. In general, the payment will not be more than 10% of the borrower's discretionary income, which is defined as the difference between earned income and 150% of the poverty guidelines for the borrower's family size. With the income-driven plans any student loan debt remaining after 20 or 25 years of payments (depending on the plan chosen) will be forgiven. At first the income-driven plans appear to be the best option but there are downsides to these plans. Since the loan payment is based on income level and not term of loan, the amount of interest will be greater on the income-driven loans than the standard, graduated, or extended loans. The total repayment will be greater. In fact, depending on income level and the interest rate, the amount of loan remaining at the end of the period, could be greater than the loan principal originally borrowed. The fact that loan forgiveness occurs after 20 or 25 years of repayment may also prompt the borrower to consider this type of repayment plan. The downside of loan forgiveness is that the balance forgiven is considered taxable income in the year forgiven. Therefore, if the borrower has a loan balance of $40,000 remaining and forgiven, the borrower will have additional taxable income of $40,000. This additional income will result in federal and state taxes that are due immediately. The income-driven plan can work for some individuals, but should be monitored throughout the repayment period. If the borrower has difficulty meeting monthly payments he should consider changing the repayment plan to an income driven plan.

Regardless of the repayment method chosen, monitor loan balance and interest accrued. Change plans to a more aggressive payment plan if possible. Aggressive repayment during the early repayment period of the loan will benefit toward the end of the loan term by diminishing interest payments. If there is a period of unemployment or medical hardship the borrower should contact the loan broker to request a deferment to avoid defaulting on the loan. Loan default can have severe long-term financial consequences. If default occurs on a federal student loan future wages maybe garnished. Garnishment typically occurs after not making a payment for 270 days or more. The borrower will receive a notice from the service provider 30 days in advance of garnishment. Once notified, if the borrower believes the garnishment decision is in error a hearing can be requested. The garnishment can be up to 15% of take-home pay. If garnishment occurs the borrower should remain in close contact with the loan provider for ongoing discussion of options to stop the garnishment. If discussions with the service provider do not stop the garnishment, the borrower may be able to enter the loan rehabilitation program provided by the Department of Education.[7] The loan rehabilitation program requires the borrower to pay an additional amount above the garnishment rate for a period of five months. This will stop the wage garnishment and the loan status will be moved from default to good standing and thus be eligible for loan consolidation or other repayment plans.

There are limited cases where the borrower can receive discharge from a portion of the student loan debt for certain public service—the Peace Corps, AmeriCorps, or serving as a teacher in specific areas or in the National Health Service Corps may offer partial relief from student loan debt. If a student becomes permanently disabled, he or she can apply for debt forgiveness. Forgiven debt is considered taxable income to the student.

Death will also forgive the student loan. If the student is the only borrower on the loan the forgiveness of the loan will not be taxable. This is the case for most federal student loans. For private loans and federal loans that require cosigners this forgiveness of debt will be taxable income. The tax will be assessed on the estate, spouse, or cosigner of the loan. This is not an easy topic to discuss at the time of loan application. The cosigners of the loan and the spouse of the student should be aware of their financial responsibility. Depending on the amount of the loan and the financial resources of the cosigner/spouse, life insurance on the student could be an option to offset future liability.

Bankruptcy may also be a way to discharge student loans. In studies that have reviewed bankruptcy cases involving student loans, only one-tenth of 1% of student loan debtors have attempted to discharge their student loans and of that group only 40% have been successful.[8]

Due to the overwhelming debt held by graduating students, there are services available to discuss debt and help manage a plan for repayment. These firms are similar to credit card debt services and delinquent tax services. Prior to choosing a consultant, obtain professional references and review their filings with the Better Business Bureau to assist with coming to a complete understanding of all fees prior to engaging services.

It is important to understand that student debt is critical to the borrower's credit rating. The credit rating influences the ability to obtain a mortgage, credit card, apartment lease, or auto loan. The credit score is not considered when applying for a federal student loan. All students receive the same interest rate on the same type of federal loan. Student debt may be the largest portion of credit experience for recent graduates. The credit rating or FICO (Fair Isaac Corporation score) is a composite and comparable score of the amount of debt owed and the prediction of ability to pay one's bills on time. The ratings range from 300 to 850. The higher the score, the more likely the borrower is to qualify for a loan and the more likely the loan will have a more favorable interest rate and terms. Student loans, if managed and paid on time, can create credit experience that will allow a recent graduate to qualify for auto loans, rental agreements, and credit cards. Be aware that credit ratings change on a monthly basis. To reiterate what has been previously written, if the borrower is late or does not pay a repayment bill the borrower must contact the lender to discuss the possibility of deferment, selection of a new payment plan, or consolidation of loans. Paying back student loans on time will create good credit history which, in the future, could save the borrower thousands of dollars with lower interest rates on future debt.

Table 12.2 Example of salary and benefits review form

	Offer one	Offer two	Offer three
Company name	Mercy Hospital		
Company address	1 Lincoln Park, Chicago, IL 55555		
Company telephone number	555 555 5555		
Contact person	John Doe		
Department	Human Resources		
Exempt or non-exempt	Nonexempt		
Base salary	$25.00/hour		
Retirement plan	401(k)		
Retirement match	50% up to $2,000/year		
Signing bonus	$1,000		
Signing bonus rules	Paid in full on 1-year anniversary		
Signing bonus value	$1,000		
Paid holidays	7 days/year		
Paid holiday value	$1,400		
Paid sick	7 days/year		
Paid sick rules	No carryover; receive all 7 January 1		
Paid sick value	$1,400		
Paid vacation	10 days		
Paid vacation rules	No carryover; receive all 10 January 1		
Paid vacation value	$2,000		
Medical plan	HMO		
Company portion of yearly premium	$2,400		
Employee portion of yearly premium	($2,400)		
Yearly deductible	($500)		
Dental plan	None		
Employee estimated dental cost/year	($500)		
Vision plan	Yes		
Company portion of yearly premium	$200		

Table 12.2 continued

	Offer one	Offer two	Offer three
Employee portion of yearly premium	0		
Life insurance	Yes		
Benefit	1X annual salary		
Company portion of yearly premium	$200		
Continuing education yearly benefit from company	$1,000		
Total salary value	$52,000		
Total benefit value paid by company	$10,600		
Total benefit value paid by employee	($3,400)		
Total value of offer	$59,200		

Note: "Offer one" included in the table is a hypothetical offer for a staff physical therapist position. Parenthetical numbers are costs paid by the employee.

12.5 Salary and Benefits Review Form

▶ Table 12.2 is an example of a salary and benefits review form. The use of the form is relatively intuitive and does provide the applicant with an objective method of comparing competing offers.

12.6 Review Questions

1. An employee who has no scheduled hours but can be "called in" when the organization requires additional manpower, is called which type of employee?
   a) Full-time employee.
   b) Per diem employee.
   c) Part-time employee.
   d) Contract employee.
2. A salaried employee is also known as which type of employee?
   a) Contract employee.
   b) Exempt employee.
   c) Nonexempt employee.
   d) Per diem employee.
3. The federal law permitting qualified employees to take up to 12 weeks of unpaid leave per year is known by which acronym?
   a) FMLA.
   b) IRA.
   c) 401(k).
   d) 403(b).
4. The type of insurance offered by employers which requires an employee to choose a primary care physician to act as a gatekeeper for services provided and often require a referral

in order to visit specialists, is known as which type of insurance?

a) Preferred provider organization.
b) Point of service plan.
c) Health savings account.
d) Health maintenance organization.

5. Most employers offer the equivalent of what number of years' salary of life insurance as a standard benefit?

a) One.
b) Two.
c) Three.
d) Four.

6. Employee performance reviews, performed by the employer, typically occur at which frequency?

a) Every 3 months.
b) Every 6 months.
c) Every 9 months.
d) Yearly.

7. A bereavement benefit provides an employee which of the following?

a) Time to grieve following a close relative's death.
b) Sick leave.
c) Retirement savings account.
d) Vacation.

8. Continuing education credits, a requirement of most physical therapists, are mandated by which organization?

a) The American Physical Therapy Association.
b) Individual state licensing boards.
c) American Medical Association.
d) American Hospital Association.

9. What is a dollar amount which must be paid by the employee for health care services before health benefits are available to offset cost of medical intervention?

a) Copay.
b) Deductible.
c) Business copay.
d) Standard deduction.

10. Which of the following is not a permitted reason for granting Family Medical Leave?

a) To care for a newborn.
b) To care for an immediate family member with a serious physical impairment.
c) For the employee to receive care for a serious physical impairment.
d) For the employee to take a sabbatical from work to earn an advanced degree such as the PhD.

12.7 Review Answers

1. An employee who has no scheduled hours but can be "called in" when the organization requires additional manpower, is called which type of employee?
b. Per diem employee.

2. A salaried employee is also known as which type of employee?
b. Exempt employee.

3. The federal law permitting qualified employees to take up to 12 weeks of unpaid leave per year is known by which acronym?
a. FMLA.

4. The type of insurance offered by employers which requires an employee to choose a primary care physician to act as a gatekeeper for services provided and often require a referral in order to visit specialists, is known as which type of insurance?
d. Health maintenance organization.

5. Most employers offer the equivalent of what number of years' salary of life insurance as a standard benefit?
a. One.

6. Employee performance reviews, performed by the employer, typically occur at which frequency?
d. Yearly.

7. A bereavement benefit provides an employee which of the following?
a. Time to grieve following a close relative's death.

8. Continuing education credits, a requirement of most physical therapists, are mandated by which organization?
b. **Individual state licensing boards.**

9. What is a dollar amount which must be paid by the employee for health care services before health benefits are available to offset cost of medical intervention?
b. Deductible.

10. Which of the following is not a permitted reason for granting Family Medical Leave?
d. For the employee to take a sabbatical from work to earn an advanced degree such as the PhD.

References

[1] United States Department of Labor. Available at: https://www.dol.gov/whd/fmla/

[2] Littler. Available at: https://www.littler.com/publication-press/publication/minimum-wage-increases-new-york-what-employers-should-know. Accessed March 31, 2017

[3] New York State Budget S6406C, A9006C (April 4, 2016) at Part SS; https://paidfamilyleave.ny.gov/ (accessed September 21, 2018)

[4] https://www.bestworkplaces.org/resource-center/qualified-transportation-fringe-benefits/. Accessed September 21, 2018

[5] Medicare. Available at: https://www.medicare.gov/forms-help-and-resources/contact/contact-medicare.html

[6] U.S. Department of Education. Available at: https://www2.ed.gov/finaid/landing.jhtml?src=ln

[7] Consumer Finance Protection Bureau. Available at: https://www.consumerfinance.gov/paying-for-college/repay-student-debt/?utm_source=bing&utm_medium=cpc&utm_term=loanrehabilitationprogram&utm_content=LoanRehabilitation&utm_campaign=CFPBStudentDebtRepayment2016

[8] U.S. News. Available at: https://www.usnews.com/education/blogs/student-loan-ranger/2014/08/13/debunking-the-student-loan-bankruptcy-myth

13 The Physical Therapist as an Effective Teacher

Stephen J. Carp

Keywords: Assessment, behavioral change, behaviorism, comprehension, domains of learning, flipped classroom, instructional method, learning theories, Piaget's theory of cognitive development, reflection, reliability, transformation, translating, universal classroom design, validity

"I am a teacher. I am an educator. I instruct my students. I assess their understanding of my content knowledge. I teach in the cognitive domain (facts), the psychomotor domain (physical skill sets), and the affective domain (feelings and perceptions). I even sometimes touch in the spiritual domain (if my students lead me down that pathway). I sometimes teach with a traditional blackboard. I lecture. I use power points. I use technology such as social media, email, and websites. I facilitate my teaching with videos, pictures, case studies, flipped classroom technique, small group discussion, and problem solving. And, I have not been in a university classroom since graduation from my entry-level Doctor of Physical Therapy (DPT) 11 years ago.

"I teach patients receiving physical therapy services at my clinic and I teach their families. My classroom is the clinic. Patients often ask me about the percentage of my day spent teaching and I cannot answer that question honestly. Teaching is such an important part of the patient–therapist alliance that there is no definitive distinction between evaluation, assessment, intervention, reevaluation, discharge planning, and teaching. All parts of my day meld together within the framework of my patient and my patient's family. This is how it should be.

"What do I teach? Perhaps it would be easier if I described what I do not teach! This morning I saw a patient scheduled to undergo a total knee arthroplasty (knee replacement) in two weeks. I was seeing him for 'prehabilitation'—rehabilitation before the surgical procedure. I taught him what to expect when he arrived at the hospital for surgery. I shared a short video about the actual surgical procedure. I discussed his postoperative physical therapy care. We practiced crutch walking and his exercises. The entire session was teaching.

"My second patient this morning was a young man with a wound on his foot. He was diagnosed with type I diabetes ten years ago and he has recently developed a wound on his toe. I taught him proper wound dressing techniques. We discussed the need to follow up regularly with his podiatrist. I taught him the extreme necessity of monitoring his blood sugars. I taught him insensate limb precautions. I taught him how to properly perform foot hygiene.

"My third patient this morning was a young athlete postanterior cruciate reconstruction. She injured her knee playing basketball and was extremely anxious to return to basketball as soon as possible. She feels wonderful and cannot understand why she is not yet allowed to play. I spent perhaps 30 minutes reviewing the physiology of ligament healing with her (translating my clinical knowledge into words a 13-year-old girl could understand) with hopes of tempering her enthusiasm to get back on the court and also to follow the rehabilitation protocol given by me.

"Below is one of my favorite quotes about teaching. It hangs on the wall over my desk:

"'The best thing for being sad,' replied Merlin, beginning to puff and blow, 'is to learn something. That's the only thing that never fails. You may grow old and trembling in your anatomies, you may lie awake at night listening to the disorder of your veins, you may miss your only love, you may see the world about you devastated by evil lunatics, or know your honour trampled in the sewers of baser minds. There is only one thing for it then—to learn. Learn why the world wags and what wags it. That is the only thing which the mind can never exhaust, never alienate, never be tortured by, never fear or distrust, and never dream of regretting. Learning is the only thing for you. Look what a lot of things there are to learn.' (T.H. White, The Once and Future King)"

—D. Gillespie, Conshohocken, Pennsylvania

13.1 Overview

The fascinating aspect of the physical therapist as a teacher is that rarely does an incoming physical therapy student consider the magnitude and importance of teaching within the scope of contemporary physical therapy practice, and rarely does an established practicing physical therapist or physical therapist assistant not consider the magnitude and importance of teaching within the scope of contemporary physical therapy practice. "Teacher," as used in this chapter, refers to a faculty member tasked with teaching in a doctor of physical therapy (DPT) or associate's degree in physical therapy assistant program, or a clinician teaching a specific target audience. "Student," as used in this chapter, refers to the target audience of the teaching session. The most obvious "student" is the patient/client. However, a physical therapist's target audience is much broader than simply the patient/client. Physical therapists and physical therapist assistants teach families, other physical therapists, representatives from insurance companies, physicians, nurses, physical therapy and physical therapist assistant students, assistants and aides, legislators, and representatives from the public (see ▶ Table 13.1). This chapter will provide the reader with a global understanding of the role of the physical therapist and physical therapist assistant as a teacher; explain what physical therapists and physical therapist assistants teach and in which arenas teaching occurs; elaborate on the pedagogy of teaching including the philosophical orientations of teaching, learning theories, and domains of learning; review the environmental variables which may impact teaching success; discuss universal classroom design; provide specific teaching techniques for the cognitive, psychomotor, and behavioral change teaching; and end with a discussion on the importance of health literacy on teaching effectiveness.

Table 13.1 Who do physical therapists teach?

Target audience	Examples
Patient/client	Information about diagnosis, prognosis, behavioral modifications, therapeutic exercise technique
Patient/client family	Transfer techniques, guarding techniques, wound care, handwashing
General public	Low back pain precautions, fall risk assessment, insensate foot precautions
Insurance company representatives	Effectiveness of particular physical therapy interventions, medical necessity of particular durable medical equipment items
Legislators	Importance of pending legislation to our patients/clients, insurance reform
Physical therapy students	Performance of specific psychomotor interventions (clinical teaching), didactic knowledge, professional behaviors, clinical interventions (classroom)
Nurses	Patient transfer and positioning techniques
Physicians	Indications and effectiveness of physical therapy science
Physical therapists	Data and content from continuing education courses attended; continuing education course presentation
Aides	Daily duties permitted under the State Practice Act
Assistants	Delegated instructions for care of a particular patient/client

13.2 What Do Physical Therapists Teach?

The three primary goals of the therapist as a teacher—regardless of arena of teaching or audience—are to enhance the student's didactic knowledge, enhance the student's psychomotor performance, and to influence behavior change. Enhancing the student's didactic knowledge is a very common goal of physical therapist teaching because members of the physical therapy profession have a complex and unique knowledge and process set which needs to be shared with the patient/client, the patent/client's family, and other cohorts. Due to its commonality, teaching didactic information is the easiest of the three goals to successfully accomplish. We have all had experiences on the receiving end of teaching these types of data and facts and have a global understanding of what makes and does not make an effective teacher. Teaching a psychomotor skill set, however—such as crutch walking up and down a flight of steps, changing a wound dressing, or the performance of a complex nerve glide exercise—is difficult and fraught with risk. Poor technique with crutch walking may result in an injurious fall. Poor sterile technique with a wound dressing change may result in an infection. The transference of verbal instruction into a physical component such as exercise is challenging. Fortunately, with newer technology such as videos, texting of reminders, and instructional software programs, teaching psychomotor activity is a bit easier now as compared with years past. Teaching behavioral change, however, is extremely difficult for most physical therapists. Health care providers ask patients to make enormous changes in their lives in order to prevent disease, diminish risk factors, and promote health. For example, physical therapists often ask patients with diabetes to lose or maintain weight by staying on a prescribed diet 365 days a year, every year, for life. Patients with diabetes must also carefully control their intake of dietary fat and cholesterol to decrease their risk of heart attacks and stroke. Constant and accurate self-monitoring of blood glucose is required by finger sticks and urine testing. Exercise is part of the treatment as well, but it must be planned to avoid causing elevations or severe drops in blood glucose levels. In addition, the patient must inject insulin several times a day or take oral medications. Self-management of diabetes is very complex, yet we ask ordinary people to take on all these extraordinary tasks and, at the same time, carry on their normal life of work, school, and social relationships. When asked by a physical therapist if he had ever attempted to quit smoking, the three pack-per-day man responded: "Quitting smoking is easy. I've done it dozens of times." Teaching behavioral change is easy; teaching behavioral change which facilitates a true change of behavior is difficult. Physical therapists teach in a number of domains to a number of different audiences. ▶ Table 13.2 provides examples of the teaching domains, audiences, and content taught.

13.3 Overview of the Teaching Process

13.3.1 Teacher Preparation

Activities and processes controlled by the teacher may be the most influential variables in obtaining a successful teaching outcome. Controllable variables by the teacher include preparation for teaching a specific content which includes teacher preparation; syllabus development; identification of the philosophical orientation of teaching and identification of preferred learning domains utilized by the student(s); teaching methods and methodology; methods of assessment or outcome measures; incorporation of a universal classroom design principles; environmental constraints; and the choosing of appropriate teaching tools and methods.

Prior to teaching didactic, psychomotor, or behavioral change information, the teacher must be prepared to teach. The teacher must possess a strong *comprehension* or understanding of the content which is to be taught. Content knowledge is typically acquired through the educational process, professional experience, or research. Good teachers have a strong understanding of the subject matter which they are to teach. A good understanding permits the material to be delivered with confidence and with creativity. Good content understanding also permits the teacher to move to the autonomous stage of teaching. A strong content understanding permits the teacher to free his or her concentration away from remembering and transforming what

Table 13.2 What do physical therapists teach?

Content	Student(s)	Examples
Didactic	Patient/client	Information related to the diagnosis
		Information related to the prognosis
		Precautions
		Potential complications of the prescribed intervention
		Diabetic foot precautions
	Families of a patient/client	Bed positioning rationale to avoid pressure ulcers
		Exercise schedule for newborn with brachial plexus injury
		Positioning of elderly relative to avoid aspiration when eating
	Physical therapists	Content from recently attended educational conference
	Nurses	Proper bed positioning to avoid pressure ulcers Rationale for early mobilization in the ICU
	Physical therapy and assist students in clinic	Required skills and content required by the educational program
	Physical therapy and assist students in the classroom	Content determine to be contemporary practice by the Commission on Accreditation in Physical Therapy Education, the university or college, and the community
	Insurance company representatives	Evidenced-based rationale for a specific number of allowable visits for an outpatient attending physical therapy
	General public	Reducing fall risk in the home Flexibility exercises prior to the golf season
	Physicians	Emerging evidence for a specific physical therapy intervention such as pelvic floor exercises and biofeedback for urinary incontinence
Psychomotor	Patient/client	Teaching an exercise program using exercise bands
	Families of a patient/client	Sterile technique to be used during wound dressing changes
Behavioral	Patient/client	Smoking cessation Daily skin checks for a new diagnosis of diabetes
	Physical therapy and assist students in the classroom	The importance of becoming a lifelong learner in the field of physical therapy

it is he planned to teach and allow his attention to be directed to other variables such as nonverbal assessment of the student's understanding of the content presented, time constraints, and use of creativity. Once comprehension of the content to be taught has been mastered, the teacher must *transform* the content into a format which can be understood by the client. Much as a carrot must be pureed in order for a toddler to eat it, the teacher must prepare the content into a format which can be understood by the student. Following transformation of content, the teacher must determine the *instructional method*. Will the method be lecture, discussion, self-learning, video, or group work? The method of instruction is determined by a number of variables which include the preferred learning style of the student, the comfort of the teacher in utilizing a specific method of instruction, and the content itself being presented. Another example of effective instructional method is service-learning. Service-learning is a required course activity which matches an altruistic opportunity with an aspect of the course content. *Reflective evaluation by the student and teacher* is often the most underutilized and underappreciated aspect of the teaching process.[1] A number of studies have validated the importance of reflection as a learning component. Schon's *The Reflective Practitioner* details the importance of reflection as a facilitator of acquiring professional knowledge.[2] Shepard and Jenson described a number of methods of incorporating reflection into student learning. Student portfolios—especially when the content is outlined by the teacher but permitting the student to determine the variety and quantity of the included elements—is a unique and interesting method of student self-assessment.[3] Reflective journaling—either based upon a limited experience such as daily entries during a clinical internship or a required element to be performed weekly during the professional program—is a very effective method of learning facilitation. Lastly, reflective learning activities associated with service-learning opportunities (reflective journal, position papers, daily peer oral reflections, oral and written interrogations, and postexperience presentations to peers) provide opportunities for the student to associate the service-learning experience with the course objectives and content.[4] Reflection is also a necessary component to the process improvement activity of improving a teacher's effectiveness. By far the simplest and easiest method of teacher reflection is taking a few minutes each day to ask oneself: "As a teacher what did I do well today and which aspects of my performance can I improve?" Formal methods of reflection include peer review evaluations by fellow teachers and administrators, the use of student feedback forms following the completion of a course, and the development of faculty portfolios.[5,6] Comprehension is when the student attains competency in the didactic, psychomotor, or behavioral change content taught which permits transformation of the content into a form which permits its utilization in real-world situations. The utilization of content learned. Comprehension is not memorization. Comprehension is fusing content, psychomotor, and behavioral knowledge with real-world situations. Memorization is a short-term recall of data. *Assessment* is the process of gathering and discussing information from multiple and diverse sources in order to develop a deep understanding of what students know, understand, and can do with their knowledge as a result of their educational experiences; the process culminates when assessment results are used to improve subsequent learning.[7]

13.3.2 Syllabus Development

A syllabus is defined as "a contract between faculty members and their students, designed to answer students' questions about a course, as well as inform them about what will happen should they fail to meet course expectations."[8] Conventionally, syllabi refers to content related to a specific course but colloquially, it can also refer to the content of a specific lecture, such as a 2-hour lecture about back pain provided by a physical therapist to members of the community. In other words, the syllabus is a document developed by the course director to communicate accountability and commitment to the students.

Over time, the notion of a syllabus as a contract has grown more literal but is not an enforceable contract. In fact, the syllabus is considered a "living" document, free to be amended throughout the course of the teaching timeline.[9] Amendments may be made to incorporate scheduling changes due to weather or travel, the addition of guest lecturers, or the addition of emerging or timely content. Any amendments should, of course, be communicated as quickly as possible to the students. Along with being a description and plan for a course the well-written syllabus may also be a tool that improves student learning, facilitates faculty teaching, improves communication between faculty members about their courses, aids in curricular review, and assists with monitoring program quality. Altman and Cashin state, "The primary purpose of a syllabus is to communicate to one's students what the course is about, why the course is taught, where it is going, and what will be required of the students for them to complete the course with a passing grade."[10] Additionally, Parkes, Fix, and Harris suggest that the syllabus serves as a nonbinding contract between the instructor and the learner.[11] Typically focused on the learner, well-written syllabi communicate to students what is expected to succeed in a course and what competencies must be mastered. Thus, syllabi assist faculty members with communicating with their learners and help learners understand what is expected of them. In the educational arena, a syllabus is a descriptive academic document that communicates course information and defines expectations and responsibilities. In community education, the syllabus provides data related to the discourse presented. ▶ Table 13.3 compares and contrasts the two types of syllabi.

The lead instructor for the course and, depending on the college/university policy, other recognized bodies (e.g., departments, supervisors, administrative bodies, program review committees, etc.) are responsible for developing and maintaining course syllabi. Typically, the lead instructor is responsible for the distribution of the most updated syllabus to all other course instructors and to the students in either printed and/or electronic formats.

As a general rule, when writing or reviewing a syllabus, the syllabus content should be so clear that it is easily understood by others who are not familiar with the course (i.e., those who have not taken the course). The syllabus should provide enough detail for students to understand what is expected of them and how the course proceeds. Optimally, the course syllabus should generate interest and motivate students to take responsibility to learn the content of the course. The syllabus content should be in compliance with the college's other documents, such as course catalog and policy documents, in order to ensure that there is consistency and a relationship with the educational program.[12]

Table 13.3 The content of a syllabus

Syllabi content	Community presentation/continuing education course	University/college course
Name of course	Name must match the educational content presented and any associated advertising materials	Name must match the educational content and the course listing in the most recent course catalogue
Dates course offered	The date the course is being held	State when the course is being offered unique to the delivery of the course (term, quarter, year)
Location	The specific location of the course may be a physical location (community center) or web-based (URL) location	The specific location of the course may be a physical location (community center) or web-based (URL) location
Semester hours/credits	List whether CEU credits will be awarded for this course and if so, by whom and how many	List the approved semester and credit hours associated with the course
Prerequisites/corequisites	List the prerequisites (a prerequisite is a course that must be successfully completed prior to enrolling in the course) and/or corequisites (a corequisite is another course that must be taken at the same time). This section should include course names and numbers in order to easily identify them	List the prerequisites (a prerequisite is a course that must be successfully completed prior to enrolling in the course) and/or corequisites (a corequisite is another course that must be taken at the same time). This section should include course names and numbers in order to easily identify them
Instructor(s) names	*Instructors' names:* clearly list the instructors' names and their function in relation to the course, such as lead instructor, laboratory instructor, and so forth. Degrees and credentials may also be included	*Instructors' names:* clearly list the instructors' names and their function in relation to the course, such as lead instructor, laboratory instructor, and so forth. Degrees and credentials may also be included
Instructor(s) contact information	*Contact information:* include information about how students should communicate with faculty. Include items such as how students make appointments (e.g., drop in, phone, and sign up). Contact information typically includes both phone number and e-mail address	Office hours and contact information: Include information about how students should communicate with faculty. Include items such as office hours, where the meeting place is located, how students make appointments (e.g., drop in, phone, and sign up). Contact information typically includes both phone number and e-mail address
Course description	A one to two paragraph summation of the course objectives, content of the course, teaching methods and tools, assessments, and expected outcomes	A one to two paragraph summation of the course objectives, content of the course, teaching methods and tools, assessments, and expected outcomes
Course objectives	Course objectives are broad, general statements related to the expectations of the student. Course objectives describe a practical purpose for a course. Objective statements describe a general learning outcome and are measurable. Well defined objectives are easily matched with course content	Course objectives are broad, general statements that are directly related to program objectives and outcomes. Course goals describe a practical purpose for a course. Typically goals relate to core. Course objectives establish the direction of the course. Objective statements describe a general learning outcome and are typically not measurable. The successful implementation of program objectives is accomplished through clear, well-defined course objectives stating the overall purpose of the course. Therefore, course objectives should be clearly linked to program goals, course content, and assessments
Teaching methods	Describe the different types of formats that will be used to facilitate student learning in the course. In what manner will the student be learning and in what particular environment (e.g., open lab small group sessions, video review in the library, MRI film review in radiology lab, online listserv discussions, taking notes in a lecture hall, etc.)	Describe the different types of formats that will be used to facilitate student learning in the course. In what manner will the student be learning and in what particular environment (e.g., open lab small group sessions, video review in the library, MRI film review in radiology lab, online listserv discussions, taking notes in a lecture hall, etc.)
Required readings	List the required text(s) including books, articles, blogs, and websites including title, author(s), publisher(s), and edition (e.g., 2nd edition). If textbooks are not required, clearly state so	List the required text(s) including books, articles, blogs, and websites including title, author(s), publisher(s), and edition (e.g., 2nd edition). If textbooks are not required, clearly state so
Recommended readings	List the supplemental text(s) including books, articles, blogs, and websites including title, author(s), publisher(s), and edition (e.g., 2nd edition). If textbooks are not required, clearly state so. Supplemental readings are adjuvant content to supplement and explain the required readings and course content	List the supplemental text(s) including books, articles, blogs, and websites including title, author(s), publisher(s), and edition (e.g., 2nd edition). If textbooks are not required, clearly state so. Supplemental readings are adjuvant content to supplement and explain the required readings and course content

(Continued)

Table 13.3 continued

Syllabi content	Community presentation/continuing education course	University/college course
Instructor-provided materials	These are materials provided by the faculty. Common materials include microscopes, dissection kits, and patient gowns. Be sure to obtain copyright permission for any materials that will be duplicated for the course	These are materials provided by the faculty. Common materials include microscopes, dissection kits, and patient gowns. Be sure to obtain copyright permission for any materials that will be duplicated for the course
Assessments	Typical assessments for community presentations and continuing education courses are pretest/posttest items, question and answer sessions, and satisfaction surveys	Assessments are a listing of required items, a description of each item, the due date, and the percentile value of the final grade for each assessment
Attire	Typically not stated for community presentations and community education courses	Courses may have required attire for lectures, laboratory, guest speakers, student presentations, and service-learning opportunities
Course plan	For community presentations and continuing educational courses which are typically of a duration of hours to a few days. The course plan for these types of activities resembles an agenda	The course plan is the course calendar, which includes what materials are covered and when. Course schedules are typically organized by week and by topic; however, they may be arranged as modules, depending on the course and program. The course plan may include the dates specific assessments are due to the teacher
Grading scale	Not applicable	Typically a restatement of the university/college grading policy (i.e., the quality point value of each letter grade)
Attendance policy	Not applicable	Attendance policy is a narrative describing the teacher's policy about attending classes, laboratories, and service-learning opportunities and policies related to missed or late assessments
Special policies	Not applicable	Special policies are typically a restatement of specific university/college policies related to items such as disability accommodation, class withdrawal, attendance, syllabi amendments, telephone use in class, notifying the teacher if the student is ill or late, grade posting, etc.

Abbreviations: CEU, continuing education unit; MRI, magnetic resonance imaging.

13.3.3 Philosophical Orientation of Teaching

Elliot Eisner, a professor of art and education in the Stanford University Graduate School of Education, developed five philosophical orientations that are now considered classic guides for curricular design: the development of cognitive processes, academic rationalism, technology, social adaptation, social reconstruction, and personal relevance.[13,14] These, according to Shepard and Jensen are orientations based upon what teachers think the aims of the curriculum, course, or class should be.[3] The orientations are "why (and how) the teachers are teaching what they are teaching."

The development of *cognitive processes* teaches the students the art of developing their ability to gather, sift through, transform and comprehend data; to pose and answer questions related to the data; how to infer and deduce conclusions based upon the data; and, to locate resources of additional data. The concern of the teacher utilizing the cognitive process is the "how" and not the "what." In a problem-based cognitive processes curriculum a large portion of the curriculum is based upon this philosophy. Case studies, competencies, standardized patients, high-frequency mannequins, clinical internships, and role play replicate situations that physical therapists and physical therapist assistants encounter. *Academic rationalism* relies on the belief that if students can comprehend the basic theories and tenets of the profession—often from a historical perspective—the students will be able to understand and appreciate the contribution of the leaders of the physical therapy profession and thus transform these ideals and principles into today's lexicon of contemporary practice. Obviously, no program can completely rely on academic rationalism to complete the journey from applicant to entry-level practice; however, understanding important topics though a historical perspective does often provide a framework of understanding and appreciation. *Social adaptation* and *social reconstruction* focuses the framework of the teaching to societal interests. Social adaptation directs the curricular content to developing physical therapists and physical therapist assistants to maintaining the social status quo—to fill those areas of practice with the greatest job vacancies as quickly and as competently as possible. Social reconstruction focuses on directing the curricular content toward identifying the predicted needs of society and how the student can meet these needs in the future. An example of content which is based upon social reconstruction may be skills working with the needs of a large immigrant population such as cultural sensitivity, language skills, and epidemiological characteristics of the immigrant population. *Personal relevance* is a philosophical orientation which focuses on what is personally relevant to the student. The prerequisite for teaching from this orientation is an empathetic and trusting relationship between the student and teacher which permits the student to share his or her relevant ideas and needs with the teacher thus to tangentially assist the teacher in developing course content. An example of content taught through personal relevance is as follows: a student shares with the teacher that his mother has been stricken with multiple sclerosis and that because of her illness, he has developed a deep interest in treating persons with multiple sclerosis and perhaps one day performing research in this area. The teacher adds additional content to the course related to multiple sclerosis and perhaps even schedules a field trip for the class to the local multiple sclerosis clinic. Personal relevance works better with smaller groups such as PhD students rather than with a large DPT or PTA class.

13.3.4 Learning Theories

Behavioral learning theorists believe that learning has occurred when changes in behavior are observed. The behavioral learning model says that learning is the result of conditioning. The basis of conditioning is that a reward following a desirable response acts as a reinforcer and increases the likelihood that the desirable response will be repeated. Reinforcement is the core of the behaviorist approach. Continuous reinforcement in every instance of desirable behavior is useful when a behavior is being introduced. Once a desired behavior is established, intermittent reinforcement maintains the behavior. Behaviorist theory approaches are frequently used in weight loss, smoking cessation, assertiveness training, and anxiety-reduction programs. The importance of regularly and consistently rewarding desired behavior immediately and not rewarding undesirable behavior is crucial to the success of a behaviorist approach to learning. Learning is broken down into small steps so that the person can be successful. The nurse provides reinforcement at each step of the process. For example, when a patient is learning how to inject insulin, the nurse looks for a positive behavior and then gives the patient immediate reinforcement by saying, "I liked the way you pulled back the syringe," or "you did an excellent job of withdrawing the insulin."

Cognitive learning theorists believe that learning is an internal process in which information is integrated or internalized into one's cognitive or intellectual structure. Learning occurs through internal processing of information. From the cognitive viewpoint, how new information is presented is important. In the first, or cognitive phase of learning, the patient learns the overall picture of what the task is and the sequences involved. In the second, or fixation learning phase, the learner begins to gain skill in performing the task. Whether a physical task is learned as a whole or part by part depends on its complexity. For example, learning how to take a blood pressure is a complex task. The student must learn how to physically manipulate the blood pressure manometer, learn how to hear and interpret blood pressure sounds, and understand the meaning of the sounds. Each of these tasks can be practiced as a separate activity, then combined. In the last phase of learning, the automatic phase, the patient gains increasing confidence and competence in performing the task.

The philosophical orientation of teaching specific content is primarily teacher driven. Learning theories and learning domains—how students learn—are primarily student driven.

Current traditional learning theories are typically pictured as a quadrilateral with the apices being behaviorism, Gestalt/problem solving, cognitive structure, and Christian humanism.

Developed by experimental psychologists I. Pavlov,[15] Watson[16] and Raynor,[17] E.L. Thorndike,[18] and B.F. Skinner,[19] *behaviorism* is a worldview that assumes the learner is essentially passive but responds to environmental stimuli. The learner starts off as a blank slate (i.e., tabula rasa) and behavior is shaped through positive reinforcement and negative reinforcement. Positive reinforcement increases the probability that the antecedent behavior will occur again; negative reinforcement increases the probability that the antecedent behavior will not occur again. In contrast, punishment (both positive and negative) decreases the likelihood that the antecedent behavior will happen again. Much of the early behaviorist research was performed with animals and generalized to humans.

Behaviorism combines elements of philosophy, methodology, and psychological theory. It emerged in the late 19th century as a reaction to depth psychology and other traditional forms of psychology, which often had difficulty making predictions that could be tested experimentally. The earliest derivatives of behaviorism can be traced back to the late 1800s where Edward Thorndike pioneered the law of effect (a process that involved strengthening behavior through the use of reinforcement).[18]

Teachers utilize behaviorism theory often in the classroom with students and in the clinic when working with patients. Exams are the classic example of positive and negative reinforcement techniques facilitating learning. The teacher instructs the student in a particular aspect of the curricular content. To assess the student's comprehension, the teacher develops an examination. Performing well on the examination results in positive reinforcement (teacher praise, self-satisfaction, praise from peers and parents) and performing poorly on the exam results in negative reinforcement (teacher disappointment, loss of self-satisfaction, and concern from peers and family). Therapists and assistants often use behaviorism techniques in the clinic. Patients are praised when completing a psychomotor task properly. Mastery of a psychomotor task or series of tasks may result in the positive reinforcement of discharge from outpatient therapy or discharge home from a rehabilitation hospital; failure to develop mastery of a psychomotor task or series of tasks may result in delayed discharge or additional days required to stay in the rehabilitation hospital.

Perhaps 40 years after the introduction of behaviorism theory, gestalt psychologists presented a novel theory—a theory nearly opposite to that of behaviorism. The principle advocates of *Gestalt* (Ger: "unified whole") *theory* were Kohler, Koffka, and Max Wertheimer.[20] Gestalt theory emphasizes higher-order cognitive processes in the midst of behaviorism and attempts to understand the laws behind the ability to acquire and maintain meaningful perceptions in an apparently chaotic world. The focus of Gestalt theory is the idea of "grouping," that is, characteristics of multiple stimuli cause us to structure or interpret a visual field or problem in a certain way.[21] The fundamental principle of gestalt perception is the law of *prägnanz* (in the German language, pithiness), which says that we tend to order our experience in a manner that is regular, orderly, symmetrical, and simple.[22] Gestalt psychologists attempt to discover refinements of the law of *prägnanz*, and this involves writing down laws that, hypothetically, allow us to predict the interpretation of sensation—what are often called "Gestalt laws."[23] The primary factors that determine grouping are[1] proximity—elements tend to be grouped together according to their nearness,[2] similarity—items similar in some respect tend to be grouped together,[3] closure—items are grouped together if they tend to complete some entity, and[4] simplicity—items will be organized into simple figures according to symmetry, regularity, and smoothness. These factors were called the Laws of Organization and were explained in the context of perception and problem-solving. The original famous phrase of Gestalt psychologist Kurt Koffka, "The whole is other than the sum of the parts," is often considered the basis of Gestalt theory.[24] The concepts of reflection-in-action and reflection-on-action, originally ascribed to Schon, are examples of the present day evolution of Gestalt theory made practical for the world of physical therapists and physical therapy assistants. Schon advanced the position that there is a fundamentally important aspect to the knowledge possessed by professionals that has been overlooked.[25,26,27,28] Initially, he develops his case by arguing that our academic institutions place undue emphasis upon "technical rationality"—the disciplines of knowledge and the methods that are believed to make formal, prepositional knowledge reliable and valid. Our society's emphasis upon technical rationality, Schon argues, has led to an undervaluing of the practical knowledge of action that is central to the work of practitioners.[26] This form of knowledge, which he calls "knowing-in-action," is the practical knowledge that professionals hold about their professional work and that cannot be formulated in prepositional terms. By exploring the elements of knowing-in-action, Schon demonstrates that professional knowledge itself has been virtually unrecognized because it appears not to be as "rigorous" as knowledge developed in the more familiar and public "scientific" research traditions.[27] In his argument, Schon proposes a fundamental reorganization of how to think about professional practice and the relationship of theory to practice. For Schon, professional knowledge is developed through the ability to reflect on one's actions so as to engage in a process of continuous learning. According to one definition it involves "paying critical attention to the practical values and theories which inform everyday actions, by examining practice reflectively and reflexively. This leads to developmental insight." A key rationale for reflective practice is that experience alone does not necessarily lead to learning; scheduled, focused, and deliberate reflection on experience is an essential component of learning.[27]

Reflective practice can be an important tool in practice-based professional learning settings where people learn from their own professional experiences rather than from formal learning or knowledge transfer. Reflection may be the most important source of personal professional development and improvement. Reflective practice can also bring together theory and practice; through reflection a clinician is able to see and label forms of thought and theory within the context of his or her clinical work. A person who reflects throughout and after his or her practice day is not just looking back on past actions and events, but is taking a conscious look at emotions, experiences, actions, and responses, and using that information to add to his or her existing knowledge base and reach a higher level of understanding and clinical practice.

Schon elaborates his position in his second book (1985), with special attention to what he calls "the reflective practicum"—the specific experiences that he believes help students to acquire knowing-in-action under the coaching of expert practitioners.[27] In a later piece, Schon defines what he means by reflective teaching—"giving the kids reason"—and argues for a reflective supervision by expert teachers that might help teachers become more reflective-in-action.[28]

Learning researcher Graham Gibbs discussed the use of structured debriefing to facilitate reflection. Gibbs presents the stages of a full structured debriefing as follows[29]:

- Experience occurs.
- Description. ("What happened? Don't make judgments yet or try to draw conclusions; simply describe.")
- Feelings. ("What were your reactions and feelings? Again, don't move on to analyzing these yet.")
- Evaluation. ("What was good or bad about the experience? Make value judgments.")
- Analysis. ("What sense can you make of the situation? Bring in ideas from outside the experience to help you. What was really going on? Were different people's experiences similar or different in important ways?")
- Conclusions (general). ("What can be concluded, in a general sense, from these experiences and the analyses you have undertaken?")
- Conclusions (specific). ("What can be concluded about your own specific, unique, personal situation or way of working?")
- Personal action plans. ("What are you going to do differently in this type of situation next time?" What steps are you going to take on the basis of what you have learned?")

13.3.5 Piaget's Theory of Cognitive Development

Piaget's Theory of Cognitive Development is a comprehensive theory about the nature and development of human intelligence. Created by the Swiss developmental psychologist Jean Piaget (1896–1980), the theory deals with the nature of knowledge itself and how humans gradually come to acquire, construct, and use it.[30] To Piaget, cognitive development is a progressive reorganization of mental processes resulting from biological and chronological maturation and environmental experience. He believed that children construct an understanding of the world around them, experience discrepancies between what they already know and what they discover in their environment, then adjust their ideas accordingly. Moreover, Piaget claimed that cognitive development is at the center of the human organism, and language is contingent on knowledge and understanding acquired through cognitive development.[31] Piaget's theory is commonly known as a developmental stage theory. The Piaget stages of development is a blueprint that describes the stages of normal intellectual development from infancy through adulthood. This includes thought, judgment, and knowledge. As Piaget himself noted, development does not always progress in the smooth manner his theory seems to predict. Furthermore, studies have found that children may be able to learn concepts and capability of complex reasoning that are supposedly represented in more advanced stages with relative ease. More broadly, Piaget's theory is "domain general," predicting that cognitive maturation occurs concurrently across different domains of knowledge (such as mathematics, logic, and understanding of physics or language). Piaget did not take into account variability in a child's performance notably how a child can differ in sophistication across several domains.[32] More recent works[33,34,35,36] have strongly challenged some of the basic presumptions of the "core knowledge" school, and revised ideas of domain generality—but from a newer dynamic systems approach, not from a revised Piagetian perspective. Dynamic systems approach harkens to modern neuroscientific research that was not available to Piaget when he was constructing his theory. One important finding is that domain-specific knowledge is constructed as children develop and integrate knowledge. This enables the domain to improve the accuracy of the knowledge as well as organization of memories. However, this suggests more of a "smooth integration" of learning and development than either Piaget or his neo-nativist critics had envisioned. Additionally, some psychologists, such as Lev Vygotsky,[37] thought differently from Piaget, suggesting that language was more important for cognition development than Piaget implied.

13.3.6 Christian Humanism

Christian humanism theorists emphasize the humanity of Jesus, his social teachings and his propensity to synthesize human spirituality and materialism as a teaching and learning tool.[38] Christian humanism regards humanist principles such as universal human dignity and individual freedom and the primacy of human happiness as essential and principal components of, or at least compatible with, the teachings of Jesus. Christian humanism can be seen as a philosophical union of Christian ethics and humanist principles. The term humanism was coined by theologian Friedrich Niethammer at the beginning of the 19th century.[39]

Christian humanism has its roots in the traditional teaching that humans are made in the image of God (Latin: *Imago Dei*) which is the basis of individual worth and personal dignity. This found strong biblical expression in the Judeo-Christian attention to righteousness and social justice. Its linkage to more secular philosophical humanism can be traced to the 2nd century CE writings of Justin Martyr, an early theologian-apologist of the early Christian church. While far from radical, Justin in his Apology finds value in the achievements of classical culture. Influential letters by Cappadocian fathers, namely Basil of Caesarea and Gregory of Nyssa, confirmed the commitment to using preexisting secular knowledge, particularly as it touched the material world. Learning is a function of the whole person—learning cannot take place unless both the cognitive and affective domains are involved. The individual's capacity for self-determination is an important part of humanist theory. For example, humanist theory is used to help patients post stroke to regain a sense of personal control over their health care management.[40]

Among other traditional forms, Salesian Christian humanism revels in the glory revealed by God, who guides history along its path toward the perfection of love and who inserts into that history the human being created in the divine image and likeness, whose fullness is the incarnate Word, Jesus Christ. Central to the spirituality of St. Francis de Sales (1567–1622) is his vision of Man as the perfection of the universe, mind the perfection of man, love the perfection of the mind, and charity (love of God) the perfection of love.[41] Interest in the human person and the positive affirmation of human life and culture which stems from faith is the hallmark of any humanism qualified as "Christian." Several salient features distinguish its world view, including[41,42]

- An understanding of human nature as dependent on one's relation to God.
- An acknowledgment of human sinfulness and faith in the power of forgiveness.
- An emphasis on human freedom as ordered to ultimate beauty, truth, and goodness.
- An emphasis on human responsibility over and against forms of determinism.
- A vision of the individual as rooted in communion with God and others through the Church.
- A vision of the universe as ordered by divine providence and oriented toward salvation.
- A conviction that human history as a purpose for which Jesus Christ is the key.

All patients grow with success and do better when achievements are recognized and reinforced. Respecting the whole person in a supportive environment can encourage learning. Learning is also fostered through structuring information appropriately and presenting it in meaningful segments with appropriate feedback.

13.3.7 Domains of Learning

Following careful consideration by the teacher of the content to be taught, the objectives of the course, the relationship of the content to be taught to the core curriculum and curricular objective the teacher can then consider the philosophical orientation in which the content will be presented, the appropriate leaning theory or theories in which to frame the content, and finally the domain of learning. Learning can generally be categorized into three domains: cognitive, affective, and psychomotor. Within each domain are multiple levels of learning that progress from more basic, surface-level learning to more complex, deeper-level learning. The level of learning we strive to impact will vary across learning experiences depending on (1) the nature of the experience, (2) the developmental levels of the participating students, and (3) the duration and intensity of the experience.

When writing learning objectives, it is important to think about which domains are relevant to the learning experience you are designing. The paragraphs below provide further information about each domain. The concept of "domain of learning" was originally discussed by Benjamin Bloom in his Taxonomy of Educational Objectives, Handbook 1: The Cognitive Domain.[43] Additional writings have been added to the domain list.[44,45,46] Along with cognitive, we now speak of affective, psychomotor, perceptual, and spiritual domains. The cognitive, psychomotor, and affective domains are well known to physical therapists and physical therapy assistants practicing in the educational arena or the clinical arena. Not coincidentally, these are the domains most rigorously studied.

The *cognitive domain* refers to how we acquire, process, and use knowledge. It is the "thinking" domain. ▶ Table 13.4 provides a conceptual framework for the most common utilized learning domains in physical therapy education. The domains include cognitive, psychomotor, and affective. The table provides elaboration on the three domains which have been fully

Table 13.4 Learning domains

Learning domains					
→→ Level of complexity →→					
Cognitive domain					
Remember	Understand	Apply	Analyze	Evaluate	Create
Retrieve relevant knowledge from long-term memory	Construct meaning from instructional messages, including oral, written, and graphic communication	Carry out or use a procedure in a given situation	Break material into its constituent parts and determine how the parts relate to one another and to an overall structure or purpose	Make judgments based on criteria and standards	Put elements together to form a coherent or functional whole; reorganize elements into a new pattern or structure
Descriptors					
Arrange	Abstract	Apply	Analyze	Argue	Assemble
Cite	Associate	Carry out	Attribute	Assess	Build
Choose	Categorize	Demonstrate	Deconstruct	Check	Combine
Count	Clarify	Determine	Differentiate	Conclude	Compose
Define	Classify	Develop	Discriminate	Coordinate	Construct
Describe	Compare	Employ	Distinguish	Criticize	Create
Duplicate	Conclude	Execute	Focus	Critique	Design
Identify	Contrast	Implement	Organize	Detect	Draft
Label	Exemplify	Operate	Outline	Evaluate	Formulate
List	Explain	Show	Parse	Judge	Generate
Locate	Extrapolate	Sketch	Select	Justify	Hypothesize
Match	Generalize	Solve	Structure	Monitor	Integrate
Name	Illustrate	Use		Prioritize	Plan
Outline	Infer			Rank	Produce
Recall	Interpret			Rate	
Recite	Map			Recommend	
Recognize	Match			Test	
Record	Paraphrase				
Repeat	Predict				
Restate	Represent				
Review	Summarize				
Select	Translate				
State					

→→ Level of complexity →→				
Affective domain				
Receiving	Responding	Valuing	Organization	Characterization
Openness to new information or experiences	Active participation in, interaction with, or response to new information or experiences	Attaching value or worth to new information or experiences	Incorporating new information or experiences into existing value system	Full integration/ internalization resulting in new and consistent attitudes, beliefs, and/or behaviors
Descriptors				
Ask	Answer	Complete	Adhere	Act
Choose	Assist	Demonstrate	Alter	Discriminate
Describe	Aid	Differentiate	Arrange	Display
Follow	Compile	Explain	Combine	Influence
Give	Conform	Follow	Compare	Listen
Hold	Discuss	Form	Complete	Modify
Identify	Greet	Initiate	Defend	Perform
Locate	Help	Join	Formulate	Practice
Name	Label	Justify	Generalize	Propose
Select	Perform	Propose	Identify	Qualify
Reply	Practice	Read	Integrate	Question
Use	Present	Share	Modify	Revise
	Read	Study	Order	Serve
	Recite	Work	Organize	Solve
	Report		Prepare	Verify
	Select		Relate	Use

Table 13.4 continued

Learning domains				
Tell Write			Synthesize	

→→ **Level of complexity** →→

Psychomotor

Imitation	Manipulation	Precision	Articulation	Naturalization
Observing and copying another's action/skill	Reproducing action/skill through instruction	Accurately executing action/skill on own	Integrating multiple actions/skills and performing consistently	Naturally and automatically performing actions/skills at high level

Descriptors

Imitation	Manipulation	Precision	Articulation	Naturalization
Adhere Copy Follow Repeat Replicate	Build Execute Implement Perform Recreate	Calibrate Complete Control Demonstrate Perfect Show	Adapt Combine Construct Coordinate Develop Formulate Integrate Master Modify	Design Invent Manage Project Specify

Source: https://www.emporia.edu/studentlife/learning-and-assessment/guide/domains.html. Accessed March 3, 2017.

described with learning steps, definitions of the learning steps, and examples of verbs which match the learning steps and can be used when writing course and curricular objectives. The cognitive domain involves using mental processes to recall, apply, and evaluate facts and information. Cognitive learning involves learning new facts or concepts, and building on or applying past knowledge to new situations. An example of learning in the cognitive domain is a patient with diabetes mellitus who is able to state the signs of hypoglycemia and hyperglycemia, or is able to plan an appropriate diet based upon caloric restrictions. When teaching a patient factual information, use teaching strategies such as discussion, programmed instruction, written information, videotapes and audiotapes, and computer assisted instruction.

The *affective domain* deals with our attitudes, values, and emotions. It is the "valuing" domain. ▶ Table 13.4 outlines the five levels in this domain and verbs that can be used to write learning objectives. The affective domain involves attitudes, beliefs, and values that influence behavior. Affective learning includes values, religious and spiritual beliefs, family interaction patterns and relationships, and personal attitudes that affect decisions and the problem-solving process. Learning in the affective domain involves a change in attitudes or emotions that will affect behaviors. Discussion, simulations, and role-playing are teaching strategies used to teach in the affective domain. The nurse uses all three domains, depending on what is to be taught. To learn or change a health behavior, the patient may need to learn in all three domains. The nurse's role is to select a combination of content from the three domains that is appropriate to meet individualized patient teaching goals.

The *psychomotor domain* deals with manual or physical skills. It is the "doing" domain. ▶ Table 13.4 outlines the five levels in this domain and verbs that can be used to write learning objectives. The psychomotor domain involves the physical skills that a person needs to perform a procedure or technique. Psychomotor

learning includes the development of manipulative or physical skills, ranging from simple movements to complex actions. A diabetic patient who learns how to operate blood glucose monitoring equipment or to inject insulin is acquiring psychomotor skills. Strategies to help a patient learn psychomotor skills are demonstration and return demonstration and practice drills.

The *perceptual domain* involves the senses. Much of what physical therapists teach, especially in the clinical setting, involves the interpretation of various sensory stimuli such as vision, hearing, touch, and kinesthesia/proprioception. Many psychologists think of knowledge and wisdom exclusively in terms of problem solving, reasoning, conceptualizing, remembering, and so on. However, the hallmarks of knowledge and wisdom begin with and mature through perception. Knowledge and wisdom are built on the foundation of the perceptual domain and together become a system of representations and beliefs about the natural and philosophical worlds.

The *spiritual domain* is the most variably utilized by educators, therapists, and assistants. The reason for the variability is comfort; some individuals are very comfortable conversing in the spiritual domain and others are not. The degree is comfort in teaching in this domain is directly related to the exploration of one's spirituality, the confidence in discussing spiritual issues in front of a patient, patient families, and students, and the support of one's colleagues and institution in teaching in his domain. The use of the spiritual domain is often encouraged in faith-based centers of learning and health care facilities.

13.3.8 Student Learning Styles

Teachers, as with their students, have a preferred learning style. Teachers also often choose to teach in that particular style because of comfort. If an individual learns best in, for instance, the psychomotor style, he or she will often decide to teach in that style—superficially assuming that his students will also learn best from that style. This is, of course, an incorrect assumption. Whether in the classroom with graduate students or in the clinic with a patient, the content taught will be more thoroughly comprehended if the presentation mode is matched to the student learning style. A number of validated learning style assessments have been developed. Learning styles refer to a range of competing and contested theories that aim to account for differences in individual learning. These theories propose that all people can be classified according to their "style" of learning, although the various theories present differing views on how the styles should be defined and categorized. The common concept is that individuals differ in how they learn.

The idea of individualized learning styles became popular in the 1970s, and has greatly influenced education despite the criticism that the idea has received from some researchers. Proponents recommend that teachers assess the learning styles of their students and adapt their classroom methods to best fit each student's learning style. Although there is ample evidence that individuals express preferences for how they prefer to receive information, few studies have found any validity in using learning styles in education. Critics say there is no evidence that identifying an individual student's learning style produces better outcomes. There is evidence of empirical and pedagogical problems related to forcing learning tasks to "correspond to differences in a one-to-one fashion." Well-designed studies contradict the widespread "meshing hypothesis" that a student will learn best if taught in a method deemed appropriate for the student's learning style.

A number of validated measures are utilized to determine student learning styles. *The Learning Style Inventory* (LSI) is connected with David A. Kolb's model and is used to determine a student's learning style.[47] Previous versions of the LSI have been criticized for problems with validity, reliability, and other issues. Version 4 of the LSI replaces the four learning styles of previous versions with nine new learning styles: initiating, experiencing, imagining, reflecting, analyzing, thinking, deciding, acting, and balancing. The LSI is intended to help patients or students "understand how their learning style impacts on problem solving, teamwork, handling conflict, communication and career choice; develop more learning flexibility; find out why teams work well—or badly—together; strengthen their overall learning."

13.3.9 The National Association of Secondary School Principals Learning Style Profile

The National Association of Secondary School Principals (NASSP) Learning Style Profile (LSP) is a second-generation instrument for the diagnosis of student cognitive styles, perceptual responses, and study and instructional preferences.[48] The LSP is a diagnostic tool intended as the basis for comprehensive style assessment with students in the sixth to twelfth grades. It was developed by the NASSP's research department in conjunction with a national task force of learning style experts. The profile was developed in four phases with initial work undertaken at the University of Vermont (cognitive elements), Ohio State University (affective elements), and St. John's University (physiological/environmental elements). Rigid validation and normative studies

were conducted using factor analytic methods to ensure strong construct validity and subscale independence.

The LSP contains 23 scales representing four higher order factors: cognitive styles, perceptual responses, study preferences and instructional preferences (the affective and physiological elements). The LSP scales are analytic skill, spatial skill, discrimination skill, categorizing skill, sequential processing skill, simultaneous processing skill, memory skill, perceptual response: visual, perceptual response: auditory, perceptual response: emotive, persistence orientation, verbal risk orientation, verbal-spatial preference, manipulative preference, study time preference: early morning, study time preference: late morning, study time preference: afternoon, study time preference: evening, grouping preference, posture preference, mobility preference, sound preference, lighting preference, temperature preference.

13.3.10 David A. Kolb's Model of Learning Style Assessment

David A. Kolb's model of learning style assessment is based on his experiential learning model as explained in his book *Experiential Learning*.[49] Kolb's model outlines two related approaches toward grasping experience: concrete experience and abstract conceptualization, as well as two related approaches toward transforming experience: reflective observation and active experimentation.

According to Kolb's model, the ideal learning process engages all four of these modes in response to situational demands; they form a learning cycle from experience to observation to conceptualization to experimentation and back to experience. Kolb postulated that in order for learning to be effective all four of these approaches must be incorporated. As individuals attempt to use all four approaches, they may tend to develop strengths in one experience-grasping approach and one experience-transforming approach, leading them to prefer one of the following four learning styles. According to this model, individuals may exhibit a preference for one of the four styles—accommodating, converging, diverging and assimilating—depending on their approach to learning in Kolb's experiential learning model.[50,51,52]

- Accommodator = Concrete Experience + Active Experiment: strong in "hands-on" practical doing (e.g., physical therapists).
- Converger = abstract conceptualization + active experiment: strong in practical "hands-on" application of theories (e.g., engineers).
- Diverger = concrete experience + reflective observation: strong in imaginative ability and discussion (e.g., social workers).
- Assimilator = abstract conceptualization + reflective observation: strong in inductive reasoning and creation of theories (e.g., philosophers).

Although Kolb's model is widely accepted with substantial empirical support and has been revised over the years, a 2013 study suggests that the Kolb Learning Style Assessment still "possesses serious weaknesses."[53]

13.4 Instructional Methods and Methodology

The methods of instruction number in the hundreds and therefore, due to space requirements, all cannot be discussed here. Universal classroom design, as discussed below, teaches us that the most effective teachers utilize a number of instructional methods during each teaching session. There are two rationales for the multiple method's approach: students vary in their learning methods and when teaching a group of students one can assume there are many preferred learning methods in the classroom, and, more directly, students become bored and attention declines when one method of instruction is used for a long period of time.

Teaching Methods

Current universal design teaching theory recommends varied teaching methods to facilitate "reaching" all students. This table provides examples of a number of teaching methods. Experience and expertise facilitate matching the appropriate teaching method to the content.

- Applying simple statistical techniques to class data.
- Assignment to outline certain supplementary readings.
- Assignment to outline portions of the textbook.
- Assist an immigrant.
- Attend council meeting, school board meeting.
- Audio-tutorial lessons (individualized instruction).
- Biographical reports given by students.
- Book reports.
- Bulletin boards.
- Choral speaking.
- Class discussion conducted by teacher.
- Class discussions conducted by a student or student committee.
- Coaching: special assistance provided for students having difficulty in the course.
- Collect colored slides.
- Collect money for a cause.
- Collect old magazines.
- Collecting and presenting artifacts.
- Compile list of older citizens as resource people.
- Conduct a series.
- Construct a drama.
- Construction of exhibits and displays by students.
- Construction of scrapbooks.
- Construction of vocabulary lists.
- Cooking foods of places studied.
- Crossword puzzles.
- Dances of places or periods studied.
- Debate (informal) on current issues by students from class.
- Detect propaganda.
- Diaries.
- Discussion groups.
- Drama, role playing.
- Draw a giant map on floor of classroom.
- Elect a "Hall of Fame" for women.
- Elect a "Hall of Fame" for men.
- Exchange program with schools from different parts of the state.
- Field trips.
- Filling out forms (income tax, checks).
- Flags.
- Flash cards.
- Flowcharts.
- Follow a world leader (in the media).
- Forums.
- Gaming and simulation.
- Group presentation of student papers.
- Hall of Fame by topic or era (military or political leaders, heroes).
- Interviews.
- Investigate a life.
- Invite senior citizen(s) to present local history to class including displaying artifacts (clothing, tools, objects, etc.).
- Jigsaw puzzle maps.
- Join an organization.
- Laboratory experiments performed by more than two students working together.
- Lecture by guest in person.
- Lecture by teacher.
- Library research on topics or problems.
- Making announcements.
- Making of posters by students.
- Maps, transparencies, globes.
- Mobiles.
- Models.
- Murals and montages.
- Music.
- Newspaper reading.
- Nondirective techniques applied to the classroom.
- Obtain free and low-cost materials.
- Open textbook study.
- Open textbook tests, take home tests.
- Pen pals.
- Photographs.
- Playing music from other countries or times.
- Portfolio development.
- PowerPoint presentation.
- Prepare an exhibit.
- Prepare editorial for school paper.
- Prepare mock newspaper on specific topic or era.
- Prepare presentation for senior citizen group.
- Presentation by a panel of instructors.
- Presentation of student papers.
- Presentations by student panels from the class: class invited to participate.
- Problem solving or case studies.
- Puppets.
- Reading aloud.
- Reading assignments in journals, monographs, etc.
- Reading assignments in supplementary books.
- Recitation oral questions by teacher answered orally by students.
- Reports on published research studies and experiments by students.

- Reproductions.
- Required term paper.
- Research local archaeological site.
- Role playing.
- Service learning activities.
- Simulation.
- Small groups such as task oriented, discussion, Socratic.
- Stamps, coins, and other hobbies.
- Start a campaign.
- Story telling.
- Student construction of diagrams, charts, or graphs.
- Students drawing pictures or cartoons vividly portray principles or facts.
- Students from abroad (exchange students).
- Studying local history.
- Supervised study during class period.
- Surveys.
- Taking part (community elections).
- Telling about a trip.
- Textbook assignments.
- Time lines.
- Tutorial: students assigned to other students for assistance, peer teaching.
- Units of instruction organized by topics.
- Use of chalkboard by instructor as aid in teaching.
- Use of community or local resources.
- Use of diagrams, tables, graphs, and charts by instructor in teaching.
- Use of dramatization, skits, plays.
- Use of exhibits and displays by instructor.
- Use of filmstrips.
- Use of pretest.
- Use of radio programs.
- Use of recordings.
- Use of sociometric text to make sociometric analysis of class.
- Use of technology and instructional resources.
- Use of television.
- Use of theater motion pictures.
- Using case studies reported in literature to illustrate psychological principles and facts.
- Video.
- Visit an "ethnic" restaurant.
- Visit an employment agency.
- Vocabulary drills.
- Volunteer (tutoring, hospital).
- Word association activity.
- Workbooks.
- Write a caption for chart, picture, or cartoon.

Direct lecture is arguably the most common and universal of teaching methods. Direct lecture is the oral presentation (often augmented by supportive techniques such as prereading selected items, pretest/posttest, videos, and power point presentations) to present didactic information to a student or group of students. Strong lecturing techniques greatly improve student comprehension. The first five minutes of the lecture provides a golden opportunity to draw the students into the lecture. Expert teachers begin with the obvious—introducing oneself,

explaining objectives for the lecture, and outlining the presentation of content. Beginning a lecture with passion and enthusiasm facilitates quick engagement and buy-in by the students. The introduction needs to engage, excite, challenge, and create expectations. Effective introductions often contain little-known facts, nonoffensive humor, or interesting graphics or videos via PowerPoint to spark curiosity. When preparing the framework of the lecture, consider the sequencing of the material and ensure that it's presented in a clear and logical manner. The pace should be well controlled and evenly presented. One of the crucial elements to a successful lecture is the planning process. The teacher needs to fully comprehend the content and transform it into verbiage the students can understand. Presentation of content has been revolutionized with the rising age of technology. With visual aids, lecture material can be broken up with visual stimulation such as educational videos, distance interviews, pictures, photographs, and class participation techniques such as "clicker voting" which are all particularly effective in conveying information in a powerful manner. Jargon, colloquialisms, and abbreviations easily disengage students. If lecturing on a specialist subject, an expert teacher does not assume that students will understand an expert's jargon from the outset. Jargon which may seem comfortable to the teacher may be foreign to the student. This is especially true in the health care arena and classroom. Professional language of clinicians is littered with abbreviations, acronyms, jargon, and technical terms. Care should always be taken to transform these data into language understood by the student.

Good lecturing is a process of continuous improvement, so expert teachers strive for best practice with presentation style. The teacher can be animated without being theatrical, informative without being dull, and interesting without being outlandish. Avoid fidgeting. Keep the body language strong and confident. Avoid space fillers such as "umm," "you know," and "sooooooo." A teacher should not be afraid to show genuine passion and enthusiasm for the subject. Conveying lecture material in an enthused and passionate manner will instantly attract attention and will help students to focus and endorse your point of view. Good teachers vary the intonation and tone of their voices during a lecture. Use nonoffensive humor (nothing political, sexual, religious, racial, or cultural is a good rule) and conversational tone to help maintain attention. Pause at regular intervals to ensure students are still engaged and attentive. Ask questions to see if they are keeping up with the pace; this will help you to organize future lectures effectively. Occasionally scan the audience to identify nonverbal feedback about your performance. Obviously, students sleeping, yawning, or daydreaming is not a good sign and may indicate a need to provide the students with either a short classroom break or a change in teaching method.

Small group discussion is another strong teaching tool. Place the students in small groups (do not permit the students to choose their own groups—they will choose their friends and the objective of the lesson will be detoured by small talk) and provide each group with a discussion question. Provide sufficient time to permit the students to adequately discuss the question and formulate an answer. Ask for a spokesperson from each group to present the answer in depth to the entire class. Encourage the students in the class to ask questions of the discussion group.

"Sticky" topic work group is an interesting method of encouraging students to reflect on what they know and do not know, and to work together to learn the unknown content. After a lecture, the teacher asks the students to write a topic on a piece of paper that was covered in the lecture but remains confusing (sticky). The teacher collects the papers and reviews them tossing out the repetitive topics. Divide the class into small groups and provide each group with a "sticky topic." Provide the groups 10 minutes to formulate a teaching tool explaining the sticky topic. Have them present the sticky topic to the class.

PowerPoints have revolutionized classroom lectures for a number of reasons. Portable electronic devices permit their development at pretty much any location, including home, school, place of employment, restaurant or coffee shop, and even public transportation. They can be easily downloaded onto educational platforms and shared with the students. They can be seamlessly edited and amended quickly and efficiently. They can be easily transported to colleagues and experts for additional content and organizational input. Students can print the presentation and take notes on the hard copy or take notes on the electronic copy. Videos, tables, figures, photographs, and graphs can be easily added to the presentation prior to the teaching episode and smart board technology permits adding content during the presentation.

The first rule of developing a PowerPoint presentation is to keep it simple. Use only one message per slide. Limit the amount of text on each slide—no one wants to read a research article embedded on a slide. Use only elements that add to the content of the message. Use graphics (tables, figures, videos, and pictures) that clearly support the message. Good graphics can significantly add to learning, bad graphics can confuse and distract the audience. Maintain a consistent design with regard to colors, font styles, and graphics. Choose the font based upon content. For serious content use a serious font; for lighter content choose an asymmetrical font such as comic sans. Always begin with an overview slide—a slide that outlines the presentation. This allows the student to mentally organize the presentation. Provide course objectives. Choose slide colors thoughtfully. Dark blue projects a stable, mature message and has a calming effect. Red or orange tend to trigger excitement or an emotional response. Greens enhance comfort. Yellow grabs the audience's attention.

When developing the presentation brainstorm these questions: Who is the audience? What is their educational level? What is the audience's attention span? What are the preferred learning styles? What do I need for the audience to learn and what do I hope they learn? What are the environmental concerns which I should address regarding the presentation room? For drier presentations choose a dark background with a white font. The eye is drawn to lighter colors on a dark background.

13.5 Methods of Outcomes

Outcomes assessments close the loop for the teacher. The teacher develops the learning objectives for the course and then develops course content which matches the learning objectives. To close the loop—to provide the teacher with feedback as to how well the student learned the content and thus met the learning objectives—the teacher typically assesses how well the student has mastered the content. Outcomes assessments provides the teacher with objective feedback about the effectiveness of student learning.

Well-developed assessments can be associated with one of the published learning objectives and with particular educational content provided to the student. Well-developed assessments, based on the principles of universal classroom design, should be numerous and of sufficient domains to meet the learning styles of the students. The most common forms of outcomes assessment are quantitative methods, qualitative methods, interviews, observations, and documents.

13.5.1 Quantitative Assessment Methods

Quantitative methods use numbers for interpreting data. The potential to generalize results to a broader audience and situations make this type of assessment design popular with many teachers. Although the assessment process can be carried out with the rigor of traditional research, including a hypothesis and results that are statistically significant, this is not a necessary component of programmatic or class outcomes-based assessment. In addition, unlike use of some quantitative methods of assessment it is not essential to have a certain classroom size in order to provide a quantitative assessment.

Quantitative assessment offers a myriad of data collection tools including structured interviews, questionnaires, quizzes, and examinations. The most commonly used tool is the structured examination. Multiple-choice test questions, also known as items, can be an effective and efficient way to assess learning outcomes. Multiple choice test items have several potential advantages:

Versatility. Multiple-choice test items can be written to assess various levels of learning outcomes, from basic recall to application, analysis, and evaluation. Because students are choosing from a set of potential answers, however, there are obvious limits on what can be tested with multiple choice items. For example, they are not an effective way to test students' ability to organize thoughts or articulate explanations or creative and novel ideas.

Reliability. Reliability is defined as the degree to which a test consistently measures a learning outcome. Multiple-choice test items are less susceptible to guessing than true/false questions making them a more reliable means of assessment. The reliability is enhanced when the number of multiple items focused on a single learning objective is increased. For this reason, many teaching experts utilize multiple smaller multiple-choice quizzes that assess just one or two learning objectives each rather than broad exams addressing many objectives. Lastly, objective scoring associated with multiple-choice test items avoids issues with scorer inconsistency that can plague scoring of essay and short answer questions.

Validity. Validity is the degree to which a test measures the learning outcomes it purports to measure. Students can typically answer a multiple-choice item much more quickly than an essay question, therefore, tests based on multiple-choice items can able focus on a relatively broad representation or narrowly focused representation of course material, thus increasing the validity of the assessment. Various statistical analyses can be employed to assess a specific question's reliability and validity.

The key to taking advantage of these strengths is construction of good multiple-choice items. A multiple-choice item consists of a problem, known as the stem, and a list of suggested solutions, known as alternatives. The alternatives consist of one correct or best alternative, which is the answer, and incorrect or inferior alternatives, known as distractors. The stem should be meaningful by itself and should present a definite problem. A stem that presents a definite problem allows a focus on the learning outcome. A stem that does not present a clear problem, however, may test students' ability to draw inferences from vague descriptions rather serving as a more direct test of students' achievement of the learning outcome. All alternatives should be plausible. Distractors should be selected by students who did not achieve the learning outcome but ignored by students who did achieve the learning outcome. Alternatives that are implausible do not serve as functional distractors and thus should not be used. Common student errors provide the best source of distractors. Item analysis software provides question and test reliability and validity measures.

13.5.2 Qualitative Assessment Methods

According to Denzin and Lincoln, qualitative research is "multimethod in focus, involving an interpretive, naturalistic approach to its subject matter."[54] Upcraft and Schuh expand this definition by stating, "Qualitative methodology is the detailed description of situations, events, people, interactions, and observed behaviors, the use of direct quotations from people about their experiences, attitudes, beliefs, and thoughts."[55] Qualitative assessment is focused on understanding how people make meaning of and experience their environment or world. This type of assessment focus, as compared with quantitative assessment, is narrow in scope, applicable to specific situations and experiences, and is not intended for generalization to broad situations.

Each primary type of data provided to the teacher from qualitative assessments offers a unique and valuable perspective about student learning. Grading qualitative assessments such as essay and short answer exams is a bit more challenging than quantitative assessments. Qualitative assessments require a complex rubric to improve the validity and reliability of the assessment but this requirement is certainly not insurmountable. A combination of quantitative and qualitative assessments provides a more complete or holistic picture of student learning than either assessment individually.

Interviews

Interviews comprise a number of open-ended questions that result in responses that yield information about people's experiences, perceptions, opinions, feelings, and knowledge.[56] It is common to engage in face-to-face verbal interviews with one individual; however, interviews may also be conducted with a group and administered via e-mail, telephone, or on the web. Though questions and format may differ, an essential component of any interview is the "trust and rapport to be built with respondents." Open-ended questions are commonly used in the clinical arena to assess the patient in having meet learning objectives. The use of the "teach back" technique is an excellent interview method.[55] Following the completion of an educational session with a patient, the therapist may ask the patient: "Please teach back to me exactly what I taught you."

Observations

Observations, often used in laboratory, practical, internship, and clinical experiences, do not require direct contact with a study participant or group. Rather, this type of data collection involves a teacher providing information-rich descriptions of behavior, conversations, interactions, organizational processes, psychomotor or any other type of human experience obtained through observation. Such observation may be either participant, in which the researcher is actually involved in the activities or distant, in which the researcher is a nonparticipating observer. Observational assessments are commonly used in student skills' check analysis, practical examinations, and to analyze performance in clinical internships. In the clinical setting, therapists utilize observation to assess the patient's psychomotor performance is such areas as gait, transfers, bed mobility, exercise performance, and precautions. In keeping a record of observations, many methods can be used. One way is to take notes during the observation; another method commonly employed is to create a checklist or rubric to use during the observation. The checklist or rubric not only gives the observer a set of criteria to observe, but it also allows the observer to show student progress over time and to correlate a number grade with a qualitative process.

Documents

Finally, documents include "written materials and other documents from organizational, clinical, or programs records; memoranda and correspondence; official publications and reports; personal diaries, letters, artistic works, photographs, and memorabilia; and written responses to open-ended surveys."[56] When assigning a document as part of the assessment process, teachers must realize that there is a direct relationship between the number and severity of constraints and requirements placed upon the finished document and the diminishment of the process of inductive discovery on the part of the student. Nonetheless, documents are a rich source of information and provide a great starting point for any assessment project in the classroom arena documents such as essays, term papers, position papers, portfolios, theses, dissertations, and field reports are the most common documents reviewed as assessments. Again, criteria checklists and rubrics can be used in the analysis of documents to identify whether outcomes are met.

13.6 Development of a Universal Classroom Design

Designing any product, service, or environment involves the consideration of many factors, including production costs, customer needs and expectations, aesthetics, engineering options, environmental issues, and safety concerns. In large scale manufacturing, design is created for the average user. As an example, stadium seats have a prescribed depth and width which accommodates the majority of the men and women—based upon mean anthropomorphic measures—in the United States. In contrast, "universal design" (UD) is, according to the Center for Universal Design (CUD), "the design of products and environments to be usable by all people, to the greatest extent possible, without the need for adaptation or specialized design."[57] The CUD believed it advantageous to design product that meet the needs of all members of a population rather than designing for the average user and retrofitting for the less common user. In the past decades, the educational sector has adapted the CUD definition to include the design of classroom, classroom and educational products, learning aids, and curricula.[58]

UD in education is an approach to designing the environment, products, and services that takes into consideration the variability in abilities, disabilities, leaning styles and domains, and other characteristics of the student body. Rather than focus on adapting the educational environment, products, and services for an individual at a later time, UD posits initial development with universal accessibility as a goal.

The principles of universal design, developed at the CUD at North Carolina State University, were originally directed toward design engineers but have been adapted for multiple settings, including education. The principles of universal design are listed below along with an example of an application in an architectural and educational setting for each.[57,59]

1. **Equitable use.** The design is useful and marketable to people with diverse abilities. *Architectural example:* Instead of steps leading to the student center's coffee shop, a gentle ramp built with Americans with Disability Act specifications allow equal access for those ambulatory, those in wheelchairs, and those utilizing assistive devices to walk. *Curricular example:* A textbook publisher also designs an electronic version of the textbook which can be viewed on a monitor and enlarged to permit students with poor visual acuity to read it.

2. **Flexibility in use.** The design accommodates a wide range of individual preferences and abilities. *Architectural example:* Bathroom stalls are all designed to meet the needs of persons with impairments. They can be used by persons with impairments or persons without impairments equally well. *Curricular Example:* An example is a campus software program that automatically records video and auditory from a guest lecturer to be viewed at a later date by students who are ill the day of the presentation.

3. **Simple and intuitive.** Use of the design is easy to understand, regardless of the user's experience, knowledge, language skills, or current concentration level. *Architectural example:* Directions to the rest rooms are written in symbols and arrows rather than a narrative permitting non-English speaking persons to locate the restroom easily. *Curricular example:* The use of concept maps for difficult content.

4. **Perceptible information.** The design communicates necessary information effectively to the user, regardless of ambient conditions or the user's sensory abilities. *Architectural example:* Crosswalks with audio and visual cures related to time to safely cross the road. *Curricular example:* An example of this principle being employed is when multimedia projected in a classroom such as power point containing a video includes captioning for the hearing impaired.

5. **Tolerance for error.** The design minimizes hazards and the adverse consequences of accidental or unintended actions.

Architectural example: An example of a product applying this principle is a classroom building door with an electronically opening door with a call bell in the event the door does not work as planned. *Curricular example:* Distance-enabled live video and audio feed from the classroom in the event of icy streets.

6. **Low physical effort.** The design can be used efficiently and comfortably, and with minimal fatigue. *Architectural example:* For example, doors that open automatically for people with a wide variety of physical characteristics demonstrate the application of this principle. *Curricular example:* The availability of lightweight notepads to students, preloaded with adaptive software for persons unable to carry a standard laptop.

7. **Size and space for approach and use.** Appropriate size and space is provided for approach, reach, manipulation, and use regardless of the user's body size, posture, or mobility. *Architectural example:* A study table which accommodates standard desk chairs and wheelchairs is an example of this principle. *Curricular example:* Unattached classroom desks and which can accommodate students of variety of sizes and weight as well as left- and right-hand dominant.

8. **Community of learners.** To create a community of learners, instructors need to be flexible, perceptive, and tolerant of different levels of prior knowledge, as well as being aware of approaches to increase students' attention and ways to use physical space. *Architectural example:* Designing classroom buildings with multiple entrances, multiple bathrooms, computer laboratories, and snack bars to reduce the need to travel. *Curricular example:* To create a positive community of learners, faculty members need to incorporate all aspects of the Universal Design for Instruction principles. The willingness to learn from the students in the class will facilitate the growth of a community of learners.

9. **Instructional climate.** One cannot have a community of learners without having a positive instructional climate. *Architectural example:* A classroom that is quiet, well-insulated, of proper temperature, and sufficiently large to permit wheelchairs and those ambulating with assistive devices to move around comfortable. *Curricular example:* Instructor response to student question and needs, willingness to adapt, and willingness to embrace change.

13.7 Theories Related to Teaching Behavioral Change

Much of what physical therapists and physical therapist assistants teach in the clinic is related to behavioral change. Behavioral change refers to any transformation or modification of human behavior. Clinically, physical therapists attempt to transform or modify behavior to improve a client's safety, to modify risk factors, to eliminate poor habits and actions determined by evidence, and to, especially in the behavioral health arenas, encourage a more socially accepted behavior.

A number of theories that can be applied to patient education originate from the disciplines of communication, organizational development, sociology, psychology, and adult education.

13.7.1 The Health Belief Model

The health belief model helps explain why individual patients may accept or reject preventative health services or adopt healthy behaviors.[59] Social psychologists originally developed the health belief model to predict the likelihood of a person taking recommended preventative health action and to understand a person's motivation and decision-making about seeking health services. The health belief model proposes that people will respond best to messages about health promotion or disease prevention when the following four conditions for change exist: the person believes that he or she is at risk of developing a specific condition; the person believes that the risk is serious and the consequences of developing the condition are undesirable; the person believes that the risk will be reduced by a specific behavior change; and, the person believes that barriers to the behavior change can be overcome and managed.[60]

The first condition in the health belief model is perceived threat. If the person does not see a health care behavior as risky or threatening, there is no stimulus to act. For example, a 59-year-old woman who smokes two packs of cigarettes per day but does not believe she will develop a lung pathology if she continues to smoke. There are two types of perceived threats: perceived susceptibility and perceived severity. Susceptibility refers to how much risk a person perceives he or she has; severity refers to how serious the consequences might be. To effectively change health behaviors, the individual must usually accept the immediacy of susceptibility and severity. This is one reason that many people "get religion" after they have been diagnosed with an illness. With susceptibly and severity being an imminent danger, people who have previously resisted or put off behavior change finally give up smoking, stop drinking, lose weight, or start an exercise program. Individuals must also have the expectation that the new behavior will be beneficial; they must feel that barriers to change do not outweigh the benefits and that they can realistically accomplish the needed changes in behavior. Unfortunately, as we know, for many desirable health behaviors, the barriers are immediate and the benefits are long-range. From this perspective, it is not hard to see why it is so difficult to get patients to change behaviors.[61]

Knowing what aspect of the health belief model patients accept or reject can help the clinician design appropriate teaching interventions. For example, if a patient is unaware of his or her risk factors for one or more diseases, you can direct teaching toward informing the patient about personal risk factors. If the patient is aware of the risk, but feels that the behavior change is overwhelming or unachievable, you can focus your teaching efforts on helping the patient overcome the perceived barriers.

13.7.2 Self-Efficacy Model of Change

Self-efficacy is an individual's self-perception of their own ability to perform a demanding or challenging task such as facing an exam, undergoing surgery, or enacting a difficult behavioral change.[61] The perception is based upon factors such as the individual's prior success in the task or in related tasks, the individual's physiological state, and outside sources of encouragement and persuasion. Self-efficacy is thought to be predictive of the amount of effort an individual will expend in initiating and maintaining a behavioral change, so although self-efficacy is not a behavioral change theory per se, it is an important element of many of the theories, including the health belief model, the theory of planned behavior and the health action process approach.

13.7.3 Theory of Reasoned Action

The theory of reasoned action assumes that individuals consider a behavior's consequences—both positive and negative—prior to assuming the particular behavior. Therefore, the active consideration of the result of a behavior is an important factor in determining initiation of behavior and potential behavioral change. Intention is shaped by peer and social pressure, history, attitude, and knowledge.[62]

13.7.4 Theory of Planned Behavior

In 1985, Ajzen expanded his theory of reasoned action to the theory of planned behavior, which also emphasizes the role of intention in behavior performance but is intended to cover instances in which a person is not in control of all variables affecting the actual performance of a behavior.[63] As a result, the updated theory states that the incidence of actual behavior performance is proportional to the amount of control an individual possesses over the behavior and the strength of the individual's intention in performing the behavior.[64]

13.7.5 Transtheoretical or Stages of Change Model

According to the transtheoretical model, which is also known as the stages of change model, behavioral change is a five-step process.[65] The five stages, between which individuals may oscillate before (or not) achieving complete change, are precontemplation, contemplation, preparation for action, action, and maintenance. At the precontemplation stage, an individual may or may not be aware of a behavioral problem and has no thought of changing their behavior. From precontemplation to contemplation, the individual begins thinking about changing a certain behavior. During preparation, the individual begins his plans for change, and during the action stage the individual begins to exhibit new behavior on a consistent basis. An individual finally enters the maintenance stage once they exhibit the new behavior consistently for a long period of time. The transtheoretical model is an attractive model for behavioral change because it accounts for the inherent fallibility of man.[66]

13.7.6 Social Learning and Social Cognitive Theory

According to the social learning theory, which is also known as the social cognitive theory, behavioral change is determined by environmental, personal, and behavioral elements.[67] Each factor is linked through the others via a codependence. For example, in congruence with the principles of self-efficacy, an individual's thoughts affect their behavior and an individual's characteristics elicit certain responses from the social environment. Likewise, an individual's environment affects the development of personal characteristics as well as the person's behavior, and an individual's behavior may change his environment as well as the way the individual thinks or feels. Social learning theory focuses on the symbiotic interactions between these factors which are hypothesized to determine behavioral change. Behavioral change outcome is predicted on the codependent relationship between these variables.

13.7.7 Health Action Process Approach

The health action process approach is designed as a sequence of two continuous self-regulatory processes, a goal-setting phase (motivation) and a goal-pursuit phase (volition). The second phase is subdivided into a preaction phase and an action phase. Motivational self-efficacy, outcome expectancies, and risk perceptions are assumed to be predictors of intentions. This is the motivational phase of the model. The predictive effect of motivational self-efficacy on behavior is assumed to be mediated by recovery self-efficacy, and the effects of intentions are assumed to be mediated by planning. The latter processes refer to the volitional phase of the model.[68]

Behavioral change theories are not universally accepted. Criticisms include the theories' emphases on individual behavior and a general disregard for the influence of environmental and societal factors on behavior.[69] In addition, as some theories were formulated as guides to understanding behavior while others were designed as frameworks for behavioral interventions, the theories' purposes are not consistent. Such criticism illuminates the strengths and weaknesses of the theories, showing that there is room for further research into behavioral change theories.

13.8 The Continuum of Learning: From Children to Adults

To provide effective patient teaching, the teacher must consider the patient's age and developmental level. Developmental level, for this chapter, is defined as the summation of the patient's or student's physical maturation and abilities, psychosocial development, and cognitive capacity.

Specific developmental issues characterize each age group. Infancy is the time from birth to the first 12 to 18 months of life. During this time, the infant is totally dependent on others to meet basic needs. The toddler period is the time from when a child begins to walk until around 3 years of age. The years between 2 and 3 are a significant time for physical and emotional development. Motor development progresses significantly, and the child begins to have a degree of physical and emotional independence while still maintaining a close relationship with the primary family unit. During the preschool period—generally between ages 3 and 6—a child shows increasing interest in and involvement with his age group peers, though there is often anxiety when placed under supervision of others. Most preschool children are able to relate to their peers and have beginning social interactions with persons of varying ages though with limited capabilities to differentiate these individuals based upon personal characteristics. From 6 to 12 years of age, the interests of school-age children turn away from their immediate family to the wider world. The school-age child has enough maturity to begin to relate to other people as individuals.

Adolescence is characterized by the onset of puberty and is associated with a significant amount of personal exploration and often rebellion against convention. Adolescence ends when the young person demonstrates his or her readiness to assume full financial, emotional, and social independence. In Western societies, this usually occurs between 18 and 21 years of age.

During young adulthood—from approximately 21 to 39 years of age—individuals focus on selecting an occupation or career, choosing and learning to live with a partner, and starting and raising a family. During middle adulthood, individuals work at establishing themselves in a marriage and mature in their career choices. Most middle-aged adults between ages 40 and 65 begin to face adjustments to physiological changes that occur with maturity. Older adults must make adjustments to decreased physical strength, diminished endurance, pain, declining health status, retirement from the work force, reduced income, decreasing independence, and the deaths of spouse, siblings, friends, and self.

Each age cohort offers the teacher unique opportunities, challenges, and variables. The expert teacher considers age of the students when considering teaching domain, presentation method, and assessment method.

13.8.1 Teaching Parents of Infants

It is important to teach parents that infancy is a time of rapid growth and development. New parents may misinterpret many normal aspects of infant development as a positive or negative deviation from the norm. New parents often overstate the importance an infant's interest or behavior positively and negatively. It is important to emphasize to the parents that development does not occur at the same rate for all infants. Unless new parents are aware of this, they may experience considerable anxiety when comparing their infant to others who may be developing more quickly. Teaching parents about normal infant development, as well as the range of individual differences, can relieve unnecessary anxiety. Other typical topics for infant development teaching include the need for immunizations, infant stimulation, infant feeding, and safety issues, and teething. Occasionally, the physical therapist must teach the parents of a child a specific psychomotor activity such as range of motion activities and positioning techniques. Adjuvant cognitive teaching about these psychomotor activities must also be considered.

13.8.2 Toddlers

Between 18 months and 3 years of age, the young child rapidly gains language skills and begins to demand increased autonomy. Therapists can help parents learn what behaviors to expect and how to effectively manage behavioral issues. Child safety is an extremely important area to teach parents of toddlers. Young parents may be unaware of safety hazards and may need help in learning ways to childproof their home. Toilet training also occurs at this age. By teaching various ways to toilet train, and by continuing to emphasize individual rates of development, nurses can help parents toilet train children with realistic expectations and lessened stress. Although toddlers are unable to reason and may take many things literally, they are capable of some degree of understanding when they have medical tests or procedures. The therapist's approach to the toddler should be calm, warm, and matter of fact. The basis of a therapist's relationship with the toddler is one of trust and fun. A strong therapist–toddler relationship must be developed prior to evaluation, assessment, and intervention. Therapeutic activities should be fun and consistent from session to session.

Planning health teaching for an infant and toddler is primarily directed toward the parents. As separation from parents often causes anxiety, parents should be included in patient care whenever possible. It is helpful for one therapist to establish a relationship with the child and family and to be consistently involved with learning activities. Reading stories and involving the young child using pictures, dolls, and puppets can stimulate learning. Because young children have no real sense of time, health teaching must occur in close proximity to the time of any event to which the teaching relates. Children this age have a very limited ability to attend to information, so plan teaching in very brief (2–5 minutes) sessions.

13.8.3 Preschool Children

In the clinical arena teaching children about interventions to be done should be a routine part of interacting with preschool children. Keep in mind, however, that the preschool child has limited reasoning abilities, so it is not helpful to explain in any detail the purpose of a procedure. Explanations should be simple and matter of fact. Most preschool children fantasize and are quite vulnerable to fear of pain and bodily harm. It is important for the therapist to help children to express their fears and to deal with them openly. Teaching topics for parents of preschool children include understanding the importance and role of play, dealing with sexual curiosity, beginning school adjustment, and handling eating and sleeping problems.

Remember that the preschool age child is just beginning contact with the larger outside word. To avoid overwhelming the preschooler with choices, give the child no more than two or three. For example, "Would you rather look at the pictures about the exercise you will be performing or have me show your dolly about the exercise?" is a choice preschoolers can make. Parents continue to provide support for this age group and can be helpful participants in the teaching–learning session. The use of play, active participation, and sensory experiences work well for this age group. Physical and visual stimuli are better than verbal ones since the language ability of the preschooler is limited.

13.8.4 School-Age Children

School-age children between ages 6 and 12 are capable of logical reasoning, following schedules, and carrying out plans. They should be included in the patient education process whenever possible, and especially before procedures that affect them. Explain procedures, as well as the reasons for them, in a simple, logical way, and with confidence and optimism. Always ask for consent prior to initiating an activity. Therapists should also plan to spend considerable time teaching the parents of school-age children. School-age children learn best through their senses. Choose activities which stimulate the senses. When possible, give the child something fun to take home. Activities such as games, role playing, showing items and objects, using puppets and artwork, and telling stories and reading books are appropriate for this age group.

13.8.5 Adolescents

Adolescence is a distinct stage that marks the transition between childhood and adulthood. Adolescents are capable of abstract reasoning. Although therapists may still include the family in education, adolescents themselves are a major focus of teaching since they have considerable independence and are, consequently, in more control of the degree to which recommendations will be carried out. Therefore, instruction should be directed toward the adolescent and not toward the parent or caregiver. Adolescents have many important developmental tasks to achieve. They are in the process of forming their own identity, separating themselves from parents, and adapting to rapidly changing bodies. Bodily changes at puberty may cause a strong interest in bodily functions and appearance. Sexual adjustment and a strong desire to express sexual urges become important. Be aware that an adolescent may be wary of this topic when their parents are nearby. Adolescents may have difficulty imagining that they can become sick or injured. This may contribute to accidents due to risk taking or poor compliance in following medical recommendations. Because adolescents have a strong natural preoccupation with appearance and have a high need for peer support and acceptance, health recommendations that they view as interfering with their concept of themselves as independent beings may be less likely to be followed.

13.8.6 Teaching Young Adults

Malcolm Knowles, author of the book *The Modern Practice of Adult Education*, proposes four assumptions about adult learning that nurses should be familiar with.[70] Adults value self-direction. They view themselves as capable of making decisions, taking responsibility for the consequences of choices, and being able to manage their own lives. Adults are motivated to learn when they perceive that they have a need to learn. Always acknowledge the adult patient's desire to express his or her own needs and to make choices. Second, adults bring a variety of life experiences to the learning situation. Acknowledge and use the adult's previous learning and knowledge base. Relate new knowledge to knowledge that has already been learned. Third, learning readiness is strongly influenced by social roles and developmental tasks. Recognizing this, therapists should relate new learning to the adult's ability to become successful in important roles, for example, parent, spouse, or worker. Fourth, adults have a very present-centered time perspective and learn best when they can apply new knowledge immediately and learn how to problem solve.

The developmental tasks of young adults include establishing and managing a home, becoming established in an occupation or career, and starting and caring for a family. All of these changes can be sources of stress. Health teaching topics that the therapist may become involved in include teaching about a new or existing diagnosis, precautions, risk factor reduction, and an exercise prescription.

13.8.7 Teaching Adults in Midlife

Midlife serves as a transition period between young adulthood and later years. During middle adulthood, many individuals have reached the peak in their careers. Because people at midlife are often confronted with recognizing their own physical changes and their parents' declining health, middle aged people may become especially aware of their own goals and values and their own mortality. Oftentimes midlife is when a patient develops his first chronic illness. Risk factor modification gains importance as diseases of aging tend to present themselves during this period. Rare is the midlife adult referred to a physical therapist who, along with the presenting diagnosis, would not benefit from risk factor modification education. This realization may either motivate the person to follow recommendations more closely or, if the prospect of mortality is especially threatening, to deny illness or abandon health promotion and prevention practices.

13.8.8 Teaching Older Adults

Health promotion is an important activity throughout the life span. Older adults are not too old to stop smoking, start exercising, or change their diets. One of the greatest challenges is to dispel misconceptions about health promotion among older adults.

It is important for the physical therapist to understand normal physiological changes that occur with age and to know how to adapt teaching strategies to accommodate for normal aging changes and concurrent functional loss. As chronic illnesses become more prevalent after the fifth or sixth decades of life, a majority of health teaching for older adults focuses on illness and disease management. Older people are often coping with varying types of loss, including the loss of a spouse, lifelong friends, and individual physical capabilities. It is important to interact with each elderly patient as a unique individual, capable of learning and changing. Patient teaching for older people should be delivered with the same enthusiasm and conviction with which it is provided to younger patients. In addition to specific disease issues or treatment recommendations, many older adults are interested in sexuality and aging, exercise, nutrition, and other topics related to preventing illness and promoting quality of life. The older patient's barriers to independence should be assessed to help him or her find ways to maximize strengths and promote independence. The therapist is often in an excellent position to help patients follow medical recommendations by providing information, considering patients' individual needs, building an awareness of community services that can help lessen social isolation, and helping them maintain their independence.

Learning capacity usually remains at an efficient level well into the 80 s. In fact, the inability to absorb new information may be the first indication of an acute or subclinical disease process such as Alzheimer's disease, vascular dementia, or metabolic encephalopathy in an aging person. Validated cognitive measures are an excellent method of screening persons for cognitive decline. Instead of using stereotypical modifications, such as shorter sessions or a slower pace, make sure to assess each older person individually. Although elderly who are ill learn with difficulty, many older people require no modification in teaching strategies. It is important to give all older learners a chance to show their inquisitiveness and lifelong experience.

During all phases of the teaching-leaning process (including the development of the patient–therapist collaborative relationship, evaluation, assessment, planning, implementation, and

evaluation), therapists should focus attention not just on the existing medical problem, but also on the potentially numerous functional, emotional, and psychosocial problems that are common to old age. A detailed history is a critical part of the assessment. If the patient is not a reliable informant, a family member or significant other should be included. Besides the medical history, a comprehensive social history can identify potential problems with the home environment, support systems, financial resources, and various stresses that may be contributing to the medical problem. An accurate diet history is especially important if the patient is being placed on any kind of diet restriction. It is good practice to ask the elderly patient to bring in all medications, both prescription and over-the-counter, for complete evaluation.

With advancing age, there is a corresponding normal decline in sensory function, including vision, hearing, and touch. Two-thirds of the frail elderly have vision and hearing deficits. In addition, there is a normal decline in physical dexterity and endurance. Eighty percent of people over 65 have some form of chronic disease. The effects of chronic diseases, together with the normal changes that occur with aging, may impede learning.

Doing a psychosocial assessment also yields important information about the patient's ability to follow a recommended treatment plan. There are many reasons why an elderly patient may not follow a treatment plan. The patient may not see that the medical regimen is pertinent to his or her well-being. The patient may simply choose not to make lifestyle changes and instead choose to continue long-standing habits and patterns. The patient may choose not to accept a new treatment regimen based on his or her perceptions of quality versus quantity of life. Finally, the patient, although willing, may be unable to carry out treatment recommendations. The single most important issue in health care management for many people of advanced age is that of personal resources, including the presence of a support person or caregiver in the home, adequate finances, availability of transportation, and a safe and accessible home environment.

13.8.9 Teaching the Very Old

Consider using specific teaching techniques when providing health teaching for the very old. Never assume but be aware that some elders have increasing difficulty understanding complex sentences, are less proficient than younger people in drawing inferences, and have problems with motor tasks. Oftentimes normal or aberrant senses decline (vision, hearing, touch, smell, taste) may appear as cognitive loss. Present new information at a slower rate than you do for younger patients. Ensure all unnecessary ambient noise is reduced. Speak in a low tone of voice and allow enough time for the patient to assimilate and integrate conceptual material. Allow plenty of time for the assimilation and integration of conceptual material, and emphasize concrete rather than abstract material. It is important to reduce environmental distractions, both to compensate for any age-related hearing loss and to help the patient with attention and concentration. Group teaching may help some elderly patients increase their health-related problem-solving abilities. When suggesting lifestyle changes, be aware that many elderly patients are cautious and may not make changes easily. The implications for patient teaching are that we must take more time in teaching and that we should deliver the educational materials in small increments so that the material can be integrated.

In order for the teaching–learning plan to be effective, it must be individualized to fit the needs and lifestyle of the older patient, and in order for goals to be mutually acceptable, the patient must participate actively in goal setting. The ability to comply with expected behavioral changes depends heavily on the changes being perceived as important by the patient, the changes being able to fit into the patient's lifestyle, and the availability of adequate resources. In planning patient teaching for an elderly person, goals must be must be individualized not only in accordance with what the patient needs, but with what he or she chooses to do. For example, an 84-year-old patient with chronic obstructive pulmonary disease and the therapist may agree that to be less short of breath with activity is a goal. The therapist can then plan a teaching program designed to help the patient feel less breathless and can tie interventions such as pursed lip breathing, exercise, activity planning, medications, and nutrition to this one goal.

If the elderly patient has impaired vision, use adequate diffused light, and avoid having the older patient face a direct source of light. If the patient has prescription glasses, make sure they are being worn, and use large print for labels and instructions. To compensate for hearing loss, use a low-pitched voice, speak clearly and slowly, and face the patient while talking. Encourage the patient who has a hearing aid to use it. Ask the patient questions to verify that he or she has understood what you have said, and give written information as backup to what you've presented orally. To compensate for limited endurance, keep teaching sessions short—no more than 10 to 15 minutes—and schedule them to allow the patient rest as needed. During the teaching of any activity or skill, the pace must be set by the patient. Remember that musculoskeletal and nervous system limitations result in joint stiffness and reduced reaction time. These changes affect the performance of simple tasks such as opening a medicine bottle, as well as complex tasks such as transferring from chair to bed. Never rush the older person and do not set time limits on task performance. Always consider the effect of the patient's current medications including indication and side effects.

With advancing age, a person's memory is better for information that is heard than it is for information that is seen. Therefore, an older person is more likely to remember information he or she hears than information that he or she reads. To increase learning for a patient with memory loss, repeat the message frequently, and question the patient regularly to determine the level of retention. Pay particular attention to the language you use. Select clear, simple, terminology, and talk on the patient's level. Some elderly patients are highly educated and will prefer that you use and explain medical terminology; others will prefer that you keep interactions short and simple. Be sure to avoid making assumptions about terms, and help the patient problem solve what to do if instructions can't be followed for any reason. For example, if a patient is taking a medication "before meals," what happens if the patient doesn't eat? Should the drug be taken anyway or skipped until before the next meal? If the patient is to change his wound dressing twice per day what should happen if the patient forgets to perform one of the dressing changes?

Keep in mind that return demonstrations are important for elderly patients to ensure that they are able to do psychomotor skills independently. As an example, a patient was discharged home from the acute care hospital in a wheelchair. The physical therapist showed his elderly wife how to do a car-to-wheelchair transfer. When they arrived home, the wife was unable to help the patient out of the car. On the subsequent visit the therapist learned of this and other difficulties and was able to remediate them with further training.

13.9 Health Literacy

The federal government maintains an excellent website on health literacy. Much of the information below originated from that particular website (https://health.gov/communication/literacy/quickguide/factsbasic.htm).

Health literacy is the degree to which individuals have the capacity to obtain, process, and understand basic health information and services needed to make appropriate health decisions. Health literacy is dependent on individual and systemic factors including communication skills of lay persons and professionals; lay and professional knowledge of health topics; culture; demands of the health care and public health systems; and, demands of the situation/context. Health literacy affects people's ability to navigate the health care system, including the filling out of complex forms and locating providers and services, sharing personal information such as health history with providers, engaging in self-care and chronic-disease management, scheduling appointments, understanding the rationale for taking medications and obtaining tests, and understanding mathematical concepts such as probability and risk.

Health literacy is highly dependent on numeracy skills. For example, calculating cholesterol and blood sugar levels, measuring medications, and understanding nutrition labels all require math skills. Choosing between health plans or comparing prescription drug coverage requires calculating premiums, copays, and deductibles.

In addition to basic literacy skills, health literacy requires knowledge of current and relevant health topics. People with limited health literacy often lack knowledge or have misinformation about the body as well as the nature and causes of disease. Lack of health literacy often translates to lack of literacy related to reading and interpreting lay media reports about current health issues, such as the emerging Zika virus and Centers for Disease Control hand-washing recommendations. Instead of searching for evidence-based answers to their health questions from reliable sources, persons with low health literacy often ask for the opinions of friends and relatives who may also have health literacy difficulties. Without this knowledge, persons with low health literacy may not understand the relationship between lifestyle factors such as diet and exercise and various health outcomes, may not understand and follow instructions from their health care practitioner, and may not even be able to schedule appointments.

The complexity of health information can overwhelm even persons with advanced literacy skills. Medical science progresses rapidly. New drugs and medical tests are introduced almost daily. Conventional beliefs about health change rapidly.

What people may have learned about health or biology during their school years often becomes outdated or forgotten, or it is incomplete. Moreover, health information provided in a stressful or unfamiliar situation is unlikely to be retained.

Only 12% of adults have proficient health literacy according to the National Assessment of Adult Literacy. In other words, nearly nine out of ten adults may lack the skills needed to manage their health and prevent disease. Fourteen percent of adults (30 million people) have below basic health literacy. These adults were more likely to report their health as poor (42%) and are more likely to lack health insurance (28%) than adults with proficient health literacy. Low literacy has been linked to poor health outcomes such as higher rates of hospitalization and less frequent use of preventive services. Both outcomes are associated with higher health care costs.

Populations most likely to experience low health literacy are those with chronic illnesses, older adults, racial and ethnic minorities, people with less than a high school degree or GED certificate, people with low income levels, and nonnative speakers of English. Education, language, culture, access to resources, and age are all factors that affect a person's health literacy skills.

The primary responsibility for improving health literacy lies with public health professionals and the health care and public health systems and, to a lesser extent, our politicians and legislators. Laws and standards must be enacted to ensure that disseminated health information be written in a manner that can be understood by all and that health literacy skill building begins during the early stages of education. Health practitioners must work to ensure health literacy becomes part of their professional educational curricula, find time to assess the patient's health literacy level prior to the educational process, and work to develop health information in various media which can be understood by all.

Physical therapists and physical therapy assistants must understand that half of the patients and families they teach every day will not be able to understand many of the written teaching materials routinely disbursed to patients and families. The Joint Commission and the American Hospital Association's Patient's Bill of Rights require that patients have current information about their diagnosis, treatment, and prognosis in terms that patients and families can understand. The Joint Commission Patient and Family Education Standards specify that health care professionals consider their patient's literacy, educational level, and language in providing health care instruction. Health organizations are now scored by accreditors on how well their patients understand the safe and effective use of medications and medical equipment, potential food–drug interactions, and when and how to obtain further treatment. Patients are also being discharged home sicker and quicker than in the past, and patients and families are expected to assume more responsibility for health care. Therefore, they must be able to read and understand the health care information we provide them.

13.9.1 Designing Low Literacy Materials

If using commercially produced educational materials, make sure the reading level of these materials is ongoingly assessed. Most companies indicate reading level on the materials. The average American reads at the eighth-grade level. Health care information constructed at the eighth-grade reading level will permit 75% of the English-speaking population to read and understand the content. Match the reading level of the handout to the reading level of the patient. A number of software programs can check reading level. Microsoft Word also can check readability levels. If there is not access to a computer program to test reading levels reading formulas such as the fry formula and the simplified measure of Gobbledygook (SMOG) are effective. These formulas, which can be found online, utilize word count, syllables, and sentence length to determine reading level.

When designing written patient teaching materials there are a few easy-to-use techniques to produce materials for patients with low literacy skills. Choose short, common words rather than medical terms. For example, use pill instead of medication, eat instead of consume, and weigh instead of measure. Avoid abbreviations and acronyms such as AM/PM, CDC, CVA, PD, and PROM. Write short sentences—no more than 10 words in length and written in the active voice. Instead of writing: "Most health care experts believe it is advisable for you to take this medication consistently," write: "You must take these pills every day." Paragraphs should be short and should present one important issue. Make the materials easy on the eyes. Type font size should be between 12 and 14 points. Larger fonts are helpful for elderly people and for others with impaired vision. Keep the right margin jagged and not justified. Reading text is easier when the right margin is not justified because the jagged right edges help distinguish one line from another. When describing a procedure, such as performing a specific exercise, place illustrations next to the related ideas in the text. Highlight or underline text which is especially important.

Additional tips for teaching patients with low literacy skills include:

- Set realistic objectives. Choose only one or two objectives per teaching session and make sure the objectives state exactly what behaviors are expected. Try to make the objective relevant for the patient, such as "to help you be able to go back to work by getting your back pain under control."
- Focus on behaviors and skills. Have the patient be able to demonstrate the performance of an exercise along with being able to verbally describe it.
- Present the context first, then give new information. For example, rather than writing: "A number of diabetic diets are recommended and include those associated with high protein, low carbohydrates. This type of diet is effective in stabilizing blood sugars," write: "To help keep your blood sugar at an even keel the high protein/low carbohydrate diet is very effective." The second example places the context (stabilizing blood sugar) in the forefront of the teaching. With the first example, the patient must comprehend complex information before being taught the context of the information.
- Break up complex instructions. Separate complex instructions into smaller parts. For most people, even those with high literacy skills, three to five novel items presented at one time is a reasonable limit.
- Make educational instructions interactive by having the patient do, write, say, or demonstrate something in response to your teaching. Interaction strategies greatly assist recall and the patient's ability to carry out directions successfully.

Therapists should not be reluctant to use these techniques with patients who read well. Literacy experts have found that simplifying written materials seems to appeal to everyone—patients with low literacy skills as well as the highly literate.

13.10 Adherence in Patient Education

Health care professionals consider a patient compliant when he or she attends appointments, is interactive during the appointment, and follows recommendations for health care management. In contrast, a person is "nonadherent" when he or she cancels or fails to appear for health care appointments, ignores treatment recommendations, or doesn't follow them correctly. The extent to which patients follow health care instructions is a major issue in health care today. Therapists and other health care professionals are frequently frustrated when patients don't follow instructions despite their best efforts to help patients maintain optimum health. When examining nonadherence issues, the health care practitioner must not only look at the patient's behavior and practices but also his own. Practitioners are often too quick to blame the patient for nonadherence—as noted by synonyms health care practitioners often use to describe nonadherence: the unmotivated patient, the difficult patient, the chronically late patient, the patient who does not follow advice. Adherence is equal parts patient and practitioner responsibility.

In making personal decisions about adherence to treatment recommendations, patients may react in any of the following ways:

- They may totally ignore the information given and continue in the current pattern of action or inaction despite the threat of and actual appearance of personal consequences to health and well-being. An example of this is the patient who continues to smoke three packs of cigarettes a day despite evidence that smoking has serious and often permanent health consequences.
- They may totally accept and adopt the recommendations given without question or hesitation.
- They may appear to have decided to follow the instructions, but actually choose to follow only selected aspects of the recommendations, delaying some suggestions, or blaming events or others for their inability to follow all the recommendations.
- They may disregard instructions that seem threatening or impossible to achieve, and search for easier solutions to problems. Often this search involves lay advice or interventions from individuals associated with nonevidence-based professions.
- They may weigh the pros and cons of instructions given, seek additional information, and make a decision of whether or not to follow the instructions based on their investigation and assimilation of the information obtained.

As mentioned, it is within the realm of possibility that the nonadherence is secondary to an omission or commission by the health care practitioner. For example, some health care professionals conduct patient education by simply handing patients information about their problems and treatments with the rather naïve belief that the patient will return home, devour the information, and incorporate it into his or her daily behavior. Information may be provided which is written at an educational level far above that of the patient. The health care practitioner may provide too much information to the patient, which makes rapid assimilation difficult. The adherence may be related to a process issue. As an example, a patient was provided a large volume of information by his doctor related to caring for his recent onset of type II diabetes. The patient read the information and had a few questions. He called the physician's office with the questions and was told by the secretary that he needed to schedule a visit with the doctor to discuss the questions. The patient did not schedule, believing the answers to his questions he would receive from the doctor were not equal to the $40 copay he would be required to pay for the office visit.

In other situations, the patient may experience difficulty making the changes recommended. It is important to keep in mind that the health behaviors health care practitioners often suggest for patients involve not just one change, but changes involving many difficult daily decisions. Many of the lifestyle changes we expect patients to make may involve pain, expense, social isolation, a perceived loss of independence, and the difficulty of breaking old habits. We all know from personal experience that changing a single behavior pattern, such as starting an exercise program or going on a low-fat diet, is difficult. Yet, we frequently ask patients to change two or more behaviors—such as going on a diet, checking blood sugars three times daily, starting an exercise program, and stopping smoking—all at the same time.

Evidence consistently demonstrates that physicians significantly overestimate what patients understand when provided with health-related instructions. Physicians in one study thought that 89% of their just-discharged patients understood the side effects of the medications they were taking and that 95% knew when to resume normal activities. However, only 57% of the patients said they actually knew the side effects of their medications, and 58% knew when they could resume normal activities.

Nonadherence has a profound effect on the individual patient's health status, on individual health care professionals, and also on the health care system. Nonadherence, especially those related to health literacy, increase health disparities. Huge amounts of health care dollars are wasted when medications are not taken correctly, when medical equipment is misused, when patients are readmitted to hospital care for preventable problems, and when a large percentage of the public continue to practice health habits that inevitably lead to serious disease.

Nonadherence involving medication use occurs in many ways. Patients may never have the prescription filled or may alter the prescribed dose—taking either too much or too little of the medication, or changing the time interval at which the medication is given. It is not uncommon for patients to save up drugs that should have been completely used, increasing the possibility that they or others may use the drugs inappropriately later. In cases in which medication is a continual, ongoing part of controlling the disease itself, such as with hypertension or diabetes, failure to adhere can have life-threatening consequences. Patients who err on the side of excess run the risk of drug interactions, drug toxicity, and a variety of other impairments from misuse or overuse of prescribed, therapeutic medications.

Nonadherence also affects dietary and other lifestyle changes suggested as part of treatment, sometimes with serious consequences. For example, a patient had circulatory problems in his lower extremities due to arteriosclerosis. When his foot became infected, he was instructed to soak it several times a day, followed by a heat lamp treatment. Unfortunately, the patient adhered only sporadically and eventually had a below-the-knee amputation.

Problems with potential nonadherence are considered a major factor in developing new forms of medications and treatments. Many advertisements by drug companies claim that their produce will "improve compliance." Various techniques have been used to assess adherence with treatments, especially drug therapy, including technical methods such as checking blood concentration and serum levels of drugs, and urine screening for drug metabolites or other biochemical markers. Other simpler methods are pill counts, checking whether prescriptions are dispensed, and direct questioning of patients. There are problems with all these methods. Blood and urine screening are affected by individual variations in metabolic and absorption rates. Pill counts may be unreliable, and direct questioning may impair the relationship between clinician and patient. In addition, none of these methods gives an indication of adherence to the treatment schedule.

Patient nonadherence also has a negative impact on health care professionals. Health care professionals have the best of intentions in helping patients learn how to care for themselves and become discouraged and even angry when patients ignore our advice. Nonadherent behavior violates the professional beliefs, norms, and expectations we have about the relationship between patients and health care professionals. Not only do therapists and other health care professionals tend to underestimate the extent of nonadherence, but also have misconceptions about who is at risk for nonadherent behavior. We may assume that patients who are uneducated or from lower socioeconomic groups are less likely to follow recommendations; however, research has shown this not to be true. Amazingly, although it seems logical that patients with the most serious health care problems would be the most adherent, this has not been found to be true. One study found that patients with less severe medical problems were actually more likely to follow through with medical advice than those with a more severe illness. In addition, patients with asymptomatic disease conditions such as hypertension often have problems with adherence. It is thought that the level of perceived threat to health for asymptomatic patients is not enough to motivate a person to adhere to treatment recommendations, while very high levels of perceived threat cause such fear that the patient is unable to act.

13.11 Review Questions

1. A characteristic of a good teacher is a teacher with strong comprehension of the content of the subject being taught. A teacher of physical therapy learns content through which of the following activities?
   a) Through his or her primary education process including continuing education.
   b) Professional experience.
   c) Clinical experience.
   d) All of the above.

2. Instructional method in the science of teaching pedagogy refers to which of the following definitions?
   a) The quality of the customer service feedback given by the student to the teacher.
   b) The tools utilized to provide didactic and experiential content to the student.
   c) The voice amplitude, inflection, and tone utilized by the teacher when in front of the class.
   d) Assessment methodology including quantitative and qualitative tools.

3. The most often underutilized and underappreciated method of teacher preparation is which of the following?
   a) Transformation of content.
   b) Instructional method.
   c) Reflective evaluation by the student and teacher.
   d) Assessment tools.

4. Which statement is "false" about syllabi?
   a) The syllabus is a contract between student and teacher.
   b) The syllabus is a living document and may be amended during the semester.
   c) The syllabus should be in accord with other university documents such as the graduate/undergraduate student bulletin and university policy documents.
   d) Students and faculty have equal responsibility in syllabus development.

5. Elliot Eisner's philosophical orientations of teaching include all of the following except?
   a) Academic rationalism.
   b) Social adaptation and reconstruction.
   c) New age theory.
   d) Personal relevance.

6. The learning theory attributed to Thorndike, Skinner, and Pavlov is which of the following?
   a) Behaviorism.
   b) Gestalt.
   c) Piaget.
   d) Conditioning.

7. Christian Humanist belief includes which of the following tenets?
   a) Cognitive.
   b) Man has been given gifts by God.
   c) Man must develop those gifts and utilize them for the betterment of man.
   d) All of the above.

8. Asking physical therapy students to participate in a laboratory in which they manipulate a goniometer to measure joint range of motion is an example of which domain of learning?
   a) Cognitive.
   b) Psychomotor.
   c) Perceptual.
   d) Spiritual.

9. Which of the following student assessment method would be considered a qualitative assessment?
   a) A written examination.
   b) Interviewing a patient seen by a student about the student's customer service behavioral skills.
   c) A laboratory practical with scoring rubric.
   d) The national physical therapy examination.

10. One of the aims of universal classroom design is which of the following?
    a) To ensure that all students receive passing grades in the course.
    b) To ensure that student grades have a traditional bell shape curve distribution.
    c) To ensure that all students have an equal opportunity to succeed in the course.
    d) To make all university classrooms eco-sensitive learning environments by limiting the carbon footprints.

13.12 Review Answers

1. A characteristic of a good teacher is a teacher with strong comprehension of the content of the subject being taught. A teacher of physical therapy learns content through which of the following activities?
   d. All of the above.

2. Instructional method in the science of teaching pedagogy refers to which of the following definitions?
   b. The tools utilized to provide didactic and experiential content to the student.

3. The most often underutilized and underappreciated method of teacher preparation is which of the following?
   c. Reflective evaluation by the student and teacher.

4. Which statement is "false" about syllabi?
   d. Students and faculty have equal responsibility in syllabus development.

5. Elliot Eisner's philosophical orientations of teaching include all of the following except?
   c. New age theory.

6. The learning theory attributed to Thorndike, Skinner, and Pavlov is which of the following?
   a. Behaviorism.

7. Christian Humanist belief includes which of the following tenets?
   d. All of the above.

8. Asking physical therapy students to participate in a laboratory in which they manipulate a goniometer to measure joint range of motion is an example of which domain of learning?
   b. Psychomotor.

9. Which of the following student assessment method would be considered a qualitative assessment?
   b. Interviewing a patient seen by a student about the student's customer service behavioral skills.

10. One of the aims of universal classroom design is which of the following?
    c. To ensure that all students have an equal opportunity to succeed in the course.

References

[1] Mann K, Gordon J, MacLeod A. Reflection and reflective practice in health professions education: a systematic review. Adv Health Sci Educ Theory Pract. 2009; 14(4):595–621

[2] Schön. Donald A. The Reflective Practitioner: How Professionals Think in Action. New York, NY: Basic Books; 1993

[3] Shepard KF, Jensen GM. Handbook of Teaching for Physical Therapists. Newton, MA: Butterworth-Heinemann; 1997

[4] Johns C. Framing learning through reflection within Carper's fundamental ways of knowing in nursing. J Adv Nurs. 1995; 22(2):226–234

[5] Newman S. Philosophy and Teacher Education: A Reinterpretation of Donald A. Schon's Epistemology of Reflective Practice., London: Avebury; 1999

[6] Pakman M. Thematic foreword: reflective practices: the legacy of Donald Schön. Cybern Hum Knowing. 2000; 7:5–8

[7] Huba ME, Freed JE. Learner centered assessment on college campuses: shifting the focus from teaching to learning. Community Coll J Res Pract. 2000; 24:759–766

[8] Wasley P. The syllabus becomes a repository of legalese. Chron High Educ. 2008; 54:27

[9] Slattery JM, Carlson JF. Preparing an effective syllabus: current best practices. Coll Teach. 2005; 54(4):159–164

[10] Altman HB, Cashin WE. Witting a syllabus. Idea Paper.. 1992; 27:114–117

[11] Parkes J, Fix TK, Harris MB. What syllabi communicate about assessment in the college classroom. J of Excellence in College Teaching.. 2003; 14:61–83

[12] Habanek DV. An examination of the integrity of the syllabus. Coll Teach. 2005; 53(2):62–64

[13] Eisner E. The Educational Imagination. New York, NY: Macmillan; 1985

[14] Eisner EW. The Enlightened Eye. Qualitative Inquiry and the Enhancement of Educational Practice. Upper Saddle River, NJ: Prentice Hall; 1998

[15] Pavlov IP, Anrep GV. Conditioned Reflexes. Courier Corporation; 2003

[16] Watson JB. Psychology as the behaviorist views it. Psychol Rev. 1913; 20:158–177

[17] Benjamin LT, Jr, Whitaker JL, Ramsey RM, Zeve DR, John B. John B. Watson's alleged sex research: an appraisal of the evidence. Am Psychol. 2007; 62 (2):131–139

[18] Thorndike E. Some experiments on animal intelligence. Science. 1898; 7 (181):818–824

[19] Skinner BF. Are theories of learning necessary? Psychol Rev. 1950; 57 (4):193–216

[20] Schultz D. A History of Modern Psychology. Burlington: Elsevier Science; 2013

[21] Jäkel F, Singh M, Wichmann FA, Herzog MH. An overview of quantitative approaches in Gestalt perception. Vision Res. 2016; 126:3–8

[22] Wertheimer M, King DB, Peckler MA, Raney S, Schaef RW. Carl Jung and Max Wertheimer on a priority issue. J Hist Behav Sci. 1992; 28(1):45–56

[23] Humphrey G. The psychology of the gestalt. J Educ Psychol. 1924; 15 (7):401–412

[24] Reyna VF. A new intuitionism: meaning, memory, and development in Fuzzy-Trace Theory. Judgm Decis Mak. 2012; 7(3):332–359

[25] Schön DA. Invention and the Evolution of Ideas. London: Tavistock (first published in 1963 as Displacement of Concepts); 1967

[26] Schön DA. Technology and Change: The New. Heraclitus. Oxford: Pergamon; 1967

[27] Schön DA. The Design Studio: An Exploration of its Traditions and Potentials. London: RIBA Publications for RIBA Building Industry Trust; 1967

[28] Schön DA. The Reflective Turn: Case Studies In and On Educational Practice. New York, NY: Teachers Press; 1967

[29] Gibbs G. Learning by Doing: A Guide to Teaching and Learning Methods. Oxford: Further Education Unit, Oxford Polytechnic; 1988

[30] Piaget J. The Moral Judgment of the Child. London: Routledge & Kegan Paul; 1932

[31] Piaget J. Origins of Intelligence in the Child. London: Routledge & Kegan Paul; 1936

[32] Piaget J. Play, Dreams and Imitation in Childhood. London: Heinemann; 1945

[33] Baillargeon R, DeVos J. Object permanence in young infants: further evidence. Child Dev. 1991; 62(6):1227–1246

[34] Bruner JS. Toward a Theory of Instruction. Cambridge, MA: Belknap Press; 1966

[35] Central Advisory Council for Education. Children and their Primary Schools (The Plowden Report), London: HMSO; 1967

[36] Siegler RS, DeLoache JS, Eisenberg N. How Children Develop. New York, NY: Worth; 2003

[37] Vygotsky LS. Mind in Society: The Development of Higher Psychological Processes. Cambridge, MA: Harvard University Press; 1978

[38] Eggenschwiler D. The Christian Humanism of Flannery O'Connor. Detroit, MI: Wayne State University Press; 1972

[39] Millán-Zaibert E. Friedrich Schlegel and the Emergence of Romantic Philosophy. Albany, NY: SUNY Press; 2008

[40] Anthony MJ, Benson WS, Eldridge D, Gorman J. Evangelical Dictionary of Christian Education. Grand Rapids, MI: Baker; 2001

[41] McDonnell E. The Concept of Freedom in the Writings of St. Francis de Sales. Berne: Peter Lang; 2009

[42] Strier R. Sanctifying the aristocracy": devout humanism" in François de Sales, John Donne, and George Herbert. J Relig. 1989; 69(1):36–58

[43] Bloom BS, Engelhart MD, Furst EJ, Hill WH, Krathwohl DR. Taxonomy of educational objectives. In: Handbook I: The Cognitive Domain. New York, NY: David McKay; 1956

[44] Bloom BS, Krathwohl DR, Masia BB. Bloom taxonomy of educational objectives. Boston, MA: Allyn & Bacon; 1984. Available at: http://www.coun.uvic.ca/learn/program/hndouts/bloom.html

[45] Krathwohl DR. A revision of Bloom's taxonomy: an overview. Theory Pract. 2002; 41(4):212–218

[46] Bloom BS. Taxonomy of educational objectives: The Classification of Educational Goals. White Plains, NY: Longman; 1974

[47] Sims RR, Veres JG, III, Watson P, Buckner KE. The reliability and classification stability of the Learning Style Inventory. Educ Psychol Meas. 1986; 46(3):753–760

[48] Murray, -, Harvey R. Learning styles and approaches to learning: distinguishing between concepts and instruments. Br J Educ Psychol. 1994; 64(3):373–388

[49] Kolb DA, Fry RE. Towards an applied theory of experiential learning. In: Cooper, CL. Theories of Group Processes. Wiley series on Individuals, Groups, and Organizations. London: Wiley; 1975

[50] Kolb DA. Experiential Learning: Experience as the Source of Learning and Development. 2nd ed. Upper Saddle River, NJ: Pearson Education; 2015

[51] Smith DM, Kolb DA. User's Guide for the Learning Style Inventory: A Manual for Teachers and Trainers. Boston, MA: McBer & Co.; 1996

[52] Manolis C, Burns DJ, Assudani R, Chinta R. Assessing experiential learning styles: a methodological reconstruction and validation of the Kolb Learning Style Inventory. Learn Individ Differ. 2013; 23:44–52

[53] Kolb AY, Kolb DA. Learning styles and learning spaces: Enhancing experiential learning in higher education. Academy of Management Learning & Education. 2005; 4(2):193–212

[54] Denzin NK Lincoln YS. The Sage Handbook of Qualitative Research. Thousand Oaks, CA: Sage; 2011

[55] Upcraft ML, Schuh JH. Assessment in Student Affairs: A Guide for Practitioners. The Jossey-Bass Higher and Adult Education Series. San Francisco, CA: Jossey-Bass Inc.; 1996

[56] Patton MQ. Qualitative Research. Hoboken, NJ: John Wiley & Sons; 2005

[57] Mcguire JM, Scott SS, Shaw SF. Universal design and its applications in educational environments. Remedial Spec Educ. 2006; 27(3):166–175

[58] Scott SS, Mcguire JM, Shaw SF. Universal design for instruction a new paradigm for adult instruction in postsecondary education. Remedial Spec Educ. 2003; 24(6):369–379

[59] Hochbaum G, Rosenstock I, Kegels S. Health belief model. United States Public Health Service; 1952

[60] Rosenstock IM. Historical origins of the health belief model. Health Educ Monogr. 1974; 2(4):328–335

[61] Janz NK, Becker MH. The health belief model: a decade later. Health Educ Q. 1984; 11(1):1–47

[62] Sheppard BH, Hartwick J, Warshaw PR. The theory of reasoned action: a meta-analysis of past research with recommendations for modifications and future research. J Consum Res. 1988; 15(3):325–343

[63] Ajzen I. The theory of planned behavior. Organ Behav Hum Decis Process. 1991; 50(2):179–211

[64] Ajzen I. Perceived behavioral control, self-efficacy, locus of control, and the theory of planned Behavior. J Appl Soc Psychol. 2002; 32(4):665–683

[65] Prochaska JO, Velicer WF. The transtheoretical model of health behavior change. Am J Health Promot. 1997; 12(1):38–48

[66] DiClemente CC, Prochaska JO. Toward a comprehensive, transtheoretical model of change: stages of change and addictive behaviors. In: Miller WR, Heather N, eds. Applied Clinical Psychology. Treating Addictive Behaviors. New York, NY: Plenum Press; 1998: 3–24

[67] Lent RW, Brown SD, Hackett G. Toward a unifying social cognitive theory of career and academic interest, choice, and performance. J Vocat Behav. 1994; 45(1):79–122

[68] Schwarzer R, Lippke S, Luszczynska A. Mechanisms of health behavior change in persons with chronic illness or disability: the Health Action Process Approach (HAPA). Rehabil Psychol. 2011; 56(3):161–170

[69] Bandura A. Social Learning Theory. Englewood Cliffs, NJ: Prentice Hall; 1977

[70] Knowles MS. The Modern Practice of Adult Education. Vol. 41. New York, NY: New York Association Press; 1970

14 Cultural and Spiritual Competence in Health Care

Peter J. Leonard

Keywords: Cultural competence, spiritual competence, servant leadership, scientism, nihilism, empathy, cultural humility, interprofessional education

"I thank the authors for the opportunity to write this First Person. Spirituality in health care is a topic of strong interest to me personally and professionally. As a spiritual person I could not consider entering the health care arena without my spiritual beliefs. Spirituality defines me and is as omnipresent in my daily life as breathing in and breathing out. In addition, as Vice President of Customer Service and Performance Improvement in a large, tertiary care hospital in a large northeastern city, the facilitation of a comprehensive pastoral care environment within the health care system is part of my job description.

"Facilitating spirituality in health care seems obvious to most but less than 50% of U.S. hospitals have a full-time pastoral care or chaplaincy program. Hospitals are often defined as a 'high-tech, low-touch' environment, meaning that for many reasons—safety, infection control, urgency, staffing, and available technology—hospitals prefer to provide technological interventions rather than "high-touch" interventions. Pastoral care/chaplaincy are examples of high-touch interventions. To me, it is intuitive that when one is seriously ill and perhaps near death there is a distinct pull to connect with the spiritual side. Hippocrates wrote: "Wherever the art of medicine is loved there is also a love of humanity.

"My role as a vice president is to ensure that every patient who has a spiritual need when in the hospital has that need met. Our policy, which I helped write, states that the inpatient must be asked at admission and once every day during the admission, if he or she has a spiritual need. If the answer is yes, a pastoral care consult is written and a member of my team visits the patient to determine what the spiritual need is and identifies potential methods to meet that need. Sometimes the need is as simple as providing a Bible or a Koran. Other times it is complex as finding and bringing to the hospital a spiritual leader from a particular faith.

"Under my tenure at the hospital we have renovated our chapel. When the chapel was built 40 years ago our hospital service area was extremely homogeneous and the chapel reflected that homogeneity. Recently, our renovations included adding religious texts, hymnals, art, and artifacts from 14 different faiths. Generic faith services are held by our chaplain twice per day. We recently received a number of requests from our day shift employees to schedule another service just prior to day shift to permit employees to attend. I am so proud of these changes. What satisfaction I feel when I walk the floors at the hospital and see our amazing professionals using technology to cure the sick. What satisfaction I also feel when I walk by the chapel and see patients, patient families, and our wonderful professionals—of many different faiths—having their spiritual needs met. We are truly a high-tech/high-touch hospital!"

—Carole S., Baltimore, Maryland

14.1 Overview

Cultural and spiritual competence in health care emerges from the human need to communicate clearly and effectively in order to arrive at a proper diagnosis, treatment plan, and patient compliance. Cultural competence has been identified as a real need in the professional literature to prevent marginalization of health care consumers who exhibit different cultural values than their providers. At present, there is little evidence linking cultural competence and direct improvement in medical outcomes; however, there is an increasing body of evidence that culturally competent providers feel more comfortable in their practice. Understanding a nonnative language speaker is a major tenet of cultural competence, but there are various other challenges which may include organizational, structural, and clinical dimensions. While some people may not describe themselves as religious, many people will describe themselves as having spiritual experiences. Since spirituality is an avenue for addressing the meaning of life and human experiences, I suggest that spiritual competence needs to be considered in a way that complements cultural competence, since a sense of wellness cannot be completely confined to a scientific study of medicine. Spiritual awareness can motivate patients to interpret their health care experiences quite differently from those who are less aware. A lack of understanding of a patient's spiritual values can lead to miscommunication between patient and provider. Effective educational programs in cultural competence that include considerations of spirituality offer promise of a better patient/provider relationship.

14.2 Introduction

Throughout human history, our natural desire to be understood has been challenged by differences in language, culture, and spiritual beliefs. Health care delivery is no exception to this challenge. Since health care is a fundamental component of our sense of wellness, the achievement of an effective relationship between patient and health care provider is essential to successful diagnosis and treatment.

The adage: "If you have your health, you have everything" reminds us of the critical value we place on health and the focus that must be placed on health care delivery that takes place in a culturally competent environment. Yet, the delivery of health care is prone to power imbalances due to the years of education required to become a provider and the technical language barriers that exist between providers and patients. All of these imbalances become increasingly prominent when cultural and spiritual differences are also in play.

The western world is becoming increasingly secular. Religious values are diverse and pluralistic, thus increasing the complexity of attaining meaningful cultural understanding. In the midst of these cultural shifts, I have observed a deep desire on the part of many people to explore the existence of spiritual values. In general conversations that I have with my students, I often hear the assertion: "While I am not religious, I am very spiritual," indicating a desire to engage in a spiritual framework, even if it does not involve an organized religion. Yet the world religions have had a profound effect on the historical development of culture.

As a first step in writing this chapter, I went to PubMed and started entering the search string: "Spirituality and...." The search engine revealed medical subject headings that pair spirituality with health, mental health, palliative care, depression, cancer, aging, addiction, and many other terms. Yet the professional literature on cultural competence approaches silence on the subject of spirituality. Our spiritual well-being has an influential effect on our daily attitudes, including our self-worth, and has a major effect on our biological homeostasis. In general, consider how mood in some circumstances affects weight gain and, in other circumstances, weight loss. Our reaction to the various stimuli around us is both varied and individually unique.

14.3 Cultural Competence Defined

Betancourt and Green define *cultural competence* as "The ability of health care professionals to communicate with and effectively provide high-quality care to patients from diverse sociocultural backgrounds; aspects of diversity include—but go beyond—race, ethnicity, gender, sexual orientation, religion, and country of origin."[1]

Because most professional communication is rooted in language, I would suggest that all forms of cultural competence must begin with considerations of language and an ability to transcend any language barrier. In our modern technological era, there are software programs that are capable of translating numerous languages and are specifically tailored to handle medical terminology. If you are interested in this type of software, enter http://www.TranslationSoftware4U.com in your web search engine for a quick orientation. While software can be very helpful in dealing with numerous diverse languages, it does lack the intonation of real human speaking and the nonverbal cues that accompany person-to-person communication. As software continues to become more complex, I would expect that digital solutions to language barriers will become increasingly useful. With that being said, there are currently no software solutions that can replace real human communication between people who understand each other's language.

Consider the role that a family member can fulfill when he or she accompanies the patient. Be certain, however, to make sure that there is sufficient trust and request permission from the patient to use a family member as a translator when dealing with protected communication, unless you are dealing with a parent accompanying a minor.

14.4 Social and Cultural Barriers to Health Care

Betancourt et al define three major social and cultural barriers to health care: organizational, structural, and clinical. Organization barriers include issues of leadership; specifically, is the diversity profile of leadership reflective of the general population being served? Structural barriers include system complexity, lack of funding, and lack of interpreter services. Clinical barriers pertain to the interactions that occur between the health care provider and the patient or family. These can range from issues of trust in clinicians to cultural beliefs about health care itself.[2] It should seem intuitive that there will be struggles in delivering effective care whenever any of these three barriers are present and the severity of the challenge will increase when more than one barrier is present simultaneously. It is easy to imagine the feeling of alienation that one would feel when being approached by a health care provider who does not understand your culture; is introducing you into a very complex situation; while not speaking your language; and deals with you in a way that does not engender trust. The negative challenge in this situation is likely to be synergistic instead of additive!

14.5 Spiritual Competence

Similar to cultural competence, *spiritual competence* is the ability of a health care provider to understand the spirituality of a patient. As a minister with over 30 years of experience, I find the notion of spiritual competence to be one of the most overlooked areas in health care training. Perhaps this is related in part to the secularization that we are experiencing in our society or proceeds from the American cultural and legal notion of separation of church and state. In many cases, I have observed that practitioners are simply uncomfortable with their own spirituality and this lack of comfortability comes across very clearly when a patient brings up a spiritual subject. Yet this is quite ironic to me since the world is rich with people who demonstrate that they are spiritually aware, and for those who possess this awareness, the values that they exhibit have a profound effect on the way they address the most important questions in life. I have met many people in my professional life who I would consider spiritually actualized. These people have an evident ability to face the most difficult challenges in life with a sense of peace and calm. What makes their view of reality so different?

Spiritually aware people understand that there is a much larger reality outside of themselves. As Americans, we value our ability to self-determine our future, but spiritual people recognize that every action of our lives has an effect on others. We do not live in a relational vacuum. We are the products of families, we have friends, and we also exist in communities of fellow workers and neighbors. Instead of asking the question, "How does this action or decision affect me?" a key question that a spiritually actualized person asks is "How do my actions and decisions affect others?" As a future health care provider, consider that every patient makes decisions about his or her health care in a social context.

Many spiritually aware people recognize the existence of a supreme being and as a result, reach the conclusion that their lives are ultimately a gift from a good God who has created everyone. In a society that makes many ethical determinations based on rights, ethical determinations based on spiritual considerations lead individuals to understand that every day of their lives are a gift from their creator. Gratitude is the most appropriate response to the joys, sorrows, and challenges of our daily life because all human experiences are the result of a gracious gift. I can recall a personal experience that I had while living in my religious community with a fellow priest. He was well into his 80 s and I would frequently inquire as to his well-being and happiness. His response was always, "Every day is a gift and it is my responsibility to make the most of that gift." Instead of complaining about the issues of aging, he focused on the positive opportunities that would be available to him on that day. Viewing life through the prism of gratitude makes each part of our day have a deeper meaning. This meaning deepens when one considers that every encounter with another person is a mutual sharing of gifts. Respect for each individual is deepened by a sense of appreciation for others that progresses from politeness, to respect and ultimately to reverence. This reverence is an acknowledgment that beyond our giftedness, the presence in our lives of other people is a mutual way of acknowledging our personal value as humans. As a health care provider, I invite you to approach the patients entrusted to your care with a deep sense of reverence and observe how this reverence is most often returned by the way they treat you.

Spiritually aware people recognize that they are not completely in control of their destinies. While it may be reasonably self-evident that our decisions regarding personal lifestyle have a notable effect on our longevity, there are also many factors that we cannot control. We may be genetically predisposed to certain diseases. We are born into a particular social stratum. Our parents often model a complex series of behaviors that consist of positive components, neutral components and negative components. In some cases, we adopt these behaviors, and in other circumstances, we reject these behaviors. In most cases, we may not even realize that we are practicing certain behaviors, yet other people are well aware of the tendencies in our personalities. Consider that every person you meet, including your future patients, will have a distinct historical upbringing that leads to spiritual and other cultural tendencies. It is always best to communicate a sense of respect and negotiate with them concerning any perceived differences, rather than simply shutting down or ignoring them.

Spiritually aware people understand that suffering is part of the human condition and that suffering is a transforming experience. The common recognition, "No pain, no gain," is a rudimentary recognition of this reality. If we remember our experience of growing up, I am sure that it was filled with trial, error, and consequences for our decisions. While each of our developmental pathways was unique, we are all unified by the common experience that earning maturity was a costly process that took place at a very dear price. Understanding that there is meaning which underlies all suffering causes us to become more proactive in understanding our challenging experiences and this recognition moves us to become more aware of those who suffer with us. Consider observations of good parenting. I have observed that the most effective parents are those who communicate to their children that life requires ongoing decision making and that all of their children's decisions result in consequences. This seems far superior to calling their children bad or good since this type of behavior makes a judgment about the child's self-worth. By extension, every patient that presents to you will be have a personal decision-making history. Each of these decisions has resulted in a consequence, but even if the consequence has resulted in suffering, there has been real learning that has occurred and that person has more often grown in adult maturity as a result of the choice. A spiritual view will allow us to recognize that we are companions on a life journey and all of us have made decisions that we later recognized to be good or bad. Most important is a recognition of the growth that has occurred.

Spiritual people see that sacrifice elevates the human condition. In most cities around the world, you will find a monument to soldiers who have participated in a war and made the ultimate sacrifice of their lives. How do you reconcile our human desire for self-preservation with their virtuous behavior? The fact that we memorialize them in this way indicates the degree of human respect we have for their actions. Many of these memorials will have the word "valor" etched into them. Consider that your future patients have personal lives that involve many different forms of suffering. They may struggle to balance a budget. They may be in a difficult job. They may have family members who are ill. In some way, they practice virtue by enduring the sacrifices of daily life. In many cases, they practice their own form of daily valor.

Spiritual people find that it is better to give than to receive. I am sure that we all know a person who is tremendously generous with his or her time. Our respect for such people increases when we consider that there are generous people who share their time freely with those who are vulnerable and in need of health care. How do you envision your future identity as a health care provider? Will you be generous with your time toward those in need?

Spiritual people understand that they are inextricably anchored in a human community. That every human who acts has some effect on others around himself or herself. Who among us could actually create a life that is completely independent? Imagine yourself transported to an island where there are no other people. Next make a list of your daily activities. How many of these could you accomplish in the absence of others? From where would you obtain your daily food, drinking water, clothing, and shelter? It should become evident that it would be difficult to exist in such a social vacuum. I look around me and recognize that I am a social being. I cannot exist and certainly cannot flourish without the presence of others in the human community. This recognition invites me to place the needs of others before my own needs. Reciprocally, I realize that I need the help of others who attend to my own needs. This is clearly evident within the health care community. Practitioners who focus on a mindset that their professional leadership is manifested in a call to serve others, witness through their actions a spiritual capacity that elevates their character to a distinctively higher level. This is particularly evident in the concept of *servant-leadership* that was first advanced in 1970 by Robert K. Greenleaf. He writes:

"The servant-leader is servant first.... It begins with the natural feeling that one wants to serve, to serve first. Then conscious choice brings one to aspire to lead. That person is sharply different from one who is leader first, perhaps because of the need to assuage an unusual power drive or to acquire material possessions... The leader-first and the servant first are two extreme types. Between them there are shadings and blends that are part of the infinite variety of human nature."[3]

The difference manifests itself in the care taken by the servant-first to make sure that other people's highest priority needs are being served. The best test, and difficult to administer, is, Do those served grow as persons? Do they, while being served become healthier, wiser, freer, more autonomous, more likely themselves to become servants? And what is the effect on the least privileged in society? Will they benefit or at least not be further deprived?

A servant-leader focuses primarily on the growth and well-being of people and the communities to which they belong. While traditional leadership generally involves the accumulation and exercise of power by one at the "top of the pyramid," servant leadership is different. The servant-leader shares power, puts the needs of others first and helps people develop and perform as highly as possible.[3]

I would suggest that health care practitioners who commit themselves to a model of servant-leadership will enrich themselves and their patients spiritually and if practiced well, they will have much more positive relationships with their patients.

14.6 Questions of Ultimate Meaning and Reality

While modern medicine can do amazing things, it lacks the ability to answer questions of ultimate meaning and reality. It remains silent on questions such as "why am I here?" or "what is the meaning of human life?" or, more intriguing for a health care professional, "what is the meaning of human sickness and death?" Answers to these questions are more effectively addressed in a spiritual context. As a future health care provider, it will be incumbent on you to realize that all patients will personally interpret the meaning of their life experiences, including those in the health care realm, based on numerous cultural and spiritual value sets. Each of these sets develop from foundational philosophical and spiritual beliefs about life and its meaning. I have observed that there is a continuum which exists which ranges from a very self-determining life view to a profoundly spiritual view. Let's examine these two poles in detail.

Scientism is a philosophical term which predicates that the only things that we can know with certainty, are those which can be scientifically validated. I deliberately avoided the term "proven" since classical science is not capable of proving anything. Scientific theories are asserted and they are held as

reasonable as long there is no evidence that refutes the theory. Once sufficient negative evidence accumulates, the theory crumbles and scientists begin to assert a new theory. Thus, there is complete fluidity of thought and there is no necessity to connect old ideas, once they are discredited by new ideas. Modern health care is profoundly influenced by science, and in many ways, this is a good thing. The contribution of science to health care has greatly improved outcomes and longevity. However, when people manifest a life view that is rooted in scientism, their appreciation of the world begins to narrow to a point that nothing exists that cannot be scientifically validated. In its most extreme form this can lead to *nihilism*. Derived from the Latin word *nihil* or nothing, people who are influenced by this radical view of reality reach a personal understanding that nothing is ultimately verifiable as real and that there is nothing that can be known with certainty. Even their own lives have no inherent value and it is fine to engage in seemingly reckless behaviors since ending their existence would represent a loss of nothing. The questions of ultimate meaning and reality are unanswerable, because they are beyond the world of physical and there is no scientific way to address these concerns.

At the other pole, spiritually actualized people possess a radically different life view. They search for meaning in everything and realize that relationships, while difficult to define scientifically, are a wonderful source of meaning in their daily lives. Even if they are ill or dying, the way that they approach these challenges can be edifying to others and have a real effect on the quality of life of those with whom they relate. Conversely, ministering to the needs of others who may be ill or dying deepens the personal self-worth of both participants in the relationship. Consider, for example, hospice care. People who engage in this form of ministry share their time and talents with those who are in the process of dying. While some people may consider the work of hospice care to be very difficult, my experience has been that these people exhibit extremely altruistic behaviors by caring for the sick. A reciprocal appreciation begins to develop as the relational life of the hospice caregiver is enriched by becoming a very intimate part of the lives of the person who is dying, as well as his or her family. The patient and family are enriched by the evident spirituality of the hospice caregiver.

In reality, most humans are not on either pole of the continuum, but I would like to suggest that wherever you fall on that scale, your efforts to move toward spiritual actualization are among the most positive ways to see life in a more meaningful way. Conversely, when you invite others to become more spiritually actualized, both you and the other person will become happier and healthier with a more positive view of life.

14.7 Empathy as a Foundation for Cultural and Spiritual Competence

From a practical level, I would define *empathy* as the ability to be sensitive to and appreciative of the emotional lives of others. While verbal and nonverbal communication is the originating point of a relationship, all human beings like to be understood and empathy is the vehicle by which a deeper form of emotional communication is established. I have been regularly involved in teaching leadership skills to adults for several decades. As an illustration of what empathy is not, I sometimes start out a presentation by thanking everyone in the group for being so generous with their time and understanding of each other. Then for the sake of an example I add: "Except for so and so, who always seems to miss the mark." Almost immediately, the person who is the target of my example will completely change his or her facial expression and body language to a negative stance. I quickly rescue the situation by admitting that this is simply a simulation about human relationships that illustrates how quickly negativity can be relationally destructive. In contrast, empathy conveys a sense that we welcome and understand each other, which is a far more positive way to invite another person into a healthy relationship.

For those who are spiritually actualized, empathy takes on an even deeper meaning. By extension, people who relate to others in a spiritually empathetic way recognize the inherent value of others in a way that transcends human emotion. As addressed above, spirituality can penetrate to the deepest dimensions of our human value and engage others in a conversation of ultimate meaning and reality. As a health care practitioner, being able to at least acknowledge the spiritual dimensions of your patient, opens the door to a deeper experience of human relationship. If you are able to go beyond simple acknowledgment and progress toward mutual spiritual understanding, your professional relationship will become mutually more empowering. Our contemporary world is organized by various forms of professional specialization. As a result, there is a limit to your ability as a health care provider to engage spiritually with your patients. It is beneficial when you understand your patient's spirituality, but it is not your role to direct the patient as a spiritual physician. Other training and experience is necessary to function in this professional role.

14.8 Is Spiritual Competence a Form of Cultural Competence?

While related, there are significant similarities and differences between cultural competence and spiritual competence. At a foundational level, both culture and spirituality are deeply manifested in human nature and have developed over centuries through a complex series of human interactions with the transcendent. This observation can be seen as an invitation for us to consider that phenomena which have developed over such a long period of human history deserve high respect and diligent consideration.

Similarities exist because of the complex interactions that have taken place over such a long time. In the western world, just look around and note the similarities between a judge's robes and some of the habits worn by clerics, or some of the more classic nursing uniforms and the habits worn by nuns. The state of Louisiana refers to its counties as parishes and many governments refer to their elected officials as ministers. While these examples may seem simplistic at first, they testify to the interrelatedness of the secular, spiritual, and religious worlds that have been in place for nearly countless generations.

Differences exist since every cultural manifestation may not be traced back to a spiritual origin. In fact, political ideologies of the past few centuries have attempted to separate themselves from spiritual sources. In general, making claims that certain things are self-evident is an indication of this tendency. Yet the reliance on notions that are self-evident may narrow one's world view in ways that exclude the spiritual, which as summarized above tends to expand, rather than narrow, the view of the world. While general notions of spirituality are less affected by these political ideologies, there is a deeper separation that has formed between politics and religion. While separation of churches from states may be a culturally entrenched political ideology, health care providers need to appreciate that their clients are persons and many of them engage in spiritual and religious practice. These practices are fundamental to their life view and well-being. They lead to practicing virtuous living and such a pursuit is elevating to human nature.

14.9 The Practice of Religion as a Form of Spiritual and Cultural Competence

At a simplistic level, religion can generally be seen as an institutional repository of both spiritual and cultural values. As one practices a religion, he or she not only becomes more spiritually actualized, but also adopts an inseparable cultural dimension which can be synergistically constructive. It should be no surprise to us that human lifestyle can be positively and negatively affected by habitual practice. We all exhibit good habits, which are very empowering. Just look at the positive effects of proper diet and exercise. On the other hand, we can also develop bad habits, which are very debilitating. I often hear my students say: "I have developed a bad habit of staying up too late and now I am having a difficult time getting up in time for class." Our religious lives are not exempt from this reality. When religion helps us to develop positive habits which promote spiritual growth, our daily lives are enhanced. On the other hand, if our religious practices lead to bad habits, we should really examine if this is a proper use of a religious practice. Historically, this has always been a challenge. The long-standing Irish practice of having a "soul friend" or a more experienced guide to help one plan and evaluate religious practice testifies to the critical nature of engaging in positive and effective religious practice. Consider fasting, for example. While many people would be tempted to conclude that fasting is something to be avoided, in a religious context fasting may represent a spiritually motivated practice that leads to a habit of better mastery over our desires. I have known many people who engage in reasonable practices of fasting who not only enjoy better health, but a better equanimity of spirit. In contrast, practicing fasting that leads to health complications would seem to be a practice that at minimum should be considered for exemption. Thus, religion is an institutional way to practice spiritual values that lead to a better sense of physical, emotional, and spiritual wellness. As such, all health care providers would benefit by respecting the religious practices of their patients. In fact, understanding these practices will lead to a more positive provider-patient relationship.

14.10 Bridging the Cultural/Spiritual Competence Gap

Education is key to bridging both the cultural and spiritual competence gap. However, no education program can prepare a health care provider for every possible cultural and spiritual sensitivity. Rather than trying to educate practitioners globally on the subject, it is far more important to help them to develop a generalized sensitivity to the importance of cultural and spiritual competence. If successful, this type of sensitivity education will prepare a practitioner for the lifelong task of becoming more aware of cultural and spiritual differences. On reviewing the professional literature, it appears that educational efforts are in a state of infancy. This is especially true when one considers the real dearth of studies directly linking cultural competence to improved patient outcomes. For example, Horvat et al attempt to assess the efficacy of cultural competence education for patients from culturally and linguistically diverse backgrounds. By developing a conceptual framework which includes educational content, pedagogical approach, structure of the intervention, and participant characteristics they attempted to map existing data against their framework. Despite their attempts to review a large volume of information, their study did not reach any generalizable conclusions.[4]

A further sign that the development of cultural and spiritual competence education is in its infancy is that there are a number of constructs that have been recently evolving. Paparella-Pitzel et al review a number of these constructs, including cultural awareness, cultural knowledge, cultural skill, cultural encounters, cultural desire, and most recently, *cultural humility*.[5] Cultural humility was originally defined by Tervalon and Murray-Garcia as "commitment and active engagement in a lifelong process that individuals enter into on an ongoing basis with patients, communities, colleagues, and with themselves."[6] Thus, they clearly recognize the ongoing nature of engaging cultural competence. Paparella-Pitzel et al further comment on the notion of cultural humility: "It blends cultural competence with a commitment to ongoing self-evaluation, addresses the power imbalances in the patient-health care provider dynamic, and promotes the development of respectful partnerships with diverse clients and communities." They suggest that five processes are inherent in the development of cultural humility: self-reflecting, dialoguing, empowering, analysis of the environment and resources that provide cultural safety. Cultural humility appears to be a more desirable goal than mere cultural competence, yet the authors admit that there is a real need to develop an advanced educational methodology to accomplish this. They present data which demonstrates that a 2-hour doctor of physical therapy class, taught by a faulty member who is comfortable with the subject matter as well as having the skill to create a safe environment, is able to move students from culturally incompetent to culturally aware and competent 1.5 years after the class was offered.[5]

Because the need for cultural competence and, by extension, spiritual competence is not confined to one particular discipline within health care, it seems intuitive that it would be an excellent candidate for Interprofessional Education (IPE). Oliveira et al took an existing cultural competence education model that had been employed successfully in a physician assistant (PA) program and piloted an IPE version using a combined group of PA and physical therapist (PT) students. Using a three-item instrument entitled Interprofessional Education Series Survey, both groups of students expressed benefits in interprofessional collaboration, cultural awareness, and overall satisfaction with the experience.[7] While this work represents a beginning of a model for cultural competence education that is delivered in an IPE modality, there will need to be future development of a more extensive program with more direct assessment of the outcomes data.

14.11 Conclusion

The health care field would benefit from improved education that leads to true cultural competence. While this is increasingly recognized, the educational resources are far from fully developed. As models of cultural competence evolve toward more advanced understanding of cultural humility, I suggest that it will be necessary to also consider the inclusion of spiritual competence as a way of relating to patients more holistically. The future development of cultural humility and spiritual awareness presents many exciting opportunities that can be conducted in an IPE format and it particularly lends itself to enrichment through health care simulation, and in particular, through the use of standardized patients. This presents opportunities for synergy since the IPE model is likely to promote better team cooperation as a benefit that goes beyond cultural and spiritual competence. At present, there is a lack of data demonstrating that cultural and spiritually competent providers will have better outcomes, despite the intuitive sense that this will be a general outcome. Well-developed IPE curricula, with clearly stated learning outcomes and directly assessed student learning, is the next step in this evolution.

14.12 Review Questions

1. A strong and trusting professional relationship is a prerequisite to the delivery of excellent health care. Confounding variables which may impact this relationship include which of the following?
   a) Language.
   b) Culture.
   c) Spiritual beliefs.
   d) All of the above.
2. Our diverse and pluralistic religious values lead to difficulty in which specific aspect of medical care?
   a) Reimbursement.
   b) Scheduling.
   c) Cultural understanding.
   d) Customer service.
3. All forms of cultural competence must begin with which consideration?
   a) Age-related physiological changes.
   b) Language.
   c) Consent prior to treating.
   d) Therapeutic touch.

4. Betancourt et al defined three major social and cultural barriers to health care. One of these, organizational barriers, has to do with which term?
   a) Leadership.
   b) Physical accessibility for the impaired to health care services.
   c) Access to high level practitioners.
   d) Ability to pay for services rendered.

5. Clinical barriers, as defined by Betancourt, pertain to interactions between the health care provider, the patient, and which entity?
   a) The insurance companies.
   b) The patient's family.
   c) Legislators.
   d) Hospital administration.

6. Spiritual competence is the ability of the health care provider to understand the spirituality of which entity?
   a) Health care lobbyists.
   b) The patient.
   c) The provider's coworkers.
   d) Hospital administration.

7. Many spiritually aware people recognize the existence of a supreme being and as a result, reach the conclusion that …
   a) Health care is a privilege and not a right.
   b) Health care is right and not a privilege.
   c) Life is a gift from God.
   d) Clinical outcomes are a random, uncontrolled event.

8. Patients with terminal illnesses often reflect on their lives in terms of "good or bad" decisions. An effective counsel to this type of statement is which of the following?
   a) God will make us all pay for our sins.
   b) We are all human and we make mistakes. The importance is not that our actions were good or bad but rather, as a result of these actions, that true learning has occurred.
   c) Let's talk about happier times.
   d) We cannot undo what has been done.

9. Which quote best examples the servant-leader?
   a) The servant-leader's primary concern is meeting the needs of others.
   b) The servant-leader's primary concern is developing effective leadership strategies.
   c) The servant-leader uses delegation as an effective tool to meet the organization's objectives.
   d) The servant-leader develops policies and procedures.

10. Which question is best answered in a spiritual context?
    a) I cannot seem to pay my hospital bill. What are my options?
    b) How will this medication improve my quality of life?
    c) My family cannot care for me at home. What are my options?
    d) Why is my grandfather suffering so much with his emphysema?

14.13 Review Answers

1. A strong and trusting professional relationship is a prerequisite to the delivery of excellent health care. Confounding

variables which may impact this relationship include which of the following?
   d. All of the above.

2. Our diverse and pluralistic religious values lead to difficulty in which specific aspect of medical care?
   c. Cultural understanding.

3. All forms of cultural competence must begin with which consideration?
   b. Language.

4. Betancourt et al defined three major social and cultural barriers to health care. One of these, organizational barriers, has to do with which term?
   a. Leadership.

5. Clinical barriers, as defined by Betancourt, pertain to interactions between the health care provider, the patient, and which entity?
   b. The patient's family.

6. Spiritual competence is the ability of the health care provider to understand the spirituality of which entity?
   b. The patient.

7. Many spiritually aware people recognize the existence of a supreme being and as a result, reach the conclusion that…
   c. Life is a gift from God.

8. Patients with terminal illnesses often reflect on their lives in terms of "good or bad" decisions. An effective counsel to this type of statement is which of the following?
   b. We are all human and we make mistakes. The importance is not that our actions were good or bad but rather, as a result of these actions, that true learning has occurred.

9. Which quote best examples the servant-leader?
   a. The servant-leader's primary concern is meeting the needs of others.

10. Which question is best answered in a spiritual context?
    d. Why is my grandfather suffering so much with his emphysema?

References

[1] Betancourt JR, Green AR. Commentary: linking cultural competence training to improved health outcomes: perspectives from the field. Acad Med. 2010; 85(4):583–585

[2] Betancourt JR, Green AR, Carrillo JE, Ananeh-Firempong O, II. Defining cultural competence: a practical framework for addressing racial/ethnic disparities in health and health care. Public Health Rep. 2003; 118(4):293–302

[3] What is Servant Leadership? Available at: https://greenleaf.org/what-is-servant-leadership/. Accessed April 3, 2017

[4] Horvat L, Horey D, Romios P, Kis-Rigo J. Cultural competence education for health professionals. Cochrane Database Syst Rev. 2014(5):CD009405

[5] Paparella-Pitzel S, Eubanks R, Kaplan SL. Comparison of teaching strategies for cultural humility in physical therapy. J Allied Health. 2016; 45 (2):139–146

[6] Tervalon M, Murray-García J. Cultural humility versus cultural competence: a critical distinction in defining physician training outcomes in multicultural education. J Health Care Poor Underserved. 1998; 9(2):117–125

[7] Oliveira KD, North S, Beck B, Hopp J. Promoting collaboration and cultural competence for physician assistant and physical therapist students: a cross-cultural decentralized interprofessional education (IPE) model. J Educ Eval Health Prof. 2015; 12:20

15 The Legal Aspects of Physical Therapy Practice

Stephen J. Carp

Keywords: Administrative law, Americans with Disabilities Act, common law, constitutional law, employment law, Equal Pay Act, Family and Medical Leave Act, Health Insurance Portability and Accountability Act, Immigration Reform and Control Act, informed consent and patient rights, liability, malpractice, Pregnancy Discrimination Act, sexual harassment, Stark, anti-kickback, false claims, statutory law, Title VII of the Civil Rights Act

"Drawing on my experience as an attorney who specializes in defending medical professionals against malpractice claims, I have been asked to write this First Person.

"In my career to date I have handled perhaps 200 malpractice claims and, of those, perhaps five involved physical therapists. I will briefly review one of those claims and highlight areas of practice concern.

"This claim involved a physical therapist working in an outpatient center owned and operated by a large rehabilitation hospital. The therapist 'Dan' was assigned a 24-year-old female patient whose chief complaint was of ankle pain. She stated that she fractured the ankle 18 months previously and the ankle "was never right," with "constant pain and stiffness." Dan evaluated her and then provided intervention. One of his interventions was an ankle manipulation—a high-velocity, small force movement indicated to restore mobility. The manipulation, however, resulted in breakage of the hardware in her ankle which later required additional surgery. The patient was suing Dan and the hospital system.

"Named to defend Dan, I interviewed Dan, his coworkers and supervisor, reviewed the outpatient physical therapy medical record and the original hospital records, and I met with local therapists to garner their clinical opinions. I advised the hospital system to settle out of court. Below are some of the clinical reasons for my recommendation. The reader of this First Person should keep these issues in mind when practicing. The summation of these decisions and actions by Dan led to a large (and public) monetary out of court settlement to the patient.

1. The outpatient center that employed Dan still used the old handwritten medical record. Dan's handwriting was illegible. I asked a number of licensed therapists to review the record and none could read Dan's handwriting. The old axiom: 'If it wasn't documented it wasn't done' should be expanded to include: 'if it can't be read it wasn't done.'
2. Dan did document the occurrence of the original ankle fracture but did not document that surgery (open reduction internal fixation) was performed on the ankle. From Dan's note it appeared the fracture was simply casted. His note did not mention the four screws and metal side plate.
3. Dan's physical examination was limited. He did not document integument (skin, pulses, tissue temperature, capillary refill, and edema)—if he had assessed these issues he would have seen the surgical scar. Dan did not document the midtarsal joint ranges of motion—he only assessed ankle dorsiflexion and plantar flexion. He did not document the patient's medical history or current medications.
4. During my fact-gathering interview Dan told me he knew of the internal fixation of the ankle with the metal screws and plate but simply forgot to document it. I then asked him if he believed manipulation was contraindicated with internal fixation and he hedged. I later interviewed six local PTs, certified specialists (OCS) in orthopedics who said that manipulation of a fixated ankle is contraindicated.
5. In reviewing Dan's human resource file, I found that he documented in his license renewal application that he had completed the required continuing education credits for the renewal. There was, in fact, no documentation of the completion. His CPR certification had also expired.
6. Lastly, in reviewing Dan's final note (the day he manipulated the ankle) Dan wrote, "Manipulation performed. Mild to moderate soreness afterward which is expected.

Improving." According to the patient's complaint the patient was in so much pain after the manipulation that she required the use of crutches to leave the clinic and went directly to the hospital for an X-ray. X-rays taken 35 minutes after the PT appointment ended showed the fracture. Dan never mentioned the crutches or the severe pain.

"Most malpractice claims I have defended could have been prevented if the medical professional simply followed procedure, performed a complete examination, followed evidence-based medicine protocols, documented the truth, wrote legibly, and practiced based upon medically accepted local guidelines. In this case, Dan, a licensed PT, erred in so many arenas that we could not defend him.

"You have chosen a career with so much opportunity to help the sick and impaired. Don't practice in a way which risks my involvement. When I get involved, things are never good."

—Abraham S., Los Angeles, California

15.1 Overview

Managers and employees in health care face a variety of ethical, moral, and legal responsibilities during clinical practice and administrative management. When most physical therapists consider the legal responsibilities and implications of his or her profession, thoughts typically migrate to malpractice and liability issues. However, the scope of legal responsibilities impacting physical therapist practice is much greater than simply those two issues. The four sources of law in the United States directly and globally impact almost all aspects of physical therapist practice: clinical, behavioral, and administrative. The practicing and administrative therapist must be fully cognizant of these laws, be able to recognize situations and events in which the law becomes an important variable, and develop a strong resource group to provide valid and reliable counsel to assist in understanding and dealing with these issues when they arise.

Many persons working in the health care arena when queried about legal issues tend to immediately consider malpractice issues. In fact, malpractice is just one small subset of the legal variables affecting the health care administrator and clinician. This chapter will provide overviews on a variety of timely legal issues facing physical therapists including wage and hour laws, the Family and Medical Leave Act, the Americans with Disabilities Act, employment law, informed consent and patient rights, the Health Insurance Portability and Accountability Act, and protecting one's license.

A number of wonderful textbooks have been written about the legal aspects of health care and every health care administrator and practitioner should consider having one on his or her shelf for reference. Relationships with mentors, experts, and legal professionals should be cultivated to provide counsel in times of legal need. Professional organizations, including the American Physical Therapy Association and the individual state boards of physical therapy, offer many resources for the administrator and practitioner related to this important subject.

15.2 The Four Sources of Law

The relationship of the four sources of law of the U.S. legal system to the health care system illustrates the complexity and far-reaching implications of this defined relationship. The law of the United States comprises many levels of codified and uncodified forms of law, of which the most important is the U.S. Constitution, which is the foundation for and the basis of most of the decisions and actions of the United States. The four sources of U.S. law are constitutions, statutes, administrative regulations, and case law:

- *Constitutions* are the laws that establish systems of government (state or federal). They set out the limits of what governments can and cannot do. Within any state, the constitution overrides any lower law that contradicts it. The U.S. Constitution is the supreme law of the land and no law (including a state constitution) can violate it.
- *Statutes* are what we often think of as law. These are the laws passed by legislative bodies. Congress passes statutes that apply to the country as a whole, state legislatures pass state laws, and local legislatures (often called city, borough, or township councils) pass laws that apply only to their own jurisdictions.
- *Administrative regulations* are rules that are written by agencies developed or recognized by the executive branch. These government agencies have the authority to write rules because the legislatures give them the right to do so. These agencies' employees are experts who possess greater content knowledge of the agency's responsible parties than the legislators and thus assumed to be better at writing detailed rules than the legislators. Any administrative regulation can be overridden and repealed by the legislature.
- *Case law* consists of decisions and opinions issued by courts in various legal cases. Courts are asked to interpret the laws. When they do so, their opinions as to what the laws mean help to shape the law. For example, the recent Supreme Court ruling on gay marriage shaped the law to say that the U.S. Constitution recognizes a right to gay marriages.

15.2.1 Constitutional Law

The Constitution, written by the founding fathers and originally comprising seven articles, delineates the national frame of government. Its first three articles define the doctrine of the separation of powers, whereby the federal government is divided into three branches: the legislative, consisting of the bicameral Congress; the executive, consisting of the President; and the judicial, consisting of the Supreme Court and other federal courts. The next three articles, four, five, and six, define the roles of and relationship of the federal and state governments. Article seven establishes the procedure subsequently used by the thirteen states to ratify the document.

Since the Constitution was ratified in March of 1789, it has been amended 27 times to meet the changing needs of a nation far different from the 18th century world in which it was created. The first 10 amendments, known collectively as the Bill of Rights, offer specific protections of individual liberty and justice and place restrictions on the powers of government. The majority of the seventeen later amendments expand and define individual civil rights protections. Other amendments address issues related to federal authority or were enacted to modify government processes and procedures. Amendments to the U.S. Constitution, unlike ones made to many constitutions worldwide, are appended to the original document.

15.2.2 Statutory Law

Statutory law or statute law are written laws set down by a body of legislature. Statutes may originate with national, state or local legislatures. The scope of statutory laws includes regulatory or administrative laws that are passed by executive agencies and the common laws—the laws created by prior court decisions.

Unlike common law, which is subject to interpretation in its application by the court, statutory laws are generally strictly construed by courts. Strictly construed implies that courts are generally not able to interpret the statute in order to liberalize its application. Rather, these laws are bound by their expressed terms.

As legislative enactments, statutory laws follow the usual process of legislation. A bill is proposed in a legislature and voted upon. If approved, it passes to the executive branch (either a governor at the state level or the president at the federal level). If the executive signs the bill it passes into law as a statute. If the executive fails or refuses to sign the bill, it can be vetoed and sent back to the legislature. In most instances, if the legislature again passes the bill by a set margin it becomes a statute.

Statutes are also recorded, or codified, in writing and published. Statutory law usually becomes effective on a set date written into the bill. Statutes can be overturned by a later legislative enactment or if found unconstitutional by a court of competent jurisdiction.

15.2.3 Administrative Law

Although many people are familiar with the U.S. judicial court system, many laws and binding legal decisions come from both state and federal administrative agencies. Administrative agencies can be basically defined as official government bodies that have the power and authority to direct, supervise, and implement certain legislative acts or statutes. Not all administrative agencies have the term "agency" in the title. Many are referred to as boards, departments, divisions, or commissions.

There are a number of ways that administrative agencies are created. At the federal level, Congress and the president have the authority to establish administrative agencies and to vest them with certain powers. An agency that is established by the president is referred to as an executive agency, while agencies established by an act of Congress are referred to as independent agencies. Overall, there are very few differences between executive and independent agencies. The primary difference between an executive agency and an independent agency is that Congress typically restricts the president from removing the head of an independent agency without just cause. The heads of executive agencies serve at the will of the president and can be removed at any time.

Some of the most widely known federal administrative agencies include the U.S. Department of Agriculture, the Federal Food and Drug Administration, and the Department of Justice.

At the state level, agencies are created in the same way and typically mirror some of the key federal agencies. For example, the federal government established the Occupational Health and Safety Administration, and almost every state has established some agency dedicated to matters involving occupational health and safety.

In 1947, Congress adopted the Administrative Procedures Act (APA),[1] which governs the process by which administrative agencies create and enact laws. The Act was implemented in order to ensure that the public has adequate notice of proposed laws, that there is an opportunity to comment on the proposed law, and that there are clear standards for agency rulemaking. The APA also specifies when and which courts may review and nullify administrative agency rules. The APA also provides standards for any administrative hearings that are conducted.

Federal agencies—both executive and independent—have to follow the rulemaking procedures outlined in the APA. First, the agency must publish a proposed rule in the Federal Register and give the public at least 45 days to review the rule and submit a public comment if they choose. Public comments can either oppose or support the proposed rule and can be submitted by almost any concerned entity, including individuals, companies, and interest groups. During this period, the agency has the option of conducting a public hearing on the proposed rule. If the agency does not hold a hearing, however, an interested party can submit a written request for a hearing at least 15 days before the close of the public review period. The agency reviews the comments and considers whether to make any changes to the proposed law. Depending on how drastic the change to the rule is, the agency may be required to permit the public 15 days to review and comment on the amended version. This cycle may occur a few times prior to the rule reaching its nearly final form. The APA also requires agencies to summarize and respond to each public comment, and each comment is to be made available to the public as part of the rulemaking record.[2]

The agency must send its proposed rule to the Office of Administrative Law (OAL), which oversees all rulemaking activities of federal agencies, within 1 year from the date the proposed rule was first released to the public. OAL reviews the law and the procedures the agency utilized to determine compliance with APA regulations. If the OAL determines that the agency followed the APA regulations appropriately, the agency receives approval to complete the process and publish a final rule which is then printed in the Federal Register and the official Code of Federal Regulations.[3]

15.2.4 Common Law

The fourth type of law is known as common law. The common law system exists in England, the United States, and other countries colonized by England. It is distinct from the civil law system, which predominates in Europe and in areas colonized by France and Spain. The common law system is used in all the states of the United States except Louisiana, where French civil law combined with English criminal law to form a hybrid system.

Anglo-American common law traces its roots to the medieval idea that the law as handed down from the king's courts represented the common custom of the people.[4] It evolved primarily from three English Crown courts of the twelfth and thirteenth centuries: the Exchequer, the King's Bench, and the Common Pleas. These courts eventually assumed jurisdiction over disputes previously decided by local or manorial courts, such as baronial, admiral's (maritime), guild, and forest courts, whose jurisdiction was limited to specific geographic or subject matter areas.[5]

Common law courts base their decisions on prior judicial pronouncements rather than on legislative enactments. Where a statute governs the dispute, judicial interpretation of that statute determines how the law applies. Common law judges rely on their predecessors' decisions of actual controversies, rather than on abstract codes or texts, to guide them in applying the law. Common law judges find the grounds for their decisions in law reports, which contain decisions of past controversies. Under the doctrine of *stare decisis*,[6] common law judges are obliged to adhere to previously decided cases, or precedents, where the facts are substantially the same. A court's decision is binding authority for similar cases decided by the same court or by lower courts within the same jurisdiction. The decision is not binding on courts of higher rank within that jurisdiction or in other jurisdictions, but it may be considered as persuasive authority.

Because common law decisions deal with everyday situations as they occur, social changes, inventions, and discoveries make it necessary for judges sometimes to look outside reported decisions for guidance. The common law system allows judges to look to other jurisdictions or to draw on past or present judicial experience for analogies to help in making a decision. This flexibility allows common law to deal with changes that lead to unanticipated controversies. At the same time, stare decisis provides certainty, uniformity, and predictability and makes for a stable legal environment.

Under a common law system, disputes are settled through an adversarial exchange of arguments and evidence. Both parties present their cases before a neutral fact finder, either a judge or a jury. The judge or jury evaluates the evidence, applies the appropriate law to the facts, and renders a judgment in favor of one of the parties. Following the decision, either party may appeal the decision to a higher court. Appellate courts in a common law system may review only findings of law, not determinations of fact.[7]

15.3 The Health Insurance Portability and Accountability Act

The Standards for Privacy of Individually Identifiable Health Information (Privacy Rule) established, for the first time, a set of national standards for the protection of certain health information.[8] The U.S. Department of Health and Human Services (HHS) issued the Privacy Rule to implement the requirement of the Health Insurance Portability and Accountability Act of 1996 (HIPAA). The Privacy Rule standards address the use and disclosure of individuals' health information—called "protected health information" (PHI) by organizations subject to the Privacy Rule—called "covered entities," as well as standards for individuals' privacy rights to understand and control how their health information is used. Within HHS, the Office for Civil Rights (OCR) has responsibility for implementing and enforcing the Privacy Rule.[9]

A major goal of the Privacy Rule is to ensure that individuals' health information is properly protected while permitting the uninterrupted flow of health information needed to provide and promote high-quality health care and to protect the public's health and well-being.[10] The rule strikes a balance that permits the clinical and administrative use of PHI while protecting the privacy of people who own this information and who seek care and healing. Given that the health care marketplace is diverse and is often practiced in a team environment (with the team, in some instances, geographically distant requiring a physical or electronic transmission of health information), the rule is designed to be flexible and comprehensive to cover the variety of uses and disclosures that need to be addressed. Entities regulated by the rule are obligated to comply with all of its applicable requirements. Practicing health professionals should not rely on this summary as a source of legal information or advice.

The Privacy Rule, as well as all the Administrative Simplification Rules, apply to health plans, health care clearinghouses, and to any health care provider who transmits health information in electronic/physical form in connection with transactions for which the Secretary of HHS has adopted standards under HIPAA (the "covered entities").[11]

Individual and group plans that provide or pay the cost of medical care are covered entities. Health plans include health, dental, vision, and prescription drug insurers, health maintenance organizations (HMOs), Medicare, Medicaid, Medicare plus Choice and Medicare supplement insurers, and long-term care insurers (excluding nursing home fixed-indemnity policies). Health plans also include employer-sponsored group health plans, government and church-sponsored health plans, and multiemployer health plans.[12]

Every health care provider, regardless of practice size, who electronically or physically transmits administrative health information in connection with certain transactions, is a covered entity. These transactions include claims, benefit eligibility inquiries, referral authorization requests, or other transactions for which HHS has established standards under the HIPAA Transactions Rule. The rule also covers the electronic or physical transmission of clinical data including the ordering and results of tests and measures, medical records, diagnoses, treatments, prescription data, and even whether or not an individual is currently or has been a patient in a specific institution. Using electronic technology, such as email, does not define a health care provider as a covered entity; the transmission must be in connection with a transaction related to PHI. The Privacy Rule covers a health care provider whether it electronically transmits these transactions directly or uses a billing service or other third party to do so on its behalf. Health care providers include all "providers of services" (e.g., institutional providers such as hospitals) and "providers of medical or health services" (e.g., noninstitutional providers such as physicians, dentists and other practitioners) as defined by Medicare, and any other person or organization that furnishes, bills, or is paid for health care.[13]

Physical therapists often routinely transmit information to professional associates such as nursing homes, health care facilities, orthotists, prosthetists, and insurance companies.[14] Many physical therapist practices are multisite indicating that patients have the opportunity of being serviced during the same episode of care at multiple sites. Transmission of PHI across sites within the same institutional umbrella is also covered by the rule. Many of these relationships are known as business associates.[15] In general, a business associate is a person or organization, other than a member of a covered entity's workforce, that performs certain functions or activities on behalf of, or provides certain services to, a covered entity that involve the use or disclosure of individually identifiable health information. Business associate functions or activities on behalf of a covered entity include administrative activities such as claims processing, data analysis, utilization review, and billing but also clinical activities such as brace or prosthetic fabrication, interpretation of tests and measures, the transmission of orders, and the current hot topic, telemedicine. Telemedicine is a broad term indicating the performance of consultations, interventions, or evaluations via the use of electronic technology rather than the typical face-to-face contact in the same examination/treatment room.[16] Business associate services to a covered entity are limited to legal, actuarial, accounting, consulting, data aggregation, management, administrative, accreditation, or financial services. When a covered entity uses a contractor or other non-workforce member to perform "business associate" services or activities, the rule requires that the covered entity include certain protections for the information in a business associate agreement (in certain circumstances governmental entities may use alternative means to achieve the same protections). In the business associate contract, a covered entity must impose specified written safeguards on the individually identifiable health information used or disclosed by its business associates. Moreover, a covered entity may not contractually authorize its business associate to make any use or disclosure of protected health information that would violate the rule.

The Privacy Rule protects a number of varied types of information related to health care. The Privacy Rule protects all "individually identifiable health information" held or transmitted by a covered entity or its business associate, in any form or media, whether electronic, paper, or oral. The Privacy Rule calls this information "protected health information (PHI)."[12]

"Individually identifiable health information" is information, including demographic data, that relates to[17]:

• The individual's past, present, or future physical or mental health or condition.
• The provision of health care to the individual.
• The past, present, or future payment for the provision of health care to the individual, and that identifies the individual or for which there is a reasonable basis to believe it can be used to identify the individual. Individually identifiable health information includes many common identifiers (e.g., name, address, birth date, Social Security Number).

There are no restrictions on the use or disclosure of de-identified health information. De-identified health information neither identifies nor provides a reasonable basis to identify an individual.[18] De-identifying health information is a complex task—often beyond the transmitter's ability to determine if the data has been completely de-identified. The most effective method of de-identifying information is to utilize the services of a trained statistician who has been formally educated in activities such as this.

There are a number of practical policies and procedures physical therapists can employee to help ensure that protected information remains protected.[19] The first step to limiting rule violations and potential leakage of PHI is with a through risk-analysis of threats to PHI. All organizational processes should be reviewed. PHI threat risk analyses are often better performed by an outside agency or consultant. Though expensive, the trained eye with no organizational bias may be a more effective evaluator than someone in-house who may have actual or perceived biases. ▶ Fig. 15.1 shows the rise in privacy complaints in recent years.

Utilizing the results of the threat analysis, the second step is the development of specific policies and procedures to assist in the protection of PHI. Specific policies should be enacted for patient identification, storage of protected health information, insurance verification, business associates, documentation, levels of protection of PHI, encryption of PHI, physical security of the facility, access to PHI, electronic communication, and so forth. Polices should be maintained in a manual and reviewed with each staff member at orientation and yearly thereafter.

Protection against a security breach begins with a policy establishing the correct identity of the patient during the initial check-in and registration process. In our experiences, we often identify patients with forged or self-amended insurance and demographic information. The rationale for forging and amending demographic information is the high cost of insurance. Obviously, "borrowing" a friend's insurance card is a very inexpensive option to purchasing insurance. My organization requires a government-sponsored photo ID prior to the provision of any nonemergent treatment.

Polices should ensure the safety of all PHI throughout the continuum of care from initial contact through the first visit, all episodes of care, discharge and finally to the short and long-term storage of the medical record. That is a big job that covers a lot of potential breach scenarios—which makes conducting a risk analysis by a consultant a practical first step to see just what coverage gaps exist, and where holes appear in the defense of patient information.

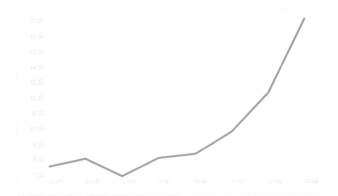

Fig. 15.1 Health care privacy complaints filed per year. The number of health information privacy complaints submitted to the Office for Civil Rights within the U.S. Department of Health and Human Services has increased dramatically in recent years, in part because of the introduction of an online complaint portal. (*Source:* HHS Office for Civil Rights, www.HHS.gov/ocr. Accessed August 15, 2017.)

Developing meaningful, effective policies and procedures that meet an organization's specific needs is crucial. Resorting to a "boilerplate" template to save time and resources is not a wise choice. Organizations must be able to show an auditor exactly how certain practices follow established policies and procedures.

Updating job descriptions is another effective method of identifying who assumes which privacy role. Job descriptions for privacy and security must be fully documented. Who will assume privacy and security roles? What are their specific responsibilities? For example, in one case witnessed by the author of this article an employee was designated as "insurance verifier," performing the important role of contacting the insurance company to obtain verification of benefits of the patient. This portion of her daily job requirements was not documented in her job description. This lack of documentation could cause problems during an eventual audit. Dual roles are not uncommon. Sometimes an IT director serves as a security officer. An HIM or compliance director may serve as a privacy officer. In such cases, descriptions must specify roles and responsibilities.

Along with the organizational suggestions to maintain compliance with the rule, a number of common sense suggestions should be offered to health care employees to further facilitate confidentiality. These items should be included in a specific organization policy. These include the following:

- Employing screen savers for all computers.
- Prohibiting the use of "hard" and electronic medical records in public areas where they may be seen by patients and patients' families.
- Reminding staff not to talk about patients or patient families in public areas such as cafeterias, stairwells, or elevators.
- Disallowing the taking home of office computers with access to PHI or any types of "hard" medical record.
- Avoiding the placement of scheduling boards in public areas.
- Prohibiting the use of cell phones in public areas.
- Employing the use of an encrypted texting system to use for interemployee communication while at work.
- Reminding all employees about the prohibition of taking photographs in the work area unless the photograph is for patient documentation and has been approved by the patient via written consent.
- Educating and documenting the HIPAA education for all volunteers and interns.

There are a number of concrete actions to help ensure compliance with privacy guidelines. Larger organizations typically have internal experts capable of developing and monitoring privacy policy. Smaller companies may need to look outside for assistance in the form of consultants.

Practical suggestions to help ensure compliance with HIPAA include:

Risk analysis. Perform a thorough risk assessment of all processes, preferably through a consultant, to identify possible sources of breach of confidentiality. Within health care facilities, all areas of the operation should be thoroughly assessed, including clinical procedures, information technology, the telephone system, human resource, record storage, virtual networks, information transmission, employee medical records, etc.

Development of privacy policies. Health care organizations must develop, implement, adopt, and routinely update privacy and security policies and procedures. These polices must be distributed and reviewed by all employees at least yearly and sooner if there are policy changes and updates. Documentation of the review should be placed in each employee's human resources file.

Appointment of privacy and security officers. Health care organizations should appoint a privacy and security officer. This could either be the same or different individuals. This person should be conversant in all HIPAA regulations and policies. Specific and routinely updated job descriptions should be maintained for the privacy and security officer.

Conducting regular risk assessments. Following the initial risk analysis, health care organizations should, on a minimum yearly basis, conduct confidentiality risk assessment analyses to identify vulnerabilities. These ongoing analyses will help ensure the confidentiality and integrity of protected health information and other data with a confidentiality import.

Adoption of electronic communication policies. With the seemingly almost monthly new methods of electronic communication, health care organizations should adopt policies regarding the use of this form of communication. What types of information can be sent electronically? Can health care workers within the same facility text information about patients to each other? Are there specific social media policies? Can employees use their cell phones at work?

Adoption of mobile device policies. Health care organizations should adopt strict policies regarding the storage of protected health information on portable electronic devices, and they should regulate the removal of those electronic devices from the premises. Most organizations only permit the use of organization-owned-and-maintained electronic devices for use at work. Most organizations prohibit these devices from leaving the building.

Virtual network. With the paradigm shift to the home office the use of a virtual network to access organization data is commonplace. Organizations need to develop polices—including oversight monitoring—related to which types of data will be available to home access.

Training. Training all employees who use or disclose protected health information must begin at orientation and be conducted on a mandatory, regular basis thereafter.

Notice of Privacy Practices. A Notice of Privacy Practices should be correctly published and distributed to all patients. The notice should also be displayed on the organization's website, posted within the facility, all customers should be provided with hard copies, and the organization should obtain acknowledgement of receipt from all of its patients.

Entering into valid agreements. Health care organizations should ensure the entering into valid business associate agreements with all business associates and subcontractors. Business agreements should be vetted by legal counsel prior to signing. Any existing business associate agreements will have to be updated to reflect any changes to HIPAA under the final rule.

Adoption of potential breach protocols. A protocol for investigating potential breaches of protected health information is a must. If a breach has been suspected to have occurred or has truly occurred, it is essential that the health care organization document the results of the investigation and notify the appropriate authorities.

Implementation of privacy policies. Privacy and security policies must be properly implemented by health care organizations, and they should sanction employees who violate them.

15.4 The Family and Medical Leave Act

The Family and Medical Leave Act (FMLA) of 1993 is a U.S. federal law requiring covered employers to provide covered employees with job-protected, unpaid leave for qualified medical and family reasons.[20] The FMLA is administered by the Wage and Hour Division of the U.S. Department of Labor.

The bill was a major part of President Bill Clinton's agenda in his first term. Rapid growth in the workforce, secondary to a large number of women joining, suggested a necessary federal regulation that would support the working class who desired to raise a family or required time off for illness-related situations. Prior to the enactment of the FMLA there was no requirement to "hold" a position for an employee required to miss work due to family or self-illness, pregnancy, adoption, and so forth. President Clinton signed the bill into law on February 5, 1993, and it became effective 6 months later on August 5, 1993.[21]

The FMLA was intended "to balance the demands of the workplace with the needs of families."[22] The act allows eligible employees to take up to 12 work weeks of unpaid leave during any 12-month period. In order to be eligible for FMLA leave (a covered employee), an employee must have been employed by the business at least 12 months, worked at least 1,250 hours over the past 12 months, and worked at a location where the company employs 50 or more employees within a 75-mile radius. The FMLA covers both public- and private-sector employees, but certain categories of employees are excluded, including elected officials and their personal staff members.

Not every employer, according to the act, is a covered employer and thus not required to provide its employees with family or medical leave. Federal law defines a covered employer as either[23]

- A state, local, or federal governmental agency; or
- A private business engaged in, or affecting, interstate commerce, that employed 50 or more employees within a 75-mile radius in twenty or more weeks in the current or prior calendar year.

This criterion may appear obtuse, but in reality, virtually every business in the United States engages in, or affects, interstate commerce. The "fifty or more employees" standard includes everyone on the employer's payroll, including part-time employees, employees on approved leave, and leased or temporary employees. The 75-mile radius rule adds employees who work from home or at local sites some distance away from the primary organization's headquarters.[24]

A covered employer must provide eligible employees with a maximum of 12 weeks of leave. The leave may be unpaid, but it may be combined with accrued paid leave (such as vacation or sick leave).

An eligible employee may take leave

- For the birth, adoption, or placement of a child;
- To care for a spouse, minor, or incompetent child, or parent who has a "serious health condition" (more on this below); or
- To handle the employee's own serious health condition that makes him or her unable to work.

A "serious health condition" is defined as an illness, injury, impairment, or condition that involves[25]

- Hospital care including acute care, skilled nursing facility, and acute medical rehabilitation facility;
- Absence from work, plus continuing treatment;
- Pregnancy;
- Treatment for a chronic condition;
- Permanent long-term supervision; or
- Multiple treatments such as chemotherapy or radiation.

Employees may be required by the employer to "apply" for FMLA—a method to ensure the provision of all relevant data to the organization and to provide a medical certification detailing the need for leave. An employer who provides health insurance is required to maintain coverage for an employee on leave on the same terms as if the employee had continued to work although in many cases the employee is responsible for the insurance premium during the period of family leave. Organizations are not required to provide the covered employee benefits while on FMLA. As an example, vacation and sick time are not accrued while on FMLA; the covered employee is not covered for bereavement leave; the covered employee is not covered by the organization's malpractice insurance.

Under some circumstances, employees may take FMLA leave on an intermittent or reduced schedule basis. This means an employee may take leave in separate blocks of time or by reducing the time he or she works each day or week for a single qualifying reason. As an example, if an employee has been diagnosed with cancer and is scheduled for 4 weeks of chemotherapy in total to be given every other week for 8 weeks, the employee may take 1-week FMLA, work a week, take another week FMLA, work a week, and so forth. When leave is needed for planned medical treatment, the employee must make a reasonable effort to schedule treatment so as not to unduly disrupt the employer's operations. If FMLA leave is for the birth, adoption, or foster placement of a child, use of intermittent or reduced schedule leave requires the employer's approval.

Under certain conditions, employees may choose, or employers may require employees, to "substitute" (run concurrently) accrued paid leave, such as sick or vacation leave, to cover some or all of the FMLA leave period. An employee's ability to substitute accrued paid leave is determined by the terms and conditions of the employer's normal leave policy.

When an employee returns from leave granted by the FMLA, he or she is entitled to be restored to his or her former job, or to an equivalent job, with equivalent pay, benefits, and other terms of employment. Taking leave may not result in the loss of any benefit to which an employee was entitled before taking leave, and may not be counted against an employee under a "no-fault" attendance policy.[26]

The FMLA entitles eligible employees of covered employers to take unpaid, job-protected leave for specified family and medical reasons, with continuation of group health insurance coverage under the same terms and conditions as if the employee had not taken leave.

Qualifying reasons for the granting of family leave[27]:

The birth of a child and to bond with the newborn child within 1 year of birth. An employee's entitlement to FMLA leave for birth and bonding expires 12 months after the date of birth. Both mothers and fathers have the same right to take FMLA leave for the birth of a child. Birth and bonding leave must be taken as a continuous block of leave unless the employer agrees to allow intermittent leave (e.g., allowing a parent to return to work on a part-time schedule for 10 weeks).

The placement with the employee of a child for adoption or foster care and to bond with the newly placed child within 1 year of placement. FMLA leave may be taken before the actual placement or adoption of a child if an absence from work is required for the placement for adoption or foster care to proceed. For example, the employee may be entitled to FMLA leave to attend counseling sessions, appear in court, consult with his or her attorney or the birth parent's representative, submit to a physical examination, or travel to another country to complete an adoption before the actual date of placement. FMLA leave to bond with a child after placement must be taken as a continuous block of leave unless the employer agrees to allow intermittent leave. An employee's entitlement to FMLA leave for the placement of a child for adoption or foster care expires 12 months after the placement.

A serious health condition that makes the employee unable to perform the functions of his or her job. An employee is "unable to perform the functions of the position" where the health care provider finds that the employee is unable to work at all, or is unable to perform any one of the essential functions of the employee's position. An employee who must be absent from work to receive medical treatment for a serious health condition is considered to be unable to perform the essential functions of the position during the absence for treatment.

To care for the employee's spouse, son, daughter, or parent who has a serious health condition. An employee must be needed to provide care for his or her spouse, son, daughter, or parent because of the family member's serious health condition in order for the employee to take FMLA leave. An employee may be needed to provide care to the family member, for example when the family member is unable to care for his or her own medical, safety or other needs, because of the serious health condition or needs help in being transported to the doctor; or to provide psychological comfort and reassurance to the family member with a serious health condition.

- Spouse: Spouse means a husband or wife as defined or recognized in the state where the individual was married and includes individuals in a same-sex marriage or common law marriage. Spouse also includes a husband or wife in a marriage that was validly entered into outside of the United States if the marriage could have been entered into in at least one state.
- Parent: Parent means a biological, adoptive, step or foster father or mother, or any other individual who stood in loco parentis to the employee when the employee was a child. This term does not include parents "in law."
- Son or daughter: Son or daughter means a biological, adopted, or foster child, a stepchild, a legal ward, or a child of a person standing in loco parentis, who is either under age 18, or age 18 or older and "incapable of self-care because of a mental or physical disability" at the time that FMLA leave is to commence.
- In loco parentis: The FMLA regulations define in loco parentis as including those with day-to-day responsibilities to care for or financially support a child. Employees who have no biological or legal relationship with a child may, nonetheless, stand in loco parentis to the child and be entitled to FMLA leave. Similarly, an employee may take leave to care for someone who, although having no legal or biological relationship to the employee when the employee was a child, stood in loco parentis to the employee when the employee was a child, even if they have no legal or biological relationship.

Any qualifying exigency arising out of the fact that the employee's spouse, son, daughter, or parent is a military member on covered active duty. Qualifying exigencies are situations arising from the military deployment of an employee's spouse, son, daughter, or parent to a foreign country. Qualifying exigencies for which an employee may take FMLA leave include making alternative child care arrangements for a child of the military member when the deployment of the military member necessitates a change in the existing child care arrangement; attending certain military ceremonies and briefings; taking leave to spend time with a military member on Rest and Recuperation leave during deployment; or making financial or legal arrangements to address a covered military member's absence; or certain activities related to care of the parent of the military member while the military member is on covered active duty.

To care for a covered servicemember with a serious injury or illness if the employee is the spouse, son, daughter, parent, or next of kin of the servicemember (military caregiver leave). Eligible family members of both current servicemembers and certain veterans are entitled to military caregiver leave.

Certain employees may be denied restoration of their jobs if returning them to their former positions would result in substantial and grievous economic harm to the employer. A "key" employee is defined as a salaried employee who is among the highest-paid 10% of the employees within a 75-mile radius. An employer must notify an employee that he or she is a key employee when the employee gives notice of intent to take leave, and must notify the employee when a decision is made to deny reinstatement.

15.5 The Americans with Disabilities Act

The Americans with Disabilities Act (ADA) became law in 1990.[28] The ADA prohibits discrimination against individuals with disabilities in all areas of public life, including jobs, schools, transportation, and all public and private places that are open to the general public. The aim of the law is to make sure that people with disabilities have the same rights and opportunities as everyone else. The ADA gives civil rights protections to individuals with disabilities similar to those provided to individuals on the basis of race, color, sex, national origin, age, and religion. It guarantees equal opportunity for individuals with disabilities in public accommodations, employment, transportation, state and local government services, and telecommunications. The ADA is divided into five titles (or sections) that relate to different areas of public life.[29]

In 2008, the Americans with Disabilities Act Amendments Act (ADAAA) was signed into law and became effective on January 1, 2009. The ADAAA clarified the definition of "disability." The changes in the definition of disability in the ADAAA apply to all titles of the ADA, including Title I (employment practices of private employers with 15 or more employees, state and local governments, employment agencies, labor unions, agents of the employer and joint management labor committees); Title II (programs and activities of state and local government entities); and Title III (private entities that are considered places of public accommodation).[30]

Glossary of Common ADA Terms

Familiarity of the terms of the ADA is a prerequisite to fully understanding the scope of the act.

- **Accessible information technology.** Technology that can be used by people with a wide range of abilities and disabilities. It incorporates the principles of universal design, whereby each user is able to interact with the technology in ways that work best for him or her.
- **Adaptive technology.** Name for products which help people who cannot use regular versions of products, primarily people with physical disabilities such as limitations to vision, hearing, and mobility.
- **American sign language (ASL).** The dominant sign language of the Deaf community in the United States, in the English-speaking parts of Canada, and in parts of Mexico.
- **Americans with Disabilities Act (ADA).** Signed into law on July 26, 1990, the ADA is a wide-ranging civil rights law that prohibits, under certain circumstances, discrimination based on disability. It affords similar protections against discrimination to Americans with disabilities as the Civil Rights Act of 1964, which made discrimination based on race, religion, sex, national origin, and other characteristics illegal.
- **Architectural barriers.** Obstacles or other features in the built environment that impede individuals with disabilities from gaining full and complete access to the goods and services being provided.
- **Architectural Barriers Act (ABA).** Addresses scoping and technical requirements for accessibility to sites, facilities, buildings, and elements by individuals with disabilities.
- **Assistive technology (AT).** Any item, piece of equipment, or product system that is used to increase, maintain, or improve functional capabilities of individuals with disabilities. Examples include message boards, screen readers, refreshable Braille displays, keyboard and mouse modifications, and head pointers.
- **Commercial facilities.** Nonresidential facilities, including office buildings, factories, and warehouses, whose operations affect commerce.
- **Damages.** Money awarded to one party based on injury or discrimination caused by the other. Money damages are not available to state employees under ADA Title I or to all plaintiffs under ADA Title III.
- **Disability.** A physical or mental impairment that substantially limits one or more major life activities, a record of such an impairment, or being regarded as having such an impairment.
- **Disability and business technical assistance centers (DBTACs).** Former name for the ten regional centers on the ADA in the ADA National Network funded by National Institute on Disability Rehabilitation and Research to provide information, training and technical assistance on the ADA in all 50 U.S. states and surrounding territories.
- **Distance learning.** Training from a remote location conducted by way of various options, including teleconference, streaming audio over the Internet, and/or real-time captioned over the Internet.
- **Equal opportunity.** An opportunity for people with disabilities to participate and benefit from programs and services that is equal to and as effective as the opportunity provided to others.
- **Equal Employment Opportunity Commission (EEOC).** Federal agency primarily responsible for enforcement of Title I of the ADA, which deals with employment discrimination.
- **Essential job function.** Fundamental job duties of the employment position the individual with a disability holds or desires. The term "essential functions" does not include the marginal functions of the position.
- **Impairment.** A physical impairment is a physiological disorder or condition, cosmetic disfigurement or anatomical loss affecting one or more of the body systems. A mental impairment is any mental or psychological disorder.
- **Individual with a disability.** A person who has a physical or mental impairment that substantially limits one or more of the major life activities of such individual or a record of such an impairment or is regarded as having such an impairment.
- **Major life activity.** An activity that an average person can perform with little or no difficulty.
- **Marginal functions.** Duties of a job that are not absolutely necessary for the job being performed.
- **Mediation.** When a third party holds an informal meeting with both sides in a dispute to promote resolution of a grievance, a compromise, or a settlement of a lawsuit. The result of the mediation, if any, is not binding on the parties. A mediator can be court-appointed or chosen by the parties.
- **National Center on Accessibility (NCA).** Organization that provides training, technical assistance and research on access to parks, recreation, and tourism.
- **National Council on Disability (NCD).** Independent federal agency making recommendations to the President and Congress on issues affecting Americans with disabilities.
- **National Institute on Disability and Rehabilitation Research (NIDRR).** Under the U.S. Department of Education, this organization provides funding for various projects, including the ten regional centers in the ADA National Network that provide information, training, and technical assistance on the ADA.
- **Office of Disability Employment Policy (ODEP).** Under the U.S. Department of Labor, provides national leadership by developing and influencing disability-related employment policies as well as practices that affect the employment of people with disabilities.
- **Office of Federal Contract Compliance Programs (OFCCP).** Part of the U.S. Department of Labor's Employment Standards Administration, responsible for ensuring that employers doing business with the Federal government comply with the laws and regulations requiring non-discrimination.
- **Personal services or personal devices.** Public entities and public accommodations are not required to provide personal services or personal devices. Examples of personal devices that entities are not required to provide include wheelchairs, prescription eyeglasses, and hearing aids. Personal assistance service need not be provided in activities such as eating, toileting, and dressing unless the service is typically provided by the entity.
- **Portable document format (PDF).** An open file format created and controlled by Adobe Systems for representing two-dimensional documents in a device independent and resolution independent fixed-layout document format. Unless

properly tagged, these documents will be inaccessible to those with visual impairments.

- **Primary function areas.** Areas housing the major activities for which a facility was intended.
- **Public accommodations.** Private entities that own, operate, lease, or lease to places of public accommodation. Places of public accommodation include places such as restaurants, hotels, theaters, convention centers, retail stores, shopping centers, dry cleaners, laundromats, pharmacies, doctors' offices, hospitals, museums, libraries, parks, zoos, amusement parks, private schools, day care centers, health spas, and bowling alleys.
- **Public entity.** A public entity covered by Title II of the ADA is defined as: any state or local government; any department, agency, special purpose district, or other instrumentality of a state or local government; or certain commuter authorities as well as AMTRAK. It does not include the federal government.
- **Qualified individual with a disability.** A person with a disability who satisfies the requisite skill, experience, education and other job-related requirements of the employment position such individual holds or desires, and who, with or without reasonable accommodation, can perform the essential functions of such position.
- **Reasonable accommodation.** A modification or adjustment to a job, the work environment, or the way things usually are done that enables a qualified individual with a disability to enjoy an equal employment opportunity.
- **Reasonable modification.** A public entity must modify its policies, practice, or procedures to avoid discrimination unless the modification would fundamentally alter the nature of its service, program, or activity.
- **Retaliation.** Individuals who exercise their rights under that ADA are protected from those who would take steps to "pay them back" for their actions.
- **Settlement agreement.** An agreement between parties to settle a lawsuit before it goes to trial. The parties agree to settle their dispute and to dismiss the lawsuit. Settlement agreements do not have the force of law.
- **Speech-to-speech (STS).** A relay service available to any telephone callers with a speech disability and to those who wish to talk with them.
- **Statute.** A law made by a legislature, such as the U.S. Congress. Federal statutes can be found in the U.S. Code.
- **Substantial limitation.** An individual who is unable to perform, or is significantly limited in the ability to perform, a major life activity that the average person in the general population can perform.
- **Summary judgment.** A ruling by a court that one party in a lawsuit is entitled to win as a matter of law before the case goes to trial. The court has to find that there are no set of facts that would allow the losing party to win.
- **Telecommunications device for the deaf (TDD).** An electronic device for text communication via a telephone line, used when one or more of the parties has hearing or speech difficulties.
- **Telecommunication relay service (TRS).** Also known as a Relay Service, or IP-Relay, this is an operator service that allows individuals who are deaf, hard-of-hearing, speech-im-

paired, and speech-disabled to place calls to standard telephone users via TDD, TTY, personal computer or other assistive telephone device.

- **Teletypewriter (TTY).** Also known as a Teletype, or text telephone, this is a device for text communication via a telephone line, used when one or more of the parties has hearing or speech difficulties.
- **Title.** A section of a statute. For example, the ADA has five titles.
- **Title I.** Of the five titles of the ADA, Title I of the ADA pertains to Employment. Under ADA Title I, covered entities shall not discriminate against a qualified individual with a disability. This applies to job application procedures, hiring, advancement and discharge of employees, worker's compensation, job training, and other terms, conditions, and privileges of employment.
- **Title II.** Of the five titles of the ADA, Title II of the ADA pertains to State and Local Government (public entities). ADA Title II requires agencies to comply with regulations similar to Section 504 of the Rehabilitation Act. These rules cover access to all services, programs, or activities offered by the public entity, and extends coverage to public transportation entities. Access includes physical access described in the Uniform Federal Accessibility Standards or the ADA Standards for Accessible Design and access that might be obstructed by discriminatory policies or procedures of the entity.
- **Title III.** Of the five titles of the ADA, Title III of the ADA pertains to Public Accommodations (private entities). Under ADA Title III, no individual may be discriminated against on the basis of disability with regard to the full and equal enjoyment of the goods, services, facilities, or accommodations of any place of public accommodation by any person who owns, leases (or leases to), or operates a place of public accommodation.
- **Title IV.** Of the five titles of the ADA, Title IV of the ADA pertains to Telecommunications. ADA Title IV addresses telephone and television access for individuals with hearing and speech disabilities. Specific requirements under Title IV include closed captioning of federally funded public service announcements, and telephone companies must establish in-state and state-to-state TRS 24 hours a day, 7 days a week.
- **Title V.** Of the five titles of the ADA, Title V of the ADA pertains to miscellaneous provisions, most of which apply to all titles of the ADA.
- **Undue burden.** Significant difficulty or expense. A public accommodation is not required to provide any auxiliary aid or service that would result in an undue burden.
- **Undue hardship.** An action that requires "significant difficulty or expense" in relation to the size of the employer, the resources available, and the nature of the operation. The concept of undue hardship includes any action that is unduly costly, extensive, substantial, disruptive, or would fundamentally alter the nature or operation of the business. Accordingly, whether a particular accommodation will impose an undue hardship must always be determined on a case-by-case basis.
- **Undue financial and administrative burden.** A public entity does not have to take any action that it can demonstrate would result in an undue financial and administrative burden.

This applies in program accessibility, effective communication, and auxiliary aids and services.

- **Universal design (UD).** Also known as "inclusive design" and "design for all," this is an approach to the design of products, places, policies, and services that can meet the needs of as many people as possible throughout their lifetime, regardless of age, ability, or situation.
- **Voice carry-over (VCO).** A call type method that allows an individual who is deaf or hard of hearing to use his or her voice while receiving responses from a hearing person via text typed by the relay operator (also known as communication assistant or relay agent). VCO, a more common call type than hearing carry-over, has many variations, including 2-Line VCO.
- **Video relay services (VRS).** Allows an individual who uses sign language to able to place a phone call by signing instead of typing. The VI (video interpreter) uses a web cam or videophone to voice the signs of the individual who is deaf or has a hearing or speech disability to the person who has hearing and sign the words of the person who has hearing to the individual who is deaf or has a hearing or speech disability.
- **Web Accessibility Initiative (WAI).** This is the effort of the World Wide Web Consortium (W3C) that pursues accessibility of the web through technology, guidelines, tools, education and outreach, and research and development.

Adapted from https://adata.org/glossary-terms and https://www.disabled-world.com/definitions/ada-glossary.php accessed July 30, 2017.

The ADA is best understood by reviewing individually its five titles, as follows.[31]

15.5.1 Title I (Employment)

This title is designed to help people with disabilities access the same employment opportunities and benefits available to people without disabilities. Employers must provide reasonable accommodations to qualified applicants or employees. A reasonable accommodation is any modification or adjustment to a job or the work environment that will enable an applicant or employee with a disability to participate in the application process or to perform essential job functions.

This portion of the law is regulated and enforced by the U.S. EEOC. Employers with 15 or more employees must comply with this law. The regulations for Title I define disability, establish guidelines for the reasonable accommodation process, address medical examinations and inquiries, and define "direct threat" when there is significant risk of substantial harm to the health or safety of the individual employee with a disability or others.

15.5.2 Title II (State and Local Government)

Title II of the ADA prohibits discrimination against qualified individuals with disabilities in all programs, activities, and services of public entities. It applies to all state and local governments, their departments and agencies, and any other instrumentalities or special purpose districts of state or local governments. It clarifies the requirements of section 504 of the Rehabilitation Act of 1973, as amended, for public transportation systems that receive federal financial assistance, and extends coverage to all public entities that provide public transportation, whether or not they receive federal financial assistance. It establishes detailed standards for the operation of public transit systems, including commuter and intercity rail (e.g., AMTRAK).

This title outlines the administrative processes to be followed, including requirements for self-evaluation and planning; requirements for making reasonable modifications to policies, practices, and procedures where necessary to avoid discrimination; architectural barriers to be identified; and the need for effective communication with people with hearing, vision and speech disabilities. This title is regulated and enforced by the U.S. Department of Justice.

15.5.3 Title III (Public Accommodations)

This title prohibits private places of public accommodation from discriminating against individuals with disabilities. Examples of public accommodations include privately-owned, leased or operated facilities like hotels, restaurants, retail merchants, doctor's offices, golf courses, private schools, day care centers, health clubs, sports stadiums, movie theaters, and so on. This title sets the minimum standards for accessibility for alterations and new construction of facilities. It also requires public accommodations to remove barriers in existing buildings where it is easy to do so without much difficulty or expense. This title directs businesses to make "reasonable modifications" to their usual ways of doing things when serving people with disabilities. It also requires that they take steps necessary to communicate effectively with customers with vision, hearing, and speech disabilities. This title is regulated and enforced by the U.S. Department of Justice.

15.5.4 Title IV (Telecommunications)

This title requires telephone and Internet companies to provide a nationwide system of interstate and intrastate telecommunications relay services that allows individuals with hearing and speech disabilities to communicate over the telephone. This title also requires closed captioning of federally funded public service announcements. This title is regulated by the Federal Communication Commission.

15.5.5 Title V (Miscellaneous Provisions)

The final title contains a variety of provisions relating to the ADA as a whole, including its relationship to other laws, state immunity, its impact on insurance providers and benefits, prohibition against retaliation and coercion, illegal use of drugs, and attorney's fees. This title also provides a list of certain conditions that are not to be considered as disabilities.

15.6 Employment Practices

A variety of antidiscrimination laws affect the employment practices of any business. Employment discrimination laws apply to all employment practices from hiring to firing employees, and all aspects of employment in between. The Federal EEOC is the agency that administers federal employment discrimination laws. In this section, the most common and most influential employment discrimination laws will be briefly reviewed.[32]

15.6.1 Title VII of the Civil Rights Act

Title VII of the Civil Rights Act of 1964, which applies to employers with 15 or more employees, prohibits discrimination on the basis of race, color, religion, sex, and national origin. Employers are not permitted to base their employment decisions on these protected characteristics when it comes to all aspects of employment, including hiring, promotions, discipline, salary, benefits, job assignments, and firing.[33]

Employers must also comply with Title VII by maintaining a workplace that is free from harassment based on a protected characteristic (such as race, sex, and so on). Employers must ensure that employees are not harassed by supervisors and coworkers, but also customers, vendors, and other third parties.[33]

15.6.2 Pregnancy Discrimination Act

The Pregnancy Discrimination Act (PDA) of 1978 is an amendment to Title VII of the Civil Rights Act. The PDA prohibits discrimination on the basis of pregnancy, childbirth, or related medical conditions, and it applies to all terms and conditions of employment, including hiring, firing, promotion, leave, and benefits. The law applies to employers with 15 or more employees.[34]

15.6.3 Age Discrimination in Employment Act

The Age Discrimination in Employment Act (ADEA) of 1967 prohibits discrimination against individuals who are 40 years of age or older. The ADEA prohibits age discrimination in all aspects of employment including hiring, firing, compensation, benefits, discipline, and job assignments. The law applies to employers with 20 or more employees.[35]

In order to comply with the ADEA, employers must avoid basing employment decisions such as hiring, firing, or promotions on age or stereotypical beliefs about older workers. For example, an employer cannot refuse to hire an older worker based on the assumption that the worker will most likely require more expensive health care services than a younger employee thus placing the employer at risk for higher health premiums due to increased utilization. Employers may not post job advertisements that could discourage older workers from applying. For example, using terms "young" or "recent graduate" in job postings would violate the ADEA.[36]

15.6.4 Equal Pay Act

The Equal Pay Act of 1963 prohibits gender based wage discrimination. Employers must pay equal wages to men and women who perform substantially equal jobs within the same company. This means that employers may not pay unequal wages to men and women who perform jobs that require substantially equal skill, effort and responsibility and that are performed under similar working conditions. The Equal Pay Act applies to virtually all employers.[37]

15.6.5 Immigration Reform and Control Act

The Immigration Reform and Control Act (IRCA) prohibits employers from discriminating against employees and applicants on the basis of citizenship or national origin. IRCA also prohibits employers from knowingly hiring individuals who are not authorized to work in the United States. The law requires employers to verify the identity and employment authorization of all employees prior to their hire.

In addition to these federal employment discrimination laws, your business may also be subject to employment discrimination laws in your state. Check with an employment attorney in your area to determine whether your business is complying with state employment discrimination laws.[38]

15.7 Staffing and Hiring

One of the five classic managerial functions is staffing.[39] Staffing includes the hiring, promotion, and termination of employees; employee orientation; ensuring employee compliance; performance appraisals; and ongoing counseling.

There are numerous federal, state, and local rules regarding hiring employees and most large companies maintain in-house legal counsel and human resource departments to deal with these rules. For most small companies, however, these are often unaffordable luxuries. For small companies, hiring a consultant to develop policy regarding staffing may be advisable. Below are general guidelines for the hiring of employees.

- Do not discriminate based on race, color, gender, religion, disability status, sexual preference, etc.
- When using current employees to interview applicants, provide a thorough orientation to the employees about what they may ask and what they may not ask the applicant based on federal, state, and local statutes.
- Respect the applicant's right to privacy: marital situation, religion, economic background, personal life, physical and emotional impairments, protected health information.
- Always be honest with the applicant regarding items such as job security, and benefits.
- Observe all laws relating to minimum wage, hiring young or immigrant workers.
- Follow the IRS guidelines for hiring independent contractors.
- Follow all IRS and state guidelines for new hiring requirements.
- Ensure that after hiring but before actual customer contact, the new employee is thoroughly oriented to the organization's policies and procedures, all reference checks and background data has been collected on the applicant and this information has been thoroughly vetted, and that the new employee's compliances (medical, legal, and job specific) have been completed and the results collated and placed in the patient's employee file.

The interview can be one of the most dangerous litigious at-risk areas an employer encounters. Many federal, state, and local laws limit the questions that can be asked about an applicant's race, gender, disability, national origin, sexual orientation, marital status, pregnancy, age, family plans, or other personal issues. These topics should be strictly avoided, as asking questions in these areas can give applicants who are not chosen grounds for a discrimination claim.

Background checks are another potential landmine that employers must address with care and content knowledge. The laws vary from state to state. Some states permit background checks for purposes of evaluating a person's qualification for hire. Other states ban all forms of background checks to prescreen applicants. Some states actually require extensive pre-employment screening requirements for certain professions such as schools and child care and health care facilities. Employers must look carefully at their state's specific statutes to determine the background check's function, applicability, and relative compliance.

Under the Fair Credit Reporting Act,[40] prior to engaging an outside agency to conduct a background check and prepare a "consumer report," the employer must obtain the applicant's written consent. The employer must give the applicant a copy of the report's findings and allow the applicant to challenge the findings before taking any adverse action.

15.7.1 Staffing—Termination

Even with the best of employees there can come a point in the employer–employee relationship where the relationship may begin to sour. The employee may no longer be performing up to the standard expected, may be having behavioral problems, or, is simply no longer able to perform certain tasks. Even when an employee is performing well, your company may need to downsize and terminate an excellent employee.

Terminating employees is an unpleasant task. Performing the task correctly, professionally, and within the guidelines of employment law can ease the process for both parties.

Perhaps the most difficult part of any manager's job is telling a subordinate that he can no longer stay with the company—that he's been fired. Knowing how being fired can impact the employee's self-esteem, financial well-being, and personal relationships, most employers find the actual act incredibly painful to perform. Firing an employee will directly or indirectly impact everyone in the office. Even though the supervisor may have had professional or personal difficulties with the employee being fired, the employee most likely has a number of good friends in the office. With the loss of the fired employee there will always be repercussions with the team associated with the delegation of work assignments, the need to work short-handed until another employee is hired and oriented, loss of a team member, and a change in the office dynamics. There is always the chance that the remaining employees may side with the fired employee and therefore begin to question the supervisor's judgment and ability to lead. Firing an employee should not be performed without extended due diligence about the pros and cons of such an action.

Given these emotional undercurrents, many managers let anxiety drive the firing process instead of intellect—choosing to quickly "rip off the band aid" to end the episode as quickly as possible and begin to move on. One rule of thumb with firing is that firing should never come as a surprise to the person being fired. Organizations must maintain a comprehensive policy related to managing employee unsatisfactory performance or behavior. Such policies contain a chronological list of activities, actions, notifications, and documentation requirements which must be performed by the supervisor prior to firing. Following the chronological list greatly diminishes the risk of successful legal action on the part of the dismissed employee. Subjectivity and impulsivity with regard to firing must be avoided; the process should be analytical, objective, and guided by the organization's policies and procedures.

The process of firing is so emotionally charged, it's easy to act counterintuitively. Impulsive firing is never good; there will always be downstream problems. To avoid those issues, below are six guidelines for those times when firing an employee becomes a necessity:

1. All organizations have (or should have) a policy related to managing employee unsatisfactory performance or behavior which instructs the supervisor about actions which must be taken in a specific chronological order and the types of documentation performed at each chronological step. Follow this policy exactly as written.

2. When an underperforming employee is identified regular meetings should be scheduled between the appropriate human resources (HR) representative, the supervisor's immediate supervisor, and the supervisor. Human resource representatives are able to provide guidance and counsel to the supervisor during these difficult times, and insisting that the supervisor's supervisor be present ensures that the organization is made aware of the underperformance by the employee and the potential of firing. This is especially true if the employee is a bargaining employee.

3. Ensure that firing the employee is the last step in a careful, thoughtful, fair, and transparent process that started long before the actual firing. In other words, if the dismissal is for poor performance, the dismissal should occur only after a series of performance discussions, plans, and documented actions. If the firing is due to reorganization or job elimination, the termination should follow conversations, announcements, and a reasonable "fair warning." The key is that, if possible, firing should not come as a surprise to anyone. If the termination is due to downsizing and the employee is a bargaining employee, the union representatives should be kept abreast of all planned actions.

4. When progressing through the chronological steps of the organization's policy related to managing employee unsatisfactory performance or behavior there will be meetings between the supervisor and underperforming employee. The supervisor needs to ensure that a human resource representative be present at the meeting to, in the event of future litigation, be a witness to what was said and discussed at the meeting.

5. Forms required by the organization's policy related to the underperforming employee must be completed as required and stored in a safe and secure location. Supervisors should also maintain meeting minutes for any counseling sessions held.

6. Come to the "firing meeting" prepared to address the practical logistical questions that the person will have about leaving

her job: When is the official end date? Are there severance arrangements? Are there opportunities elsewhere in the company? Is career counseling available? What happens with benefits? You may need help from HR to make sure that these answers are available.

7. At the meeting, be ready to listen but not react. Losing a job can be traumatic, and your employee may display a range of emotions—from passivity to outright anger—which may be directed toward the supervisor. Do not attempt to argue with emotional responses. A better response is via an "'I' message." For instance, if an employee becomes emotionally upset, simply reply with "I see you are angry," or, "I see you are upset." These benign comments often permit the employee to vent without raising the emotional level of the conversation. Listen with respect and then direct the person toward the practical realities of moving on. Offer to talk again later when the emotions are not so raw, or ask a trained HR counselor to join you. Many organizations require security to be present to escort the fired employee immediately out of the building. Security's presence is typically required to ensure the terminated employee does not steal organization property or sabotage computer programs or data files.

8. After the firing, talk to your team about the process, the reasoning, and the implications for them (within the limits of confidentiality). In some cases, they will fully understand the decision. In others, they may have a very incomplete picture. In either case, you need to be sensitive to their emotions, and then help redirect their focus back on work.

Firing a subordinate is one of the most difficult and painful tasks a supervisor will ever have to do; and for most of us it never gets easier. Unfortunately, avoiding the anxiety associated by acting with impulsivity rather than professionally and through the organization's policies will only make things worse.

15.8 Informed Consent and Patient Rights

Most industrialized countries have organized their health care systems under the tenet that citizens have a right to medical care.[41] These countries' health care systems are organized as either governmental or governmental–private industry partnership directed for the provision of care. In the United States, at the printing of this text, there remains a forceful debate as to whether medical care is a right or a privilege of citizens. Perhaps to ensure consistency among the many health care players in the U.S. system, much debate and practical consideration has historically been on rights that individuals may exercise in the medical-care context. Only in recent decades with the impetus and successes of governmental-sponsored health care programs such as Medicare, Medicaid, and the Affordable Care Act have discussions begun to focus on the right of citizenry to medical care. Even with these changes, "patient rights" continue to be a very active topic of discussion. From "informed consent" to the "right to abortion" to the "right to die," patients' rights have become both a political slogan and a part of broader political, socioeconomic, and religious agendas.[42]

Although the trend toward recognizing patients' rights initially concentrated on the institutional setting in which medical care was delivered and focused on issues such as natural childbirth and informed consent, by the 1990s the trend was visible throughout the health care system in the United States. Facilitating the trend toward recognizing these rights were accreditation standards enforced by large agencies such as The Joint Commission (TJC) and the Commission on Accreditation of Rehabilitation Facilities.[43,44]

The historic path toward patient rights in the United States has been a rather tortuous route but one worth summarizing here. The doctor–patient relationship historically has been based on location, convenience, and trust rather than on the monetary considerations evident in the more typical business transaction. In the early days of our country and up to the mid-1950s America was primarily a rural country with limited transportation options and thus limited health care options. Citizens frequented the "town doctor," the "town pharmacist," and the "town hospital." As transportation became more available, location became less of a consideration in choosing a physician and hospital. In addition, increased outcome expectations and the higher out-of-pocket cost to the patient transformed the patient from a "consumer" of health care services into a "customer." In recent decades as insurance paid smaller and smaller percentages of health care charges and these debts were assumed by the patient, the patient naturally demanded improved customer service, responsiveness, and rights.

The recognition of patients' rights flowed from two fundamental premises[1]: The health care consumer possesses certain interests, many of which may be described as rights, that are not automatically forfeited by entering into a business relationship with a physician or a health care facility; and[2] many physicians and health care facilities failed to recognize the existence of these interests and rights, failed to provide for their protection or assertion, and frequently limited their exercise without recourse.

In 1969, the Joint Commission on Accreditation of Hospitals (now known as The Joint Commission [TJC])—a private, voluntary accreditation organization which accredits most inpatient (and inpatient-owned outpatient facilities in the United States) composed of members from the American Hospital Association (AHA) and the American Medical College of Surgeons—issued its annual proposals for revisions in its standards.[43] The National Welfare Rights Organization (NWRO), a grassroots consumer organization spawned during the activist 1960s, responded in June 1970 by drafting a document containing 26 demands; this was the first comprehensive statement of "patients' rights" from the consumer perspective.[45] Included were provisions for items as grievance procedures, community representation on hospital governing boards, nondiscrimination on the basis of source of payment, restrictions on transfer from one facility to another, provisions on privacy and confidentiality, and prompt attention to patients' requests for nursing assistance. After months of negotiation, a number of these items were specifically written into the revised accreditation standards of TJC. By the late 1980s, issues of access to care, of respect and dignity, privacy and confidentiality, consent, refusal of treatment, and patient transfer to another facility were specifically addressed in a new section of its accreditation manual called "Rights and Responsibilities of Patients."

In late 1972, the American Hospital Association (AHA), realizing the shift of the patient from a "captive audience" to "consumer," adopted a Patient Bill of Rights based on the premise that "[the] traditional physician–patient relationship takes on a new dimension when care is rendered within an organizational structure ... the institution itself also has a responsibility to the patient."[46] The text of the AHA bill of patient rights called for acknowledgment of the rights to[1] respectful care[2]; current medical information[3]; information requisite for informed consent[4]; refusal of treatment[5]; privacy[6]; confidentiality[7]; response to requests for service[8]; information on other institutions touching on the patient's care[9]; refusal of participation in research projects[10]; continuity of care[11]; examination and explanation of financial charges; and[12] knowledge of hospital regulations. In 1992, additional rights detailing access to services, patient and family access to the medical record, and use of advance directives were added. Although the listing remains vague and incomplete, and there is no enforcement mechanism, it moves in the direction of more adequately informing patients of their rights.

Between 1974 and 1988, many states, including Arizona, California, Illinois, Kentucky, Maryland, Massachusetts, Michigan, Minnesota, New Hampshire, New York, Pennsylvania, Rhode Island, and Vermont, adopted a patients' bill of rights by regulation or statute. All 50 states have since adopted some form of advance health care directive document, such as a living will or durable power of attorney, in which people can express their wishes regarding medical care should they become incompetent.[47] These directives are binding to most health care workers in most health care arenas.

The American Medical Association (AMA), probably because of its traditional paternalistic philosophy of the patient–doctor relationship, did not seriously consider adopting its own version of the patients' bill of rights until 1989.[48] Five of the six provisions of its proposal—the rights of patients to access information in the medical record and to make treatment decisions and the rights to respect, to confidentiality, and to continuity of care—seem to have been noncontroversial. The bill of rights was rejected by the AMA House of Delegates, however, because of its sixth provision: "The patient has the right to essential health [medical] care." Under current legislation and the absence of a comprehensive U.S. national health care program there is no existing mandate for the patient to have the right to essential health care unless the patient is experiencing an emergency medical condition (although opinion polls taken since 1948 show that most physicians and Americans believe this right either exists or should exist).[48]

The structure and function of a delineated list of patient rights guarantees specific rights to those persons receiving medical care and, in many cases, the families of patients receiving care. With the many sources of patient rights: accreditation standards, administrative groups such as the AMA and APTA, and statute, patient rights may take the role of law or of a nonbinding declaration. With multiple sources of patient rights enforcement may be based on civil, administrative, or criminal law; by nonlegal entities such as peer pressure, the court of public opinion, or social media; or, not at all. A patients' bill of rights was considered by the U.S. Congress in 2001. The law's proposed title was the "Bipartisan Patient Protection Act." It was known officially as Senate Bill S.1052 and informally as the "McCain-Edwards-Kennedy Patients' Bill of Rights." The bill was an attempt at providing comprehensive protections to all Americans covered by health insurance plans. The bill was passed by the U.S. Senate by a vote of 59–36 in 2001. It was then amended by the House of Representatives and returned to the Senate. However, passage ultimately failed.[49]

The Association of American Physicians and Surgeons adopted a list of patient freedoms in 1990, which was modified and adopted as a "patients' bill of rights" in 1995.[50] This list is commonly published in literature provided to patients on entry into one of the levels of the health care continuum:

All patients should be guaranteed the following freedoms:

- To seek consultation with the physician(s) of their choice.
- To contract with their physician(s) on mutually agreeable terms.
- To be treated confidentially, with access to their records limited to those involved in their care or designated by the patient.
- To use their own resources to purchase the care of their choice.
- To refuse medical treatment even if it is recommended by their physician(s).
- To be informed about their medical condition, the risks and benefits of treatment and appropriate alternatives.
- To refuse third-party interference in their medical care, and to be confident that their actions in seeking or declining medical care will not result in third–party-imposed penalties for patients or physicians.
- To receive full disclosure of their insurance plan in plain language, including
  1. *Contracts*: A copy of the contract between the physician and health care plan, and between the patient or employer and the plan.
  2. *Incentives*: Whether participating physicians are offered financial incentives to reduce treatment or ration care.
  3. *Cost*: The full cost of the plan, including copayments, coinsurance, and deductibles.
  4. *Coverage*: Benefits covered and excluded, including availability and location of 24-hour emergency care.
  5. *Qualifications*: A roster and qualifications of participating physicians.
  6. *Approval procedures*: Authorization procedures for services, whether doctors need approval of a committee or any other individual, and who decides what is medically necessary.
  7. *Referrals*: Procedures for consulting a specialist, and who must authorize the referral.
  8. *Appeals*: Grievance procedures for claim or treatment denials.
  9. *Gag rule*: Whether physicians are subject to a gag rule, preventing criticism of the plan.

One of the hallmark items of any list of patient rights is informed consent. Informed consent is the process by which the treating health care provider discloses appropriate information to a competent patient so that the patient may make a voluntary choice to accept or refuse treatment. The concept of informed consent originates from the legal and ethical right the patient has to direct what happens to his body and from the ethical duty of the health care practitioner (including the physical therapist) to involve the patient in his health care. (It is interesting to note that the historical development of the patient informed consent process paralleled the development of the research subject informed consent process. As with medicine where informed consent was an inconsistent practice until recent decades, informed consent in the research community was also inconsistent as evidenced by many examples, including the disheartening and unethical Tuskegee syphilis experiments that mercifully ended in 1972.)

The goal of informed consent is that the patient has an opportunity to be an informed participant in his health care decisions. Informed consent typically includes a discussion of the following elements[51]:

- The nature of the decision/procedure.
- Reasonable alternatives to the proposed intervention.
- The relevant risks, benefits, and uncertainties related to each alternative.
- Assessment of patient understanding.
- The acceptance of the intervention by the patient.
- The right to refuse the intervention.

In order for the patient's medical consent to be valid, the patient must be considered competent to make the decision at hand and the consent must be given voluntarily. Special situations which still require consent (and one's legal counsel should be consulted to assist with writing policy) are when the patient is less than the age of consent or deemed incompetent of rendering a valid assent to care.

Coercive situations frequently arise in medicine. Patients often feel powerless and vulnerable. Patients also feel at a disadvantage talking to a content expert. To encourage voluntariness, the health care practitioner can make clear to the patient that he is participating in a decision-making process, not merely signing a form. With this understanding, the informed consent process should be seen as an invitation for the patient to participate in health care decisions rather than an affirmation permitting whatever the health care practitioner proposes doing. Comprehension on the part of the patient is equally as important as the information provided. Consequently, the discussion should be carried on in layperson's terms and the patient's understanding should be assessed along the way.

Basic or simple consent entails letting the patient know what the health care practitioner prefers as the best course of intervention action. This is performed by providing to the patient the basic information about the procedure and ensuring that the patient assents or consents to the intervention. Assent, by signature or witnessed verbal response, implies a patient's willing acceptance of a treatment, intervention, or clinical care. From a physical therapist perspective consent is required for the evaluation, assessment, and intervention. In inpatient settings, the organization's consent frequently covers the patient's assent to receive care but does not eliminate the need for the physical therapist to provide to the patient a thorough explanation of the care to be delivered and the decision process which led to this decision.

How does a practitioner know that she has provided to the patient sufficient information about a proposed intervention? Most of the literature and law in this area suggest one of three approaches[52]:

- **Reasonable health care professional standard:** *What would a typical health care practitioner acting in the role of the practitioner typically say about this intervention?* In other words, for a physical therapist, the question is: What would a physical therapist, practicing in this geographic area and state, with

a patient such as this, in an arena of medical care such as this, say about this evaluation, assessment, and intervention? This standard allows the health care practitioner to determine what information is appropriate to disclose. However, this standard is often inadequate, because most research shows that the typical health care practitioner informs the patient very little as compared with best practice.

- **Reasonable patient standard:** *What would the average patient need to know in order to be an informed participant in the decision?* This standard focuses on considering what a typical patient would need to know in order to understand the decision at hand.
- **Subjective standard:** *What would this particular patient need to know and understand in order to make an informed decision?* This standard is the most challenging to incorporate into practice, because it requires tailoring information to each patient.

Additional variables may play a part in the context of the informed consent. These variables include the stark, anti-kickback, and false claims laws and are addressed later in this chapter.

Most states have legislation or legal cases that determine the required standard for informed consent. The best approach to the question of how much information is enough is one that meets both the practitioner's obligation to provide the best care and respects the patient as a person, with the right to a voice in health care decisions.

15.9 Sexual Harassment

Sexual harassment is bullying or coercion of a sexual nature or the unwelcome or inappropriate promise of rewards in exchange for sexual favors.[53] As defined by the United States' EEOC, sexual harassment is "the (unlawfulness) to harass a person (an applicant or employee) because of that person's sex."[54] Harassment can include "sexual harassment" or unwelcome sexual advances, requests for sexual favors, and other verbal or physical harassment of a sexual nature.[53] The legal definition of sexual harassment varies by jurisdiction.

Although laws surrounding sexual harassment exist, they generally do not prohibit simple teasing, offhand comments, or minor isolated incidents—that is, sexual harassment laws do not impose a general civility code. In the workplace, harassment may be considered illegal when it is so frequent or severe that it creates a hostile or offensive work environment or when it results in an adverse employment decision (such as the victim being fired, demoted, given nonpreferred work assignments, or when the action prompts or forces the victim to voluntarily leave the job). Complicating the understanding of sexual harassment is that the legal definition of sexual harassment varies by jurisdiction and that the social definition of sexual harassment is defined by culture.

In the context of U.S. employment, the harasser can be the victim's supervisor, a supervisor in another area, a coworker, or someone who is not an employee of the employer, such as a client or customer. The harassers or victims can be of any gender. Within the professional physical therapy educational program, the harasser can be a faculty member, another student, clinical instructor, patient, employee at a clinical site, or a patient's family member. In the physical therapy professional employment arena, the list expands exponentially.

Sexual harassment includes a range of actions from mild transgressions to sexual abuse or sexual assault. For many businesses or organizations, preventing sexual harassment, and defending employees from sexual harassment charges, have become key goals of legal decision making.

There are five types of sexual harassment[55]:

- Gender harassment: Generalized sexist statements and behavior that convey insulting or degrading attitudes about women. Examples include insulting remarks, sharing of offensive pictures or websites, offensive graffiti, and obscene jokes or humor about sex or about a specific sexual class of persons.
- Seductive behavior: Unwanted, inappropriate, and offensive sexual advances. Examples include repeated unwanted sexual invitations, insistent requests for dinner, drinks, or dates, persistent letters, phone calls, and other invitations, and the continued placement of untoward cards and letters on a desk or car.
- Sexual bribery: Solicitation of sexual activity or other sex-linked behavior by promise of reward; the proposition may be either overt or subtle.
- Sexual coercion: Coercion of sexual activity or other sex-linked behavior by threat of punishment; examples include negative performance evaluations, withholding of promotions, threat of termination, unequal or unfavorable work assignments.
- Sexual imposition: Gross sexual imposition (such as forceful touching, feeling, grabbing) or sexual assault.

Of these five types of behavior, gender harassment is by far the most common, followed by seductive behavior. The "classic" forms of sexual harassment (bribery and coercion) are in fact relatively uncommon, while other forms of sexual imposition happen more frequently than most people think. Recent court decisions have also found that certain types of offensive visual displays in the workplace, such as pornography, can be considered sexual harassment.

The defining characteristic of sexual harassment is that it is unwanted. It's important to clearly let an offender know immediately that certain actions are unwelcome. The perpetrator can be anyone, such as a client, a coworker, a parent or legal guardian, relative, a teacher or professor, a student, a friend, or a stranger. The victim does not have to be the person directly harassed but can be a witness of such behavior who finds the behavior offensive and is affected by it. The place of harassment occurrence may vary from school, university, workplace, and other. There may or may not be other witnesses or attendances. The perpetrator may be completely unaware that his or her behavior is offensive or constitutes sexual harassment or may be completely unaware that his or her actions could be unlawful. The incident can take place in situations in which the harassed person may not be aware of or understand what is happening. The incident may be one-time occurrence but more often it has a type of repetitiveness. Adverse effects on the target are common in the form of stress and social withdrawal, sleep and eating difficulties, overall health impairment, etc. The victim and perpetrator can be any gender. The perpetrator does not have to be of the opposite sex.

Companies that do business globally often have a code of conduct that supersedes local law in some cases. Americans working overseas are often surprised that local jurisdictions often do not have laws governing sexual harassment.

Below are a series of practical steps a worker should consider taking if there has been a perception of sexual harassment.

1. Read the company policy and the law on sexual harassment (if any) in the state or jurisdiction where the infraction supposedly occurred very carefully and print them. The company policy will usually include employee rights, protections against retaliation, and an outline of the steps an employee should follow in the event a claim is to be reported.
2. Determine if the company has a policy that protects whistleblowers from retaliation. If there is one, read it carefully and print it.
3. Identify the person, based on the organization's policy, to whom the claim should be taken. If the policy does not specifically mention an individual determine who in the chain of command is the most mature, reasonable, and capable of being objective in handling something as sensitive as a harassment claim.
4. Do not share comments about the perceived indiscretion with coworkers. Do not make public accusations.
5. Write down what you plan to say to report the harassment. Have as many specifics as possible including dates, locations, witness names and length of the specific episode. Attempt to document exactly what was said or done. Ensure there is a mention of how the perceived harassment has affected the victim's ability to perform his or her job. Date and sign your recollections of the harassment. Make two copies and keep one for yourself in a safe and confidential location. Most likely the person the violation is reported to will ask for a copy of the reflections. Practice your talk with someone you trust outside the company who will keep this confidential. Reporting a perceived sexual harassment can be extremely awkward, uncomfortable, and stressful. Practicing will help the victim be calm when making the claim.
6. If there are trusted witnesses ask them confidentially for confirmation and support. This is a delicate and risky step that the victim may not want to take unless there is a strong belief that this person will keep the issue confidential until and if they are interviewed as part of a formal investigation.
7. Ask for a meeting with the person you choose in your chain of command and invite the appropriate executive from HR. Bring a pen and a notepad to take notes during the meeting. File these notes with the recollection notes.
8. Explain the situation, give examples, give the names of witnesses, and tell them the impact this has had on you. Let them know that you did your homework: You were subject to what you believe violates the company's sexual harassment policy and/or the law, and show them your printed evidence. Tell them that you want the behavior to stop in order to work in a safe and supportive environment.
9. Once you have laid out your complaint, ask: "Do you think this behavior is acceptable at this company?" If you get them to admit it's wrong, make sure you write it down in your notes.
10. Listen to what they say and write everything down. Let them see you are documenting, and ask them to slow down if necessary.
11. Thank them and ask what the next steps are, who will conduct the investigation, who they will talk to, how long will it take to complete it, etc.

Once the allegation of sexual harassment has been raised with human resources, the human resource leader should meet with the victim privately and explain the organization's policy with regard to these types of allegations. The first action the human resources' leader should do is to initiate a highly confidential investigation of the allegation while protecting the alleged victim from retaliation. If the first thing the human resources' leader does is try to support the alleged offender, make excuses for that person, or diminish the impact of the harm done to the victim, the victim should politely but directly inform the human resources' leader that you strongly disagree, and that if they do not conduct a proper investigation, you will be given no choice but to seek justice through an attorney who can provide proper representation.

Speaking out can carry a huge price to the victim. The victim cannot be assured that there will not be retribution by the organization for bringing forth the complaint through being fired, punished, or blackballed. The U.S. EEOC reported that charges of retaliation linked to sexual discrimination claims grew to about 40,000 in 2015, which is more than double the number in 1997.[55] In addition, the risk of retaliation by the accused—who has much to lose if the allegation has merit—cannot be dismissed.

15.10 Stark, Anti-Kickback, and False Claims

Health care is an incredibly large, broad, diverse, and dynamic industry where much money changes hands among providers, insurance companies, vendors, and patients. Sadly, with so much money involved in such a complex industry there is ample opportunity for unethical and illegal practice.[56] Medicare estimates billions in fraudulent payments made to providers in 2016 (the exact number cannot be known due to the scope and pervasiveness of the fraud committed).[57] There are several key health care laws that every provider should understand to assist in the prevention of inadvertent fraud. Below are short summations of three of the laws:

Stark Law. The Stark Law is a federal self-referral statute that prohibits a provider from referring Medicare and Medicaid patients for designated health services if the provider (or his immediate family member) has a financial relationship with the entity to which the patient is referred, unless an exception is met.[58] Below are a few examples of actions which may be considered violations of the Stark Law:

- A "patient recruiter" is employed by Dr. Jones, DPT, on a cash basis to identify and drive homeless persons to his practice for physical therapy care. For every patient brought to the clinic Dr. Jones paid the recruiter $50. The recruited homeless patients underwent a variety of medical treatments, many of which were not medically necessary, and the interventions were billed to federal health care programs.
- Pneumatic devices may be used to treat persons with lymphedema. A pneumatic device manufacturer paid kickbacks to Dr. Jones in order to obtain pneumatic device orders. The device manufacturer paid Dr. Jones $100 for every patient referred for a device.
- Dr. Jones' sister is a psychologist with her practice in the same building as Dr. Jones' physical therapy practice. Dr. Jones "identifies" many of his patients as having impairments requiring psychological intervention. He refers these patients to his sister.

Under the Stark Law, "financial relationship" is a broad term that includes ownership, investment interest, and compensation arrangements.[59] Designated health services do not include all health care services, but do include the following: clinical laboratory tests; physical therapy services; occupational therapy services; radiology services including magnetic resonance imaging, computerized axial tomography scans, and ultrasound services; radiation therapy services and supplies; durable medical equipment and supplies; parenteral and enteral nutrients, equipment, and supplies; prosthetics, orthotics, and prosthetic devices; home health services and supplies; outpatient prescription drugs; and inpatient and outpatient hospital services.

The Stark Law prohibits a provider from requesting that a patient receive any of these services or treatments from a facility with which the referring provider (or immediate family member) has a financial relationship or establishing a plan of care that includes a designated health service by a provider with which the referring provider has a financial relationship.

Penalties for violating Stark can be severe. They include denial of payment, refund of payment, imposition of a $15,000 per service civil monetary penalty and imposition of a $100,000 civil monetary penalty for each arrangement considered to be a circumvention scheme.

Anti-kickback statute. The federal anti-kickback statute is a criminal statute that prohibits the exchange of anything of value in an effort to induce the referral of Medicare or Medicaid business. The anti-kickback statute is broadly drafted and establishes penalties for both the giving and the receiving individuals.[60] Conviction of an anti-kickback statute violation results in mandatory exclusion from participation in Medicare and Medicaid programs. Absent a conviction, individuals who violate the anti-kickback statute may still face exclusion from federal health care programs at the discretion of the secretary of HHS.

Following are examples of anti-kickback statute violations:

- Mercy Hospital agrees to pay Dr. Jones' physical therapy clinic for every referral for X-ray that he makes to the hospital-employed radiologists.
- Clinical Laboratories, Inc. agrees to pay Dr. Jones for utilizing its transcutaneous nerve stimulators in his clinic hoping that the patients will order Clinical Laboratories' devices for future home use.

False Claims Act. The False Claims Act imposes liability on persons and companies that defraud governmental programs. Common violations in health care include upcoding for medical procedures and performing or ordering of unnecessary procedures.[61] The law includes a "qui tam" provision that allows people who are not affiliated with the government to file actions on behalf of the government (informally called "whistleblowing").

The following are examples of a violation of the False Claims Act:

- Dr. Jones is found by Medicare investigators that he regularly upcodes his bills to Medicare clients by adding ultrasound therapy to the client's regular interventions. The Medicare audit revealed that 94% of Medicare bills uploaded to Medicare for the previous month contained a charge for ultrasound.

- Dr. Jones, during a routine Medicare audit, was found to be upcoding Medicare bills. The audit determined that Dr. Jones was preferentially billing "therapeutic activities" codes for all persons receiving therapeutic exercise. The therapeutic activities code reimburses the provider at a higher rate than therapeutic exercise. The documentation examined did not support the inclusion of a therapeutic activities charge code.

Physical therapy has been a targeted profession by the Office of the Inspector General (OIG) due to the number of false claims identified over the past few years.[62] Physical therapists must be extremely cognizant of providing only indicated interventions, documenting well in the medical record what was provided to the patient, and billing only for items supported by the documentation.

15.11 Protecting Your Professional License: Criminal, Civil, and Administrative Law

Regarding legal proceedings there are three basic types of law: criminal, civil, and administrative. Criminal law deals with crimes and their prosecution. Each jurisdiction (federal, state, county, local) has a criminal code. Violation of the criminal code prompts criminal action. Civil law is the law governing the relations between private persons or organizations. Administrative law is the law regarding the rules or regulations made and enforced by governmental agencies.

15.11.1 Criminal Law

Criminal cases involve charges brought by the jurisdiction under that jurisdiction's criminal laws. The goal is to punish offenders for violating the criminal laws by assessing the offenders with fines, imprisonment, or probation. Thus, crimes are offenses against the jurisdiction and not against individuals. The individual suffering from the crime is the "victim." Victims are witnesses. The party bringing the case to court is the "jurisdiction," represented by the prosecutor. The prosecutor's party name is the "prosecution." The jurisdiction may also be the "people" or the "commonwealth." Bringing a criminal charge to court and carrying it through is called "prosecuting" the defendant.

Criminal offenses are almost always violation of written laws. They are labeled for identification, (e.g., "murder" and "manslaughter") but defined by parts, called "elements," each of which the prosecution must prove to get a guilty verdict. Failure to prove just one element of the crime results in the defendant's acquittal of that criminal charge. For example, to prove "negligent homicide," the prosecution might have to prove that the defendant[1] negligently[2] caused[3] the death of another[4] by means of a dangerous weapon, material, or instrument.

Crimes fall into two general categories, misdemeanors and felonies. Misdemeanors are crimes typically punishable by fines or jail sentences of 1 year or less. Felonies are crimes punishable by jail sentences typically exceeding 1 year. States divide related offenses into degrees of severity. The higher the degree, the less "serious" the crime, and lighter the sentence.

Knowledge of the legal definitions of misdemeanor and felony is an important concept for physical therapists and physical therapist assistants. In most states therapists can obtain and maintain a professional license if convicted of a misdemeanor but conviction of a felony results in an inability to obtain a professional license or, if one has already been obtained, the forfeiture of the license.

The burden of proof in a criminal proceeding is "beyond a reasonable doubt," which means being firmly convinced that the defendant is guilty. Judges, in instructing juries, often attempt to quantify reasonable doubt as being "99% sure the defendant committed the crime."

Below is a partial list of misdemeanor and felonious activities for which a physical therapist could be accused of perpetrating during clinical or administrative activities:

- Sexual assault of a patient.
- Physical assault of a patient.
- Robbing a patient.
- A pattern of purposeful improper billing to Medicare to enhance reimbursement.
- Intentionally falsifying a medical record in order to enhance Medicaid reimbursement.

15.11.2 Civil Law

Civil law deals with relations between private persons or organizations. A plaintiff in a civil case sues to redress a lost personal interest, be it money, property, or liberty. Licenses and certificates are property. Relief might include the enforcement of a contract, compensation from the defendant for the plaintiff's physical or economic harm, or a court order telling the defendant to do or not do something (e.g., an injunction). Thus, in a civil proceeding, the question for the court is not guilt or innocence, but liability for the defendant's injury, or whether to grant some equitable ("fair") relief where money is not the object.

In physical therapy, most civil suits filed against physical therapists and physical therapist assistants relate back to harm either done or perceived to be done by the therapist to the patient. Harm may occur based on physical injury or emotional injury, or loss of ability to work or enjoy the benefits of life. Examples of possible civil lawsuits against physical therapists are as follows:

- Pain and disability following a burn caused by improper application of a thermal modality by the physical therapist.
- Pain and disability following a physical therapist permitting a patient to fall when being trained in elevations (stair climbing).
- Failure by the physical therapist to provide evidence-based care in accordance with the local standard of care, resulting in permanent disability or pain.
- Sexual harassment toward an employee or patient. (Note: sexual harassment may potentially be considered a violation of a criminal statute and also be cause for a civil suit because there may be, in the jurisdiction, criminal laws against sexual harassment and the victim may perceive there has been a permanently injury related to the harassment; thus, the civil suit as well.)

In civil proceedings, the standard of proof is most often "preponderance of the evidence" (also known as "the greater weight" or

50.1%). But in some cases where fraud or criminal conduct is alleged in a civil court or a license is at stake, a "clear and convincing" standard may apply. There is no presumption for or against either party, though the plaintiff bears the burden of proving the defendant's liability. A person can be sued civilly after being tried criminally for the same behavior, whether acquitted or convicted in the previous criminal trial.

One can never be jailed for being found liable in a civil lawsuit, though a party in a civil case may be jailed for contempt of court. Contempt of court means intentionally interfering with the administration of justice (e.g., not following a court order).

Civil cases involve six basic types of disputes with an explanation of each below:

1. Lawsuits for damages ("torts").
2. Requests for court orders (injunctions, restraining orders, etc.).
3. Civil rights actions.
4. Requests for declaratory judgments (e.g., an order declaring a law unconstitutional).
5. Disputes over contracts or other agreements.
6. Appeals from administrative decisions.

Lawsuits for Damages (Torts)

The torts most likely to be brought against physical therapists are claims for negligence. Negligence includes claims of wrongful death, physical or emotional injury (professional negligence), and gross negligence. Negligence is the[1] breach of a duty[2] directly causing[3] damages to the plaintiff. A licensed physical therapist owes a client a fiduciary (professional) duty; that is, a duty of a special trust and care. To show the defendant breached that duty—in a legal state—the plaintiff usually must get testimony from other qualified physical therapists that the physical therapist's actions fell below the established standard of care for physical therapists in the local physical therapy community of practitioners.

Requests for Court Orders (Injunctions)

The most common court order one seeks in a civil case involving physical therapy is a type of restraining order called an "injunction." An injunction seeks to stop an individual from performing some action. For example, a state board might seek an injunction ordering a physical therapist found to be impaired due to opioids at work from "practicing physical therapy." In turn, the physical therapist may seek an injunction ordering a state board to refrain from enforcing a law or regulation.

Civil Rights Actions

Civil rights actions are lawsuits brought against a governmental authority, or agent acting under that authority, for harming the plaintiff by violating the U.S. Constitution or other federal law. The claim is brought under a specific federal statute, 42 U.S.C. 1983, enabling the plaintiff to sue in federal court. For example, a physical therapist from a minority group may have standing to bring a civil rights' claim against an organization which has demonstrated a pattern of refusal to hire qualified members of that minority. States have civil rights statutes also, letting plaintiffs sue in state court when the governmental authority or agent under that authority has violated plaintiffs' constitutional rights. Civil rights actions often involve declaratory actions. There are many cases in the federal courts of appeals, not to mention the Eleventh Amendment to the U.S. Constitution, which greatly restricts the ability to sue state and local governments for monetary damages. There are also legal doctrines that usually require that state and local governments be sued in state courts and not federal courts.

Declaratory Actions

A declaratory action asks the court to declare the plaintiff's right or legal status under a law, contract, or other instrument. This can include a constitutional clause or amendment. For example, a physical therapist may seek a judgment declaring that a licensing regulation or state practice act standard is unconstitutional. Declaratory actions usually come with requests for injunctions to prevent the losing party from enforcing the law or regulation.

Disputes over Contracts or other Agreements

A physical therapist who owns her own practice and is practicing legally may have a contract with an insurance company. Thus, a civil case may include a civil action to enforce the contract (e.g., about payment, etc.). Note that the same contract that strengthens a claim in civil court may create evidence useable in criminal court.

Appeals from Administrative Decisions

A separate administrative tribunal hears an administrative case. Appeals from cases heard administratively are brought in a general county civil court.

15.11.3 Administrative Law

Administrative law, as it relates to the profession of physical therapy, is that law dealing with various organs of the state government that let commissions or boards regulate professions. Each state empowers its state board of physical therapy to oversee the practice of physical therapy in that state. The state legislature creates a state board of physical therapy and then passes general laws about how the board will conduct its activities. Similar boards in a given state may be named "The State Board of Pharmacy," "The State Board of Dentistry," or "Board of Medical Examiners." The legislature gives these boards or commissions authority to make its own rules and regulations and enforce their compliance. The rules and regulations are valid provided they do not oppose, modify, overly extend, or overly restrict the legislature's original laws. In enforcing their rules and regulations, administrative agencies can investigate suspected noncompliance and hold hearings to decide relevant controversies. On finding a violation, administrative agencies have several possible remedies. They can suspend, revoke, or cancel licenses or certificates, pursue criminal charges, seek court orders, or issue "cease and desist" orders to nonlicensed offenders of the rules and regulations.

Actions by physical therapists and physical therapist assistants may be found to be in violation individually or in combination of criminal, civil, or administrative laws and regulations.

Recent decades have witnessed an increase in the number of criminal, civil, and administrative lawsuits filed against health care practitioners and health care entities. Physical therapists are included in this cohort. The reason for the increased filing of lawsuits against physical therapists is multifactorial and includes an expanded scope of clinical practice, increased autonomy, an increased number of practicing physical therapists and physical therapist assistants, and the litigious climate in the United States. A recently published report by the Healthcare Providers' Service Organization (HPSO)—a major malpractice insurer of physical therapists and physical therapist assistants—detailed that between the years 2011 and 2015 payments for malpractice claims against physical therapists and physical therapist assistants rose to $42 million.[63] A previous HPSO study, published in 2011, reported a total of $44 million in malpractice claim payments against physical therapists and physical therapist assistants, but the older study period spanned 10 years, not five. Comparing these two reports appears to indicate a twofold increase in malpractice payment for claims against physical therapists and physical therapist assistants during 2001 and 2015.[64]

In terms of the root causes of allegations made against physical therapists and physical therapist assistants, claims of improper management over the course of physical therapy treatment nearly doubled during the study period. "Management" can best be defined as clinical decision making. Therapists, using best-evidence and clinical experience as guidelines, make thousands of clinical and administrative decisions per day. Most of these decisions, such as whether to order a patient a wheelchair with extended or standard brake levers, are considered low-risk decisions. However, some decisions, such as whether to ambulate a postoperative day number one patient status post-total knee replacement who presents with redness, swelling, and pain in his operative calf, are rightfully considered high-risk and problem-prone due to the potential of a catastrophic adverse event (in this case pulmonary embolism). HPSO's additional examples of improper management include failure to follow practitioner orders, failure to obtain informed consent, failure to complete a proper patient evaluation and assessment, failure to cease treatment following excessive/unexpected pain, and failure to report the patient's condition to the referring practitioner.[62]

Now at 22.5% of all paid claims, the management category represents the largest percentage of paid civil claims against physical therapists and physical therapist assistants. Additional frequent paid claims against therapists include those related to manual therapy, failure to supervise or monitor the patient during an evaluation or therapeutic intervention, the improper use of therapeutic exercise resulting in patient injury, and improper use of a biophysical agent.[65]

As physical therapists increase their visibility through enlarging the profession's scope of practice and through increasing autonomous practice via direct access legislation, the potential of medical error becomes a greater concern for public safety and for the public's perception of the profession. Sandstrom described malpractice by physical therapists in the United States based on physical therapist malpractice reports in the National Practitioner Data Bank between January 1, 1991, and December 31, 2004.[66] A frequency analysis of data related to physical therapist malpractice reports was performed. The relationship between size of malpractice payment and public policy related to access to physical therapist services and malpractice experience was explored. A total of 664 malpractice reports were found in the study period (mean: 47.73 events annually). California had 114 malpractice events, while Maine and Wyoming had none. The median payment amount for physical therapist malpractice was $10,000 to $15,000. According to Sandstrom, "treatment-related" events and events related to "improper technique" were the most common reasons for successful malpractice claims against physical therapists and physical therapist assistants. Incidence of malpractice by physical therapists is low (estimated at 2.5 events/10,000 working therapists/year), and the average malpractice payment is small (< $15,000). Sandstrom also concluded that most physical therapist malpractice involves a direct clinical intervention by an early to mid-career therapist in an urban location. Cumulative physical therapist malpractice incidence in a state was unrelated to public policy related to direct patient access to physical therapy services.

15.12 Legal Aspects of Human Resources Documentation

With the overwhelmingly strong emphasis on the quality and scope of medical record documentation taught in professional programs, most physical therapists have a broad understanding of the medicolegal aspects of documentation. These aspects include the rationale for complete documentation performed in a timely manner, the various accreditation standards for documentation, state board requirements of documentation, the importance of legibility, et al. In addition, actual or fear of malpractice lawsuits have added to the practitioner's appreciation of strong, accurate, and complete medical documentation. How often have we been told in professional school or on our clinical internships that "if it isn't documented it hasn't been done."

In recent years employment documentation, also known as human resource documentation, has gained an importance close to or even exceeding the importance of medical record documentation. As with medical record documentation, the increasing importance of human resources documentation is driven by medicolegal concerns and accreditation standards. In addition to these two drivers "good business practices" has also been an impetus to improve human resource documentation. Along with the incorporation of legal and accreditation standards, human resources directors intuit good human resource documentation practices—either as commonsense practices or as prospective actions to offset potential future legal issues—and these practices eventually become *de rigueur* of the human resources community.

Human resources documentation can be classified as formal, informal, and supporting. Formal documentation consists of documentation required by law, regulatory, or accrediting agency. Informal documentations are those items not required by law, regulatory, or accrediting agency. These documents include items such as memoranda, productivity statistics, yearly business plans, and emails (see ▶ Table 15.1). The accumulation and maintenance of supportive documentation of meeting compliance and regulatory standards is a common practice

Table 15.1 Examples of formal, informal, and supportive human resources documentation

Formal documentation	Informal documentation	Supportive documentation
Employment application	Memoranda	Letters from patients
Resume	Yearly business plans	Time card records
Copy of professional license	Productivity reports	Work schedules
License verification	Program pro forma	Holiday schedules
Records of medical compliance	Contracts developed	Earned certifications or specializations
Records of clinical compliance	Customer satisfaction reports	Publications
Letters of employment reference	Peer review assessments	Research projects
Cardiopulmonary resuscitation certification		Grant applications
Continuing education documentation		Meeting agendas and minutes
Citizenship documentation		Lists of internal and external committee membership
Yearly performance appraisals		Records of service and volunteerism
Family Medical Leave applications		
Americans with Disabilities accommodation records		
Employment counseling records		
Notation of yearly review of policy manual		

among well-run organizations. These data aid in helping to assure meeting compliance and regulatory standards and also help ensure a safe and effective workforce. Supportive documentation often undergirds formal documentation. These items support or provide evidence for the formal documentation. Examples include yearly pay records, bonus documentation, reference letters, and letters of support.

There are a number of considerations which must be addressed related to human resource documentation. These considerations include the following:

- Developing an administrative mindset that the importance of maintaining complete, thorough, and inclusive human resource documentation should equal that of maintaining clinical documentation.
- That the medicolegal import of human resource documentation equals or exceeds the import of clinical documentation. Human resource documentation is often subpoenaed for civil,

administrative, and criminal lawsuits and lack of completeness or missing or misplaced data can negatively impact the outcome of these cases.

- Smaller organizations should utilize consultants to develop policies of inclusion for aspects of human resource documentation. As with clinical documentation the rules regarding how long to save human resource documentation vary with type of document.
- Many aspects of human resource documentation are time sensitive. For instance, documentation related to cardiopulmonary resuscitation certification is often valid for 2 years. Every 2 years the employee is required to be recertified. Recertification should be performed just prior to the expiration of the prior certification. There should never be gaps in the documentation. A policy should be established and circulated that no employee may work if there are gaps in the human resource documentation.
- Frequent audits of the human resource documentation should be performed to ensure compliance with policy.
- Human resource data for health care employees can be generally divided into medical and nonmedical documentation. Medical documentation includes immunization records, records of tuberculosis testing, and medical evaluations. Nonmedical documentation includes all other data such as the employment application and performance appraisals. Best practice indicates that these two records—medical and nonmedical documentation—should be maintained separately in two distinct files to limit the risk of loss of confidentiality. For instance, if an auditor is looking for hepatitis C documentation for a particular employee there is no need to risk him accidently viewing a warning letter from the employee's supervisor; or, if the auditor is looking for employment references there is no need to risk having him accidently reading the employee's medical history.

References

[1] Blachly FF, Oatman ME. Federal Administrative Procedure Act. Geol J. 1945; 34:407

[2] Gellhorn W. The Administrative Procedure Act: the beginnings. Va Law Rev. 1986; 72:219–233

[3] Yackee JW, Yackee SW. Administrative procedures and bureaucratic performance: is federal rule-making "ossified"? J Public Adm Res Theory. 2009; 20 (2):261–282

[4] Langbein JH, Lerner RL, Smith BP. History of the Common Law: The Development of Anglo-American Legal Institutions. Austin, TX: Wolters Kluwer; 2009

[5] Gordon RW. Introduction: J. Willard Hurst and the common law tradition in American legal historiography. Law Soc Rev. 1975; 10:9–55

[6] Douglas WO. Stare decisis. Columbia Law Rev. 1949; 49(6):735–758

[7] Cantor NF. (1997). Imagining the Law: Common Law and the Foundations of the American Legal System. New York, NY: HarperCollins

[8] Centers for Disease Control and Prevention. HIPAA privacy rule and public health. Guidance from CDC and the US Department of Health and Human Services. MMWR Morb Mortal Wkly Rep. 2003; 52 Suppl. 1:1–17

[9] Annas GJ. HIPAA regulations—a new era of medical-record privacy? N Engl J Med. 2003; 348(15):1486–1490

[10] Mercuri RT. The HIPAA-potamus in health care data security. Commun ACM. 2004; 47(7):25–28

[11] Benitez K, Malin B. Evaluating re-identification risks with respect to the HIPAA privacy rule. J Am Med Inform Assoc. 2010; 17(2):169–177

[12] Hash J, Bowen P, Johnson A, Smith CD, Steinberg DI. An introductory resource guide for implementing the health insurance portability and accountability act (HIPAA) security rule. Gaithersburg, MD: US Department of Commerce, Technology Administration, National Institute of Standards and Technology; 2005

[13] Kulynych J, Korn D. The new HIPAA (Health Insurance Portability and Accountability Act of 1996) medical privacy rule. Circulation. 2003; 108(8):912–914

[14] Thomas RJ, King M, Lui K, et al. AACVPR, ACC, AHA, American College of Chest Physicians, American College of Sports Medicine, American Physical Therapy Association, Canadian Association of Cardiac Rehabilitation, European Association for Cardiovascular Prevention and Rehabilitation, Inter-American Heart Foundation, National Association of Clinical Nurse Specialists, Preventive Cardiovascular Nurses Association, Society of Thoracic Surgeons. AACVPR/ACC/AHA 2007 performance measures on cardiac rehabilitation for referral to and delivery of cardiac rehabilitation/secondary prevention services: endorsed by the American college of chest physicians, American college of sports medicine, American physical therapy association, Canadian association of cardiac rehabilitation, European association for cardiovascular prevention and rehabilitation, inter-American heart foundation, national association of clinical nurse specialists, preventive.... J Am Coll Cardiol. 2007; 50(14):1400–1433

[15] Choi YB, Capitan KE, Krause JS, Streeper MM. Challenges associated with privacy in health care industry: implementation of HIPAA and the security rules. J Med Syst. 2006; 30(1):57–64

[16] Terry M. Medical identity theft and telemedicine security. Telemed J E Health. 2009; 15(10):928–932

[17] Liu V, Musen MA, Chou T. Data breaches of protected health information in the United States. JAMA. 2015; 313(14):1471–1473

[18] Fetzer DT, West OC. The HIPAA privacy rule and protected health information: implications in research involving DICOM image databases. Acad Radiol. 2008; 15(3):390–395

[19] Buckovich SA, Rippen HE, Rozen MJ. Driving toward guiding principles: a goal for privacy, confidentiality, and security of health information. J Am Med Inform Assoc. 1999; 6(2):122–133

[20] Rotondi JA. Family Medical Leave Act. Regulation. 2007; 30(1):4

[21] Waguespack GM, Cremer K. Family Medical Leave Act. Employment Law. 2008; 18(1):7–11

[22] Waldfogel J. Family and medical leave: evidence from the 2000 surveys. Mon Labor Rev. 2001; 124:17

[23] Grossman JL. Job security without equality: the Family and Medical Leave Act of 1993. Wash. UJL & Pol'y. 2004; 15:17

[24] Hayes EA. Bridging the gap between work and family: Accomplishing the goals of the family and medical leave act of 1993. Wm. & Mary L. Rev.. 2000; 42:1507

[25] Bornstein L. Inclusions and exclusions in work-family policy: the public values and moral code embedded in the Family and Medical Leave Act. Colum. J. Gender & L.. 2000; 10:77

[26] Aalberts RJ, Seidman LH. The Family and Medical Leave Act: does it make unreasonable demands on employers. Marq. L. Rev.. 1996; 80:135

[27] U.S. Department of Labor. Available at: https://www.dol.gov/whd/regs/compliance/whdfs28f.pdf. Accessed August 31, 2017

[28] Larson LK. Employee health—AIDS discrimination. In: Larson on Employment Discrimination. Vol. 10; 2017

[29] Lowder JL, Montoni LM. Americans with Disabilities Act. In: Encyclopedia of Aging and Public Health. New York, NY: Springer; 2008: 115–116

[30] Madorsky JG. Americans with Disabilities Act. JAMA. 1992; 268(15):2031–2031

[31] Acemoglu D, Angrist JD. Consequences of employment protection? The case of the Americans with Disabilities Act. J Polit Econ. 2001; 109(5):915–957

[32] Selmi M. The value of the EEOC: reexamining the agency's role in employment discrimination law. Ohio St. LJ. 1996; 57:1

[33] Act A. (1964). Civil Rights Act of 1964. Title VII. Equal Employment Opportunities

[34] Greenberg JG. The Pregnancy Discrimination Act: legitimating discrimination against pregnant women in the workforce. Me. L. Rev.. 1998; 50:225

[35] Eglit H. The Age Discrimination in Employment Act, Title VII, and the Civil Rights Act of 1991: three acts and a dog that didn't bark. Wayne Law Rev. 1992; 39:1093

[36] Neumark D. The Age Discrimination in Employment Act and the challenge of population aging. Res Aging. 2009; 31(1):41–68

[37] Gitt CE, Gelb M. Beyond the Equal Pay Act: expanding wage differential protection under Title VII. Loy. U. Chi. LJ. 1976; 8:723

[38] Donato KM, Durand J, Massey DS. Stemming the tide? Assessing the deterrent effects of the Immigration Reform and Control Act. Demography. 1992; 29(2):139–157

[39] Carroll SJ, Gillen DI. Are the classical management functions useful in describing managerial work? Acad Manage Rev. 1987; 12(1):38–51

[40] Fair Credit Reporting Act. (2016). Flood Disaster Protection Act and Financial Institute

[41] Scowen P. Patients' rights and responsibilities. The Bulletin of the Royal College of Surgeons of England. 2006; 88(5):152–154

[42] Kerr A. Rights and responsibilities in the new genetics era. Crit Soc Policy. 2003; 23(2):208–226

[43] Joint Commission on Accreditation of Healthcare Organizations; Joint Commission Accreditation Hospital. Comprehensive Accreditation Manual for Hospitals: The Official Handbook: CAMH. Joint Commission Resources; 2016

[44] Ruef M, Scott WR. A multidimensional model of organizational legitimacy: hospital survival in changing institutional environments. Adm Sci Q. 1998; 43:877–904

[45] Banting K, Kymlicka W, eds. Multiculturalism and the Welfare State: Recognition and Redistribution in Contemporary Democracies. Oxford, Oxford University Press; 2006

[46] Annas GJ, Healey JM, Jr. The patient rights advocate: redefining the doctor-patient relationship in the hospital context. Vanderbilt Law Rev. 1974; 27(2):243–269

[47] Zelinsky EA. Against a federal patients' bill of rights. Yale Law Policy Rev. 2003; 21(2):443–472

[48] American Medical Association. Available at: https://www.ama-assn.org/ama-history. Accessed August 29, 2017

[49] Kaestner R. You get what you pay for: consumer choice and employer-sponsored health insurance. Consumer Choice: Social Welfare and Health Policy. 2011; 1:69

[50] Association of American Physicians and Surgeons. Available at: http://aapsonline.org/resources/. Accessed August 29, 2017

[51] O'Neill O. Some limits of informed consent. J Med Ethics. 2003; 29(1):4–7

[52] Faden RR, Beauchamp TL. A History and Theory of Informed Consent. Oxford: Oxford University Press; 1986

[53] Wasti SA, Cortina LM. Coping in context: sociocultural determinants of responses to sexual harassment. J Pers Soc Psychol. 2002; 83(2):394–405

[54] U.S. Equal Employment Opportunity Commission. Available at: https://www.eeoc.gov/laws/types/sexual_harassment.cfm. Accessed August 29, 2017

[55] Fitzgerald LF, Drasgow F, Hulin CL, Gelfand MJ, Magley VJ. Antecedents and consequences of sexual harassment in organizations: a test of an integrated model. J Appl Psychol. 1997; 82(4):578–589

[56] Satiani B. Exceptions to the Stark law: practical considerations for surgeons. Plast Reconstr Surg. 2006; 117(3):1012–1022, discussion 1023

[57] Medicare. Available at: https://www.medicare.gov. Accessed September 1, 2018

[58] IRS. Available at: https://www.irs.gov/compliance/criminal-investigation/examples-of-healthcare-fraud-investigations-fiscal-year-2015. Accessed August 29, 2016

[59] Levin DC, Rao VM, Kaye AD. Why the in-office ancillary services exception to the Stark laws needs to be changed—and why most physicians (not just radiologists) should support that change. J Am Coll Radiol. 2009; 6 (6):390–392

[60] Paulhus ME. The Medicare Anti-Kickback Statute: In Need of Reconstructive Surgery for the Digital Age. Wash. & Lee L. Rev., 59, 677; 2002

[61] Krause JH. Promises to keep: health care providers and the Civil False Claims Act. Cardozo Law Rev. 2001; 23:1363

[62] Kalb PE. Health care fraud and abuse. JAMA. 1999; 282(12):1163–1168

[63] Physical Therapy Claims Study. Available at: http://www.hpso.com/Documents/Risk%20Education/individuals/Physical_Therapy_Claims_Study.pdf. Accessed August 30, 2017

[64] HPSO. Available at: http://www.hpso.com/risk-education/individuals/claims-reports. Accessed August 30, 2017

[65] American Physical Therapy Association. Available at: http://www.apta.org/APTAMedia/Handouts/PT2016/ProfessionalLiabilityExposures_Flynn.pdf. Accessed August 30, 2017

[66] Sandstrom R. Malpractice by physical therapists: descriptive analysis of reports in the National Practitioner Data Bank public use data file, 1991–2004. J Allied Health. 2007; 36(4):201–208

16 The Future of Physical Therapy

Susan Wainwright and Stephen J. Carp

Keywords: Transformation, Vision 2020, technology, data-driven health care, Innovation 2.0, patient-centered care

Chapter Outline

"I am a high school senior in Minneapolis. I am the future of physical therapy.

"For as long as I have been aware, I have been drawn to serving the sick and impaired. My only question was 'in which arena—as in, which type of profession—do I wish to do this?' With the help of my guidance counselor and my parents, I spent many months reading about each helping profession and volunteering alongside various professionals in my local hospital to see and learn what they do on a daily basis. I learned that each profession is unique in its scope of care but each professional is similar in his or her desire to serve and enrich those without. I shadowed a PT named Grace who permitted me to watch her evaluations and interventions on the acute care floor of our local hospital. Within a week I knew I wanted to become a PT. I loved the ability of the therapist to develop a relationship with the patient. I loved the medical complexity of her clientele. I loved the physicality of the job. I loved working with Grace performing what she called systematic reviews (I am still not sure what they are) to improve her care. I saw her use technology (especially apps) to augment her care. I am so proud I was recently accepted to the University of Minnesota as a physiology major. I start in August. My plan is to complete my bachelor's degree and then apply to a PT curriculum. The journey is long but I am strong and motivated.

"Every generation is unique but mine, due to technology, faces even more changes than its predecessors. I am technology and data driven. I have four electronic devices capable of connecting to the internet. I am the first generation raised on computers. They are as natural to me as television and the calculator were to my parents. Technology allows me to connect to mentors all over the world. I have emailed PTs in Canada and New Zealand asking for clarification about articles they have written. I am the first generation who experience the technological classroom changes seen over the past few years: the 'flipped classroom,' clickers, clinical simulation, simulated anatomy dissection, bringing experts into the classroom via electronic media, and using social media not as entertainment but as an educational tool.

"I am also the first generation to learn that technology has its limits. I have seen friends so deep into their devices they have forgotten the 'common touch'—the need to verbally, socially, and physically interact with peers. I am the first generation since Abner Doubleday invented baseball where we do not get off the school bus and grab our bats and gloves and head to the baseball field. Most of my friends run directly to their computers. This is not right.

"My epiphany moment was hearing a local physical therapist talk about the PT profession at a job fair at my school. He reminded us that the core behavior common to all the great therapists is being a reflective servant-leader. And that does not require technology."

—Elliott M., Minneapolis, Minnesota

16.1 Introduction

Historically, major disruptive changes in health care appear in approximately 50-year cycles.[1] In the late 1870s the concept of the germ theory of disease, coupled with sterile technique and advances in surgical and postsurgical care, made life-saving surgeries not only possible but expected. In the early 1920s the paradigm shift from the home to the hospital as the locus for clinical care became widely accepted.[2] This shift, along with the near-simultaneous development of the standardized 4-year medical school curriculum, medical school accreditation, physician licensure, and postgraduate educational requirements, greatly improved clinical outcomes and, tangentially, the public's faith in medicine as a true science.[3] The 1940s and 1950s saw the adoption of the randomized controlled trial (RCT) as the gold standard for the acquisition of evidence and as basis for the initiation of systematic, ongoing, and directed process improvement activities. These two events added immeasurably to advances in the clinical care offered to patients.[4,5] The results of the efforts of a series of U.S. presidents beginning with Theodore Roosevelt to establish national, universal health coverage for all Americans was partially fulfilled in the mid-1960s with the Medicare and Medicaid Acts.[6] (At the time of the publication of this text there appears to be great uncertainty in the United States whether the idea that health coverage is a right or privilege will gain acceptance.) The most recent paradigm shift began in the past decade and continues to gain momentum. This shift is toward the incorporation of emerging technologies into the clinical care of patients, epidemiology, health care administration, training and education, and research. For years health care was the technological laggard of U.S. industry and has only begun, somewhat unwillingly, to enter the digital age.

On a recent service trip to the rural, undeveloped highlands of Guatemala, I was able to enter a bodega and use the automatic teller machine to instantaneously access my checking account balance in my small, home town bank in Pennsylvania. In contrast, if I travelled to Philadelphia—just 30 miles from my home —for a meeting and required emergency health care services, the physician in Philadelphia may need to wait until the next work day for my primary physician's office to open to obtain my medical history. Banks talk to each other; medical records do not—even 30 miles from home.

In many ways, the changes occurring within the practice of physical therapy mirror those of health care in general, with some basic differences. Like physicians, nurses, and other health professions, physical therapists are struggling to incorporate evidence-based care into our evaluative and interventional algorithms.[7] Physical therapists also struggle to obtain appropriate reimbursement for services without bankrupting our clients. All health care workers struggle with assimilating the mountains of outcome data into cogent and useable information that will drive clinical and clerical practices to excellence. And all physical therapists are excited and energized as emerging assistive technologies make such a functional difference in our clients' lives.

Uniquely, physical therapists are unlike other health professionals in that, as members of a relatively novel profession, we struggle to modernize and standardize educational curricula, to convince payers (especially insurers) of the positive impact and absolute necessity of our interventions, and to enlarge and strengthen our scope of care to offset actual and potential inroads from other professional and nonprofessional entities.

The aim of this chapter is to briefly discuss the impact of technology—the current 50-year cycle of change—on health care in general and physical therapy in particular, and to discuss how physical therapy—especially the American Physical Therapy Association—is attempting to drive changes which will advance our profession and our professionals. The authors will also attempt to "crystal ball" the next era of change and its impact on physical therapy.

16.2 The Future of Health Care

16.2.1 Technology

The future of health care is here and its name is technology. Technology affects all aspects: clinical, administrative, research, education, and legislative associated with health care. Recent years have seen the development of scores of diagnostic tools utilizing advanced technologies which have greatly improved the overall accuracy and timeliness of diagnosing. Equally impressive is the use of technology to improve interventions. There are now intravenous pumps with microprocessors which deliver the exact prescribed volumes of medication to the patient (I wonder what the nurses of the 1990s would think of this programmable technology as compared with "the counting of drops" measurement used back then). Radiation accuracy is now precisely directed by microprocessors which eliminate much collateral damage to healthy tissue. Gallbladders and appendixes are removed through a small portal incision. Heart valves are replaced through an artery in the leg. Cancers are being treated using

gene-modifying infusions rather than systemic chemotherapy. Devastating long-term use of corticosteroids is being replaced with immune system-modifying chemicals for the treatment of many autoimmune inflammatory disorders. Newer scans develop three-dimensional representations of internal anatomy with exceptional resolution.

The performance of clinical research and the distribution of research data is enhanced by computing power. Huge quantities of data, heretofore manipulated and statistically evaluated by hand, can now be analyzed in seconds utilizing statistical programs. Research journals once accessed through painstaking medical library searches are now available in seconds from one's home personal computer or electronic device. Technology has greatly impacted the professional training of future health care workers. Computer simulations, videoconferencing, the use of high-frequency manikins and standardized patients, and online training have all added to teaching effectiveness.[8] Global health, recently more of a goal than a process, is now being realized through the improved ability to communicate data between nations and between colleagues worldwide. Recent global outbreaks of Ebola and Zika were mediated not by local action but rather through global action.[9] Even the clerical side of health care—scheduling, billing, hiring, compliance training, payroll, and benefits— is directed through technology.

The enabling technology for this data transformation fell into place over the past two decades with the emergence of massive, ubiquitous, and increasingly inexpensive processing power and the variety and portability of electronic devices capable of performing the processing. The joy and privilege of purchasing one's first personal computer a decade or two ago now seems rather quaint as each of us now possesses numerous connection devices with thousands of times more computing and storage power than similar devices 5 years ago. These trends—coupled with advances in analytic software, mobile technologies, and acquisition device receptors—have made it possible to capture and analyze vast amounts of data about individual patients, populations, and the environments in which they live.

16.2.2 Data-Driven Health Care

Collectively and individually these technological advances have laid the foundation for a core component of the current paradigm shift—data-driven health care. Data-driven health care can be defined as the effective use of vast amounts of data collected in the process of researching and managing the health and wellness of billions of patients worldwide in a continuous effort to improve the quality, access, efficacy, efficiency, outcomes, safety, and cost of care. Data-driven health care drives process change, which drives clinical decision making, which in turn drives outcomes.[10] Improved outcomes are not limited to those from the clinical side. As access to health care has improved over the past decades the issue of provider choice has become a variable which needs to be addressed. Data has improved customer service, safety, access, and responsiveness.

The following is an example of how data can drive customer service. Patients are typically not required to align with a particular primary care practitioner or hospital. Decades ago, when the United States was a predominantly rural country, citizens typically sought care from the "town doctor" and from the "local hospital." This decision was based more on convenience and ease of access rather than outcome variables. With urbanization and improved transportation, the freedom to choose the primary care practitioner and hospital has led to increased attention to customer service practices. An often-used statement in health care is "no margin, no mission," meaning that without a profit or at least a neutral budget of expenses to income, the mission of the organization cannot be accomplished. Health care is a business and a business must have customers to succeed. If not convinced, simply look at the inordinate number media adds on television, radio, and social media for local hospitals. Customer service data is as cherished by primary care practitioners and hospitals as clinical outcome data. Data-driven health care creates the possibility of delivering care that is highly personalized and customer service-oriented to each individual patient. Highly personalized, customer service-oriented care decreases recidivism and improves outcomes and the bottom line.

Data-driven technology can also shift more control and responsibility from the health care team to the largest untapped health care workforce in the country—patients and their families. Home monitoring technology, distance patient and family teaching, and the judicious use of assistive technology can improve health with only indirect and ancillary involvement of the health care team.[11] Unconvinced? Ponder the clinical outcome and cost savings impact of the home glucose monitor.

The RCT will always remain a key element of evidence-based care.[4] However, as we are seeing, the availability of vast amounts of clinical and operational data collected in the process of delivering care also creates an enormous opportunity to advance care via process improvement and epidemiological studies in addition to the historically utilized RCT. In fact, there is a beautiful synergy between the RCT approach and large population process improvement/epidemiological studies.[12] RCTs are a slow and often expensive process that can take years to complete, and there are always concerns about validity due to study controls placed in order to limit the impact of confounding variables and the small number of subjects. RCTs do have three determined advantages over nonrandomized studies for the evaluation of therapeutic procedures:

- In all probability, the randomization inherent in RCTs renders the groups comparable not only in respect to known prognostic factors, but also with regard to heretofore unidentified factors, which may affect the outcome.
- When groups in an RCT with a sufficiently high number of subjects are treated differently, any differences in the event rates can be attributed to the various treatments—provided the data are free of threats to reliability such as selection bias.
- Randomization is also beneficial in terms of statistical analysis. The statistical test of significance is readily interpretable and provides strong evidence to support the researchers' hypothesis.

Though the RCT is an extremely powerful tool at comparing the effectiveness of distinct variables, and there are often questions about how generalizable the findings of an RCT are because of the very small sample populations typically studied and research constraints employed by the researcher. On the other hand, analyzing large amounts of data collected via process improvement and epidemiological studies while delivering care to patients with a specific disease (e.g., diabetes, asthma, congestive heart failure) can help determine the generalizability of RCT findings while also improving outcomes. Furthermore, the effective analysis of large amounts of data obtained in all clinical care environments—including the patient's home—creates the opportunity for health care providers to better understand and manage the environmental and behavioral factors that influence health.[13]

Data-driven health care creates the possibility of turning every arena of health care into a learning environment—an environment in which clinicians operate in a highly supportive and evidence-directed care improvement system. These systems allow optimal patient management while simultaneously collecting ongoing, predetermined data in a variety of environments: home, hospital, outpatient, ambulatory, hospice, and school.

16.3 Unexpected Drivers of the Technology/Data Revolution

When queried about the impact of reimbursement, insurance schemas, the health care regulatory environment, and licensure requirements on daily activity in the clinic, most health care workers will scoff and give a big "thumbs down." At best, many health care workers will consider these variables the unwelcome background noise of clinical practice. At worst, most health care workers believe that these ancillary variables are generally obstructionist in nature, a nuisance to clinical practice, and something that must be endured by clinicians. A few health care workers may admit to some small levels of beneficence from these variables.

The question of beneficence aside, there is no doubt that reimbursement, insurance schemas, the regulatory environment and licensure requirements are currently and will continue to be a driving force in data-driven health care. As with the clinical arena, emerging technology enables the data collection in these ancillary, nonclinical arenas. The current legislative activity in Washington and at the state level about the provision, accessibility, and cost of health care is not only due to the ongoing debate as to whether health care is a right or privilege of Americans but also, and perhaps just as importantly, that the current climate of escalating health care costs is unsustainable. Unless something is done to curb costs, there is a real possibility of the system collapsing.

Nonclinical data collection is now a primary determinant of health policy.[14] Effectiveness data is driving the American Medical Association's yearly review of the Current Procedural Terminology (CPT) reimbursement codes.[15] Those codes lacking evidence of efficacy are being removed and those with evidence of efficacy are being added. Congress is proportioning the reimbursement dollars for the CPT codes (Medicare Fee Schedule) also based on outcome data.[16] The Joint Commission (TJC) and the Commission on Accreditation of Rehabilitation Facilities (CARF)—two of the largest health care accreditation commissions—have become extremely data driven. As an example, TJC's National Patient Safety Goals initiative is derived from ongoing systematic, preplanned review of health care safety data.[17] Not surprisingly, many of the standards required of U.S. health care facilities require mandatory data collection. State licensure standards, also based on data, require continuing educational for each discipline in specific areas deemed important by data. Over the next few years the increasing focus on the quality and cost of care, evolving state and federal regulations, and the growing emphasis on reimbursing for value rather than transactions will most certainly aggressively push the data-driven health care trend forward.

Though in its nascent stages, data-driven health care has had a number of moderate successes. There is universal agreement that the TJC's National Patient Safety Goals have improved safety in the nation's hospitals.[18] Published outcome statistics now provide the health care customer with objective data in order to assist with making cogent decisions related to the choosing of hospitals and specific practitioners for specific procedures and interventions.[19] The availability and reliability of epidemiological data has assisted in controlling worldwide epidemics such as Zika and Ebola and has shown that even a country as advanced and homogeneous as the United States continues to have significant health disparities related to age, location, ethnicity, and ability to pay.[20] Clinical practice guidelines, derived from data, provide clinicians with a framework of evaluation and intervention for a number of diagnoses across many disciplines. Data-driven areas that are lagging include the lack of universality of the electronic medical record, the confusion of medical benefits and the medical bill, the reliance on patient-to-practitioner face-to-face meeting for physiological monitoring and the delivery of health care, and inability for all these data to drive down health care costs.[21]

It is imperative that health care practitioners master the "system skills" that are necessary to meet the demands of this data revolution within our evolving health care system. This transition to systems thinking is novel to physical therapy practice and education, which to this point has focused on the individual patient-practitioner interaction. Atul Gawande identified three necessary system skills of using data to identify problems and then implement and solutions to identified problems.[22] The first system skill is to identify and appreciate nontechnology innovations. For instance, what are the 10 physiological indices that every physical therapist (PT) should check prior to getting a postoperative patient out of bed? This is the skill that was common on the early days of the aviation world, when it was just a basic set of checklists. Once health care learns to appreciate the nontechnological innovations, we must appreciate that the important resource for improving the ability of teams to follow through on those really critical things is data. Information is our most valuable resource, yet we treat it like a byproduct. The technology data systems are improving but are presently not particularly efficient at helping health care teams accomplish outcome objectives. Health care workers have to build systems around those systems. The third insight is that, for the most part, the issues have less to do with systems than with governance. Most health care process flowcharts, if documented separately by administrators and the people who actually carry out the processes, will have little in common. The people who are buying these systems, installing these systems, and determining how they're to be used, do not always understand what the systems are expected to accomplish. The system administrator may be thinking: "wow, this system will help me obtain data to aid in reimbursement" while the employee may be thinking: "this expensive system does not permit me to chart vital signs." Therefore, adjunct systems and workarounds are added to perform the needed work efficiently. What are employee's objectives? What are the administrator's objectives?

We need to figure out how to get quality and outcomes higher on the list of priorities of everybody running health systems.

In the 43rd McMillan Lecture, Dr. Alan Jette urged us as physical therapists to recognize the importance of developing and attending to these systems skills.[23] He expounded on these skills, advising physical therapists to become interested in data —developing data collection systems, actually collecting the data, analyzing data, and translating the data into clinical practice. Emphasizing data would allow physical therapists to identify solutions for system problems, and then implement these solutions at a meaningful scale along the health care delivery continuum.

16.4 The Future of Physical Therapy

As an integral part of the U.S. health care system, any facilitators, inhibitors, paradigm shifts, or algorithmic changes impacting the U.S. health care system will immediately impact physical therapy. The vision statement for the physical therapy profession—"transforming society by optimizing movement to improve the human experience"—was approved at the American Physical Therapy Association (APTA) House of Delegates in 2013.[24] Eight guiding principles that support this vision statement serve as the framework to inform actions of the APTA that shape the future of the profession. These principles are identity, quality, collaboration, value, innovation, consumer centricity, access/equity, and advocacy (see ► Table 16.1). A vision statement is an organization's road map indicating what the company wants to become and guiding initiatives by defining direction for the company's growth. In 2016, the APTA developed and approved a strategic plan to achieve its vision. ► Fig. 16.1 details the three elements of this strategic plan.

This vision statement and guiding documents communicate to all members of the profession (as well as to the numerous stakeholders with whom we interact) the direction of the APTA, and ultimately physical therapist practice. The strategic plan of the APTA includes three primary objectives:

1. Transform society: Barriers to movement will be reduced at population, community, workplace, home and individual levels.
2. Transform the profession: Physical therapists will deliver value by utilizing evidence, best practice, and outcomes.
3. Transform the association: APTA will be a relevant organization that is entrepreneurial, employing disciplined agility to achieve its priorities.

16.4.1 Transform Society

Inherent in the profession's commitment to this objective is an implied social contract that is the responsibility of physical therapists as professionals.[25] The importance of this social contract in the physical therapy profession was elucidated by Swisher and Page.[26] They identified the elements that defined physical therapy as a profession as "a body of theoretical knowledge, some degree of professional autonomy, an ethic that the members enforce, and accountability to society." The importance of our social contract with society is evident in its inclusion in the first of the three primary aims of the strategic plan.

Table 16.1 Guiding principles of the vision statement for the physical therapy profession

Identity	The physical therapy profession will define and promote the movement system as the foundation for optimizing movement to improve the health of society. Recognition and validation of the movement system is essential to understand the structure, function, and potential of the human body. The physical therapist will be responsible for evaluating and managing an individual's movement system across the lifespan to promote optimal development; diagnose impairments, activity limitations, and participation restrictions; and provide interventions targeted at preventing or ameliorating activity limitations and participation restrictions. The movement system is the core of physical therapist practice, education, and research
Quality	The physical therapy profession will commit to establishing and adopting best practice standards across the domains of practice, education, and research as the individuals in these domains strive to be flexible, prepared, and responsive in a dynamic and ever-changing world. As independent practitioners, doctors of physical therapy in clinical practice will embrace best practice standards in examination, diagnosis/classification, intervention, and outcome measurement. These physical therapists will generate, validate, and disseminate evidence and quality indicators, espousing payment for outcomes and patient/client satisfaction, striving to prevent adverse events related to patient care, and demonstrating continuing competence. Educators will seek to propagate the highest standards of teaching and learning, supporting collaboration and innovation throughout academia. Researchers will collaborate with clinicians to expand available evidence and translate it into practice, conduct comparative effectiveness research, standardize outcome measurement, and participate in interprofessional research teams
Collaboration	The physical therapy profession will demonstrate the value of collaboration with other health care providers, consumers, community organizations, and other disciplines to solve the health-related challenges that society faces. In clinical practice, doctors of physical therapy, who collaborate across the continuum of care, will ensure that services are coordinated, of value, and consumer centered by referring, comanaging, engaging consultants, and directing and supervising care. Education models will value and foster interprofessional approaches to best meet consumer and population needs and instill team values in physical therapists and physical therapist assistants. Interprofessional research approaches will ensure that evidence translates to practice and is consumer centered
Value	Value has been defined as "the health outcomes achieved per dollar spent." To ensure the best value, services that the physical therapy profession will provide will be safe, effective, patient/client centered, timely, efficient, and equitable. Outcomes will be both meaningful to patients/clients and cost-effective. Value will be demonstrated and achieved in all settings in which physical therapist services are delivered. Accountability will be a core characteristic of the profession and will be essential to demonstrating value
Innovation	The physical therapy profession will offer creative and proactive solutions to enhance health services delivery and to increase the value of physical therapy to society. Innovation will occur in many settings and dimensions, including health care delivery models, practice patterns, education, research, and the development of patient/client-centered procedures and devices and new technology applications. In clinical practice, collaboration with developers, engineers, and social entrepreneurs will capitalize on the technological savvy of the consumer and extend the reach of the physical therapist beyond traditional patient/client–therapist settings. Innovation in education will enhance interprofessional learning, address workforce needs, respond to declining higher education funding, and, anticipating the changing way adults learn, foster new educational models and delivery methods. In research, innovation will advance knowledge about the profession, apply new knowledge in such areas as genetics and engineering, and lead to new possibilities related to movement and function. New models of research and enhanced approaches to the translation of evidence will more expediently put these discoveries and other new information into the hands and minds of clinicians and educators
Consumer centricity	Patient/client/consumer values and goals will be central to all efforts in which the physical therapy profession will engage. The physical therapy profession embraces cultural competence as a necessary skill to ensure best practice in providing physical therapist services by responding to individual and cultural considerations, needs, and values
Access/Equity	The physical therapy profession will recognize health inequities and disparities and work to ameliorate them through innovative models of service delivery, advocacy, attention to the influence of the social determinants of health on the consumer, collaboration with community entities to expand the benefit provided by physical therapy, serving as a point of entry to the health care system, and direct outreach to consumers to educate and increase awareness
Advocacy	The physical therapy profession will advocate for patients/clients/consumers both as individuals and as a population, in practice, education, and research settings to manage and promote change, adopt best practice standards and approaches, and ensure that systems are built to be consumer centered

Source: http://www.apta.org/.

Full commitment to this social contract means that as professional we develop moral agency, which is the capacity to act in a moral manner to effect change.[27] As moral agents, physical therapists make clinical and ethical decisions in collaboration with patients and health care team members, and within the framework of health institutions and guiding policies. Recent revision of our physical therapy code of ethics has recognized the importance of addressing health inequities and social injustice. Literature indicates that there is a "disconnect" between societal obligations and aspirations expressed in the revised codes, and the actions and perspectives within clinical practice.[28] Such disconnect should motivate each physical therapist to explore how they embody this in practice. As members of a profession we have a responsibility to take action in a moral manner.

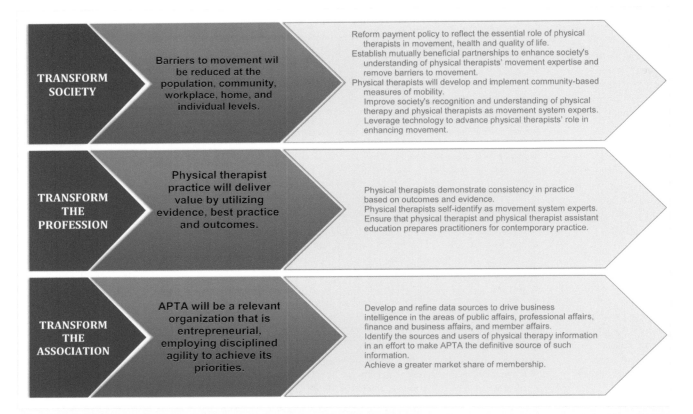

Fig. 16.1 2016 American Physical Therapy Association strategic plan.

16.4.2 Transform the Profession

The second aim of the strategic plan focuses on the profession, inclusive of education and practice. Trends in preparation of physical therapists for practice include entry-level as well as postprofessional practice.

The evolution of physical therapy practice has driven rapid and expansive changes in physical therapy education. The most visible transition has been to the doctor of physical therapy (DPT) as the entry-level degree. Students in physical therapy entry-level education programs complete part-time integrated and full-time clinical education experiences to meet program requirements for the DPT degree. Use of low- and high-fidelity simulations and standardized patients has become relatively commonplace in physical therapy education. Through these experiential learning experiences students demonstrate acquisition of knowledge, skills and behavior consistent with entry-level practice. DPT graduates enter practice on securing licensure through successful completion of the national physical therapy examination. The evolving and complex health care environment challenges physical therapists to engage in ongoing learning to meet the clinical, regulatory demands and regulatory constraints of the practice environment.

And as with all professions, education does not stop on completion of entry-level education. The APTA espouses a commitment to excellence and lifelong learning as one of our core values. A growing trend in physical therapy practice is to pursue residency and/or fellowship education. A relatively recent development in postprofessional education has been the proliferation of residency and fellowship programs. Postprofessional clinical residencies are designed to advance the skills and knowledge in patient/client management within a defined body of clinical knowledge. At present, there are 242 clinical residencies in the following practice areas: cardiovascular and pulmonary, clinical electrophysiology, geriatrics, neurologic, orthopedic, pediatrics, sports and women's health. The minimum requirements of residency programs include a minimum of 1,500 hours and in no fewer than 9 months and no more than 36 months.[28,29] Recently a nonclinical residency focused on development of the knowledge and skills consistent with DPT faculty has received accreditation.[28]

The purpose of clinical fellowship programs is to advance physical therapy practice in one of the following areas of subspecialty: critical care, hand therapy, higher education leadership, movement system, neonatology, orthopedic manual physical therapy, spine, sports division I, and upper extremity athlete.[29] The minimum expectations for fellowship requires that they encompass a minimum of 1,000 hours and be completed in no fewer than 6 months and no more than 36 months. Postprofessional fellowship programs include advanced study beyond residency and the description of specialty practice. Physical therapists eligible for fellowship have either completed a residency program in a related specialty area, hold board certification in the related area of specialty, or have demonstrable clinical skills within a particular specialty area.

While postprofessional residency is relatively new in our profession, there has been study exploring the outcomes of residency training on the professional development and leadership activities of those completing residency. Self-report comparison between residency and nonresidency trained orthopedic physical therapists indicated that residency graduates were more likely to participate in postgraduate fellowship programs, achieve board certifications in a physical therapy specialty, serve as a clinical instructor for PT students, participate in professional or postprofessional PT educational, and serve as a clinical faculty member in a PT residency or PT fellowship program when compared to nongraduates of residency programs.[30]

Traditionally residency and fellowship education have been exclusively developed to address development of clinical skills and knowledge in a specialty area. As indicated earlier, there is one nonclinical fellowship, the Educational Leadership Institute (ELI), and one nonclinical residency program. These nonclinical training programs focus on advancing the knowledge and skills of a physical therapist's career outside of their clinical practice. The ELI fellowship focuses on developing forward thinking and innovative academic leaders.[31]

Aspiring and novice PT and physical therapist assistant (PTA) educators are the target audience for this fellowship. The nonclinical faculty residency strives to develop and mentor licensed physical therapists who wish to pursue careers in academic physical therapy. Both residency and fellowship programs incorporate didactic content, competency expectations, within the subspecialty of study.

Since 2007 there has been a proliferation of both residency and fellowship postprofessional programs (see ▶ Fig. 16.2). Postprofessional residency and fellowship programs are accredited by the American Board of Physical Therapy Residency and Fellowship Education.[32,33] Currently the demand for postprofessional residency and fellowship placements exceeds the number of available slots.[33,34,35] Practitioners choosing to pursue postprofessional clinical residency do so with the goal of sitting for and securing clinical specialization. On completion of a clinical residency, you can apply to sit for the specialty examination administered by the American Board of Physical Therapy Specialties.[29] Practitioners who do not complete residency are also eligible to sit for specialty examination on completion of criteria set by each specialty council. Clinical specialization recognizes the advanced knowledge, skills, and experience of physical therapy practitioners. This credential is explicit affirmation that

a physical therapist will use to market their services to patient as well as referral courses.

There has been study of the outcomes of clinical residency and fellowship on physical therapist practice. Comparison of the clinical outcomes in patients with musculoskeletal diagnoses and efficiency of care delivery was studied across three groups of physical therapists: those who had not completed residency or fellowship training, had completed a residency program, or completed a fellowship program.[36,37] Statistical analysis of measures revealed that the fellowship-trained group of physical therapists achieved functional status changes and efficiency that were greater than those of the other groups. Residency training did not appear to contribute to improved patient functional status change or efficiency on the measures analyzed. The authors were not able to determine if these statistically significant results reflect meaningful clinical outcomes.

Continuing postprofessional training is just one way of advancing physical therapy practice. The APTA has also concentrated efforts on advancing practice by developing innovative care delivery models. There are have been numerous initiative sponsored by the APPTA to advance the professional and practice. A few of these are highlighted here.

- Physical Therapy and Society Summit (PASS). *Imagination. Inspiration. Innovation.* That's what the PASS, a first-of-its-kind event for APTA and the physical therapy profession held in February 2009, was all about. *Vitalizing Practice Through Research and Research Through Practice*—This conference asked its participants "to develop recommendations, to be published in PTJ, which would allow for creation of an environment in a number of different practice settings that would enable researchers to conduct translational research and clinicians to provide patient care based on the results of that research" in the hopes of enhancing patient care.[38]

- In 2013, the APTA sponsored the first *innovation summit*: Collaborative care models to bring together physical therapists, physicians, large health systems, and policy makers. Experts and innovators came together to discuss the role that the physical therapy profession can and should have across the health care continuum.[39] Presenters provided examples of best practice in physical therapy that is meeting the Tripe Aim—reducing cost, improving access and maximizing patient outcomes. This summit served as the platform to support development and study of emerging physical therapy care delivery.

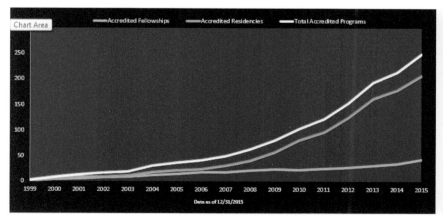

Fig. 16.2 Growth chart of residency and fellowship (www.apta.org). The number of accredited postprofessional education programs has grown over the past decade. Still, there remains concern about meeting the needs of the graduates of the growing number of entry-level programs.

- Innovation 2.0: It was launched by the APTA in 2014 to support and refine innovative physical therapy care delivery models including accountable care organizations, bundled payment, direct access, pay for performance, patient-centered medical homes, prevention and health promotion, and value-based purchasing.[40] Four models were selected and implemented. In 2016, the results of these inaugural delivery models were disseminated through Learning Labs. The Learning Lab was developed to provide resources for practitioners seeking to develop models within their own health care delivery systems.
- More recently, at the CoHSTAR (Center on Health Services Training and Research) 2017 Summer Institute, discussion of developing research focused on implementation science to demonstrate the value, efficacy and appropriate allocation of findings from innovation and discovery research. Engaging in research along this continuum of innovation and implementation will contribute in a meaningful way to demonstrate the value of physical therapy.

16.4.3 Transform the Association

It is not uncommon for students to be required by their academic program to join the APTA. As students and early career members entering the profession, the association offers many benefits to you as an individual. These benefits include resources to the best evidence and practice, publications and news, opportunities to get involved in the APTA, financial aid and insurance benefits, and employment resources.[41] Educational materials in the Learning Center, access to the research in *PTNow*, and the *Guide to Physical Therapist Practice* are often incorporated into entry-level education.

Licensed PTs can access the Learning Center to pursue continuing education units (CEUs). Continuing education courses are offered at reduced cost or in some cases no cost to APTA members. The member costs for reduced registration fees to APTA sponsored meetings such as the annual Combined Sections Meeting and NEXT meetings. Courses offered through the APTA's Learning Center and Conference meet CUE requirements to maintain/review your physical therapy license.

An important goal of the APTA's strategic plan is to increase overall membership. There is an early member plan for membership dues, offering reduced cost of membership for those renewing the first year out of school. In addition, discounted membership continues for PTs who are engaged in residency or fellowship training, or academic graduate education. It is concerning that 100% of students and early career members do not take advantage of these member benefits. Sustaining membership is the easiest way to engage in the profession and reap all of the benefits of membership.

16.5 Direct Access to Physical Therapy Services

One of the tenets of Vision 2020 was that physical therapists would become providers of choice. Consumers would be able to directly access physical therapists who would determine "… diagnosis of, interventions for, and prevention of impairments, activity limitations, participation restrictions, and environmental barriers related to movement, function, and health."[42] Lobbying efforts to secure direct access allowing patients to seek evaluation and intervention from a licensed physical therapist without referral from a physician have achieved just that in all 50 states.[43] The scope of direct access and the restrictions placed on physical therapists practice varies by state. Efforts continue to educate legislators, third-party providers, members of other health professions, and consumers. The goals are to amend existing state laws and regulations that place arbitrary and unnecessary limitations on direct access to physical therapy services.

One way that the professional is demonstrating the value of physical therapy as direct access providers is through lobbying efforts, public education efforts, and health services delivery research. Direct access to physical therapy services demonstrates value through improved access to care while containing health care costs through effective patient management of individuals with neuromusculoskeletal conditions. Through the education and training that physical therapists receive, they are qualified and have the expertise to determine if and what physical therapy services are indicated or if referral to another heath care provider is indicated. The APTA has fostered and supported research in this vein through their Innovation 2.0 program.[44] One of the four supported projects from Innovation 2.0 is evaluating the role and effectiveness of early access to physical therapy for individuals with low back pain. In this study, physical therapists are participants in a Medicare shared saving program who are frontline providers with the goal of delivering evidence-based care to maximize patient outcomes for those with low back pain.[45]

This study is but one example of physical therapists practicing at the peak level of licensure to achieve autonomy. Physical therapists achieve this level of autonomy when they provide care to consumers through direct access. As we embrace this level of autonomy we can meet the explicit obligations we have to secure society's trust in our profession. It is important to recognize that we are independent decision makers, but we do not practice isolation. Rather, as autonomous practitioners we are interdependent with members of a patient-centered health care team.[46]

16.6 Patient-Centered Care

As health care has evolved with an eye toward achieving optimal patient outcomes, team-based care has set the standard in practice to achieve this. This trend toward interprofessional practice assumes that health care providers will come together practicing at a top of their licensure. Team-based care is characteristic of interprofessional practice. This type of care delivery requires skills of us as practitioners. The four Cs of team-based care include collaboration, credibility, compassion, and coordination.[47] These skills are the building blocks of the four core competencies of interprofessional practice: values/ethics for interprofessional practice, roles/responsibilities of different health professions, interprofessional communication, and teams and teamwork.[48]

Thus, the evolution of practice is driving physical therapist education. This team-based model of care requires physical therapist to learn to assume the numerous roles and develop more than hands on clinical skills.

16.7 Practice Arena

What does the future hold for physical therapists currently entering practice? The education for students in professional DPT programs is shaped by practice—both current practice and preparation for the practice of the future. As health care delivery transitions out of inpatient setting to community-based care, physical therapists are assuming broader roles in determining what care is delivered, how the care is delivered, and to whom the care is delivered. Changes in the health care system offer extraordinary opportunity and unique challenges for the contemporary practice of physical therapy. This broadening scope of practice includes attention to prevention of injury and wellness care. The APTA proposes clients have annual movement screenings just as they have annual physical and dental examinations. Within the health care team along the continuum of care, we as physical therapists are the movement system experts. Recognizing the autonomy of each member of the health care team, physical therapists are poised to lead the team alternately with other team members to most effectively meet the patient's needs.

16.8 Prevention, Wellness, and Disease Management

Many of the population health crises that we face today are chronic health conditions. Research in the management of chronic conditions such obesity, diabetes, and cardiac disease (to name just a few) demonstrates the benefits of lifestyle changes that include physical activity. There has been increasing awareness in the health care community and general population about the importance of the prevention of disease and injury, wellness, and disease management. Physical therapists are uniquely positioned to provide services to individuals with such chronic health conditions to improve overall health, well-being, fitness and quality of life. Engaging in physical activity and physical fitness can minimize or slow decline in physical function as well as minimize risk for development of impartments and functional limitations that impact participation. The APTA has developed a variety of initiatives to educate the public, the health care community, policy makers, and their party providers about the role of physical therapists in prevention and wellness. Preventive care is primary, secondary, and tertiary dependent on which stage of health versus disease that a physical therapist encounters a client.

The APTA launched a primary prevention initiative, encouraging individuals to have an annual checkup with a physical therapist.[49] The goal of this evaluation is to determine overall health status and identify potential health risks. Through the screening process, physical therapists can determine not only potential issues, but make referrals to other health care professionals for identified issues requiring attention beyond the scope of our practice. Such annual examinations provide patients with an opportunity to ensure their overall health and wellness to fully participate in their daily activities. Physical therapists who provide this service develop a portfolio of services along the continuum of wellness and prevention service to delivery of care to ameliorate injury. Doing so serves to expand the potential client base beyond an episode of care (injury-related) to ongoing wellness and prevention consultation and services. For many practitioners this model of care provides an alternative revenue stream outside of traditional third-party payment.

Patients' chronic health conditions often receive physical therapy intervention at the time of onset or in response to an acute flare-up of a condition. On completion of these services patients can be challenged to maintain and/or enhance their wellness. Recognizing the important role of physical therapy in secondary prevention minimizes the potential for injury or illness through physical activity. Community patients should be encouraged to engage in physical fitness activity that meets their physical and psychological needs, sparks their interest, and is accessible to the patient. Numerous physical fitness activities have been developed for individuals managing progressive diseases (such as Parkinson's disease).[50] The APTA provides numerous resources for physical fitness programs for individuals with progressive and nonprogressive chronic health conditions. Community-based adaptive sports programs are available and growing in number.

A large part of physical therapist practice is on tertiary prevention, minimizing the impact of a chronic condition, ongoing illness or injury that has lasting effects. Physical therapists work with patients to help them manage (often) complex health problems and injuries that result in impairments and disability. The goal is to improve as much as possible their ability to function and participate as members of society, and subsequently improve their quality of life. One health issue facing many older adults, particularly those with one or more chronic health conditions, is falls. Morbidity and mortality rates from unintentional falls in adults over 65 years of age have increased steadily for the past 10 years. The direct medical costs related to the consequences of fall (fracture, head injury) is estimated to be $31 billion annually.[51] Physical therapists' expertise in the neuromuscular and musculoskeletal systems can decrease risk of fall through care that addresses impairments and guidelines for environmental modification as appropriate.

One community health initiative that has gained momentum over the past several years is National Falls Prevention Awareness Day, which occurs on the first day of fall in September. Physical therapists, and many academic programs, provide screening to community members to identify those at risk for falls and education about how to minimize risks for falls. Referral for services with a physical therapist or other health care provider may be identified in such a screening process. Community initiatives such as this may ultimately address prevention across the continuum to meet a health care issue.

16.9 Movement Systems

As movement system specialists, we are uniquely poised to meet the needs of patient through the evaluations, assessments, screenings, and interventions that we provide to patients. Our interventions can effect improvement at both the micro and macro levels.

16.10 Evolving Perspectives on Practice: Genetics

In the 48th Mary McMillan Lecture, Richard Shields, PT, PhD, FAPTA, stated that as physical therapists we "reset the aging clock of the human body" through the interventions we apply to our patients. Dr. Shields indicates that physical therapy interventions "are powerful regulators of genes that activate the energy systems." And while the beneficial effects of movement and exercise have been recognized as essential components of health, wellness, and quality of life at a macro level, these micro effects are equally potent to individual's health and well-being.[52]

Frequent movement, then, promotes the expression of healthy genes and represses the expression of genes that can damage tissues. And while the effect is to slow biological aging in cells and tissue, the benefits are not for only the already aged; they can be applied across the lifespan. Shields said that although PTs and PTAs "most often think about strength, endurance, coordination, and function, the cellular changes that we trigger are the most fundamental ways that we improve the health and well-being of humankind." These effects of exercise can reduce the rate at which cells and tissues age.

It is novel for us as practitioners to think of the exercises that we prescribe as changing the molecular functioning of cells. Contraction of skeletal muscle produces proteins into the bloodstream that subsequently regulate genes. Pathologic conditions and disease can block the function of health genes. Exercise and muscle activity facilitates health-promoting genes to be active and repeated activity and movement creates "molecular memory."

Just as we have prescribed physical therapy at a macro level to include length and duration of a treatment session, as well as specific interventions to be performed, our clinical reasoning should incorporate the micro level factors as well. Physical therapists can apply their knowledge and expertise about the movement system to promote molecular memory. This molecular memory is achieved through prescription of optimal dosages of exercise to effect the micro changes at the cellular level that are evidenced in clinical practice as reduction in neuromusculoskeletal impairments, improved function and engaged participation.

Blending what we know about the human genome and the evolving precision in collecting individualized data will foster the identification of the most effective doses of movement for each patient, based on biological genetic regulators, environmental factors, and lifestyle influences that affect frequency, duration, and types of treatment prescribed. In summary, Dr. Shields predicts that "precision physical therapy will emerge side-by-side with precision medicine."

16.11 Review Questions

1. Historically, major disruptive changes occur in health care approximately every how many years?
   a) 10 years.
   b) 20 years.
   c) 30 years.
   d) 50 years.
2. The sentinel health care change which occurred in the 1960s is which of the following?
   a) Introduction of penicillin.
   b) Use of sterile technique.
   c) The Medicare and Medicaid Act.
   d) Introduction of magnetic resonance imaging scanning.
3. Most health care researchers feel that the future of health care is summed up in which word?
   a) Technology.
   b) Antibiotics.

   c) Universal health.
   d) Customer service.
4. The use of data to evaluate health care processes has led to changes in which aspect of health care?
   a) Clinical.
   b) Customer service.
   c) Safety.
   d) All of the above.
5. The current vision statement for the physical therapy profession is which of the following?
   a) All for one and one for all.
   b) The patient comes first.
   c) Transforming society by optimizing movement to improve the human experience.
   d) Wellness and prevention: forever!
6. Which specialty does not currently have an associated American Physical Therapy Association-sponsored residency program?
   a) Geriatrics.
   b) Clinical electrophysiology.
   c) Palliative care.
   d) Neurology.
7. Direct access, a hallmark of Vision 2020, permits access to physical therapy service without which item?
   a) Referral.
   b) Insurance.
   c) Functional deficit.
   d) Laboratory data.
8. Tertiary prevention is concerned with which of the following?
   a) Fall-risk modification.
   b) Care of the patient with diabetes.
   c) Minimizing the impact of a chronic medical condition.
   d) Maximizing aerobic endurance.
9. The primary care prevention associated with physical therapy is best described by which statement?
   a) Clients should visit their physical therapist yearly for an evaluation.
   b) Physical therapists encouraging clients to take their medication as prescribed.
   c) Advocacy toward legislators to encourage fair reimbursement for physical therapy services.
   d) Methods to prevent physical therapists and physical therapist assistants from being injured on the job.
10. The National Patient Safety Goals, a data driven program to reduce health care errors and to improve patient, employee, and public safety, is associated with which agency?
    a) Commission on Accreditation of Rehabilitation Facilities.
    b) American Physical Therapy Association.
    c) Joint Commission.
    d) American Bar Association.

16.12 Review Answers

1. Historically, major disruptive changes occur in health care approximately every how many years?
   d. 50 years.
2. The sentinel health care change which occurred in the 1960s is which of the following?
   c. The Medicare and Medicaid Act.

3. Most health care researchers feel that the future of health care is summed up in which word?
   a. Technology.

4. The use of data to evaluate health care processes has led to changes in which aspect of health care?
   d. All of the above.

5. The current vision statement for the physical therapy profession is which of the following?
   c. Transforming society by optimizing movement to improve the human experience.

6. Which specialty does not currently have an associated American Physical Therapy Association-sponsored residency program?
   c. Palliative care.

7. Direct access, a hallmark of Vision 2020, permits access to physical therapy service without which item?
   a. Referral.

8. Tertiary prevention is concerned with which of the following?
   c. Minimizing the impact of a chronic medical condition.

9. The primary care prevention associated with physical therapy is best described by which statement?
   a. Clients should visit their physical therapist yearly for an evaluation.

10. The National Patient Safety Goals, a data driven program to reduce health care errors and to improve patient, employee, and public safety, is associated with which agency?
    c. Joint Commission.

References

[1] Carroll JS, Rudolph JW. Design of high reliability organizations in health care. Qual Saf Health Care. 2006; 15 Suppl 1:i4–i9

[2] Rosenberg CE. The care of strangers: The rise of America's hospital system. New York, NY: Basic Books; 1987

[3] Mueller PS, Stone MJ, Olsen TW, Horton MEK. History of Medicine. Philadelphia, PA: The Blakiston Company; 1947

[4] Carey RG, Lloyd RC. Measuring Quality Improvement in Healthcare: A Guide to Statistical Process Control Applications. New York, NY: ASQ Quality Press; 1995

[5] Solberg LI, Mosser G, McDonald S. The three faces of performance measurement: improvement, accountability, and research. Jt Comm J Qual Improv. 1997; 23(3):135–147

[6] Zarabozo C. Milestones in Medicare managed care. Health Care Financ Rev. 2000; 22(1):61–67

[7] Jette DU, Bacon K, Batty C, et al. Evidence-based practice: beliefs, attitudes, knowledge, and behaviors of physical therapists. Phys Ther. 2003; 83(9):786–805

[8] Rose DH, Meyer A. Teaching Every Student in the Digital Age: Universal Design for Learning. Alexandria, VA: Association for Supervision and Curriculum Development; 2002: 22311–1714

[9] Ferguson NM, Cucunubá ZM, Dorigatti I, et al. Epidemiology. Countering the Zika epidemic in Latin America. Science. 2016; 353(6297):353–354

[10] Zeger SL, Liang KY. Longitudinal data analysis for discrete and continuous outcomes. Biometrics. 1986; 42(1):121–130

[11] Stankovic JA, Cao Q, Doan T, et al. Wireless sensor networks for in-home healthcare: Potential and challenges. In: High Confidence Medical Device Software and Systems (HCMDSS) Workshop. Philadelphia, PA: Navigator Publishing; 2005

[12] Minkman M, Ahaus K, Huijsman R. Performance improvement based on integrated quality management models: what evidence do we have? A systematic literature review. Int J Qual Health Care. 2007; 19(2):90–104

[13] Humpel N, Owen N, Leslie E. Environmental factors associated with adults' participation in physical activity: a review. Am J Prev Med. 2002; 22(3):188–199

[14] Pope C, Ziebland S, Mays N. Qualitative research in health care. Analysing qualitative data. BMJ. 2000; 320(7227):114–116

[15] Thorwarth WT, Jr. From concept to CPT code to compensation: how the payment system works. J Am Coll Radiol. 2004; 1(1):48–53

[16] Centers for Medicare & Medicaid Services (CMS), HHS. Medicare program; revisions to payment policies under the Physician Fee Schedule, Clinical Laboratory Fee Schedule, access to identifiable data for the Center for Medicare and Medicaid Innovation Models & other revisions to Part B for CY 2015. Final rule with comment period. Fed Regist. 2014; 79(219):67547–68010

[17] Chang A, Schyve PM, Croteau RJ, O'Leary DS, Loeb JM. The JCAHO patient safety event taxonomy: a standardized terminology and classification schema for near misses and adverse events. Int J Qual Health Care. 2005; 17(2):95–105

[18] Leape LL, Berwick DM. Five years after To Err Is Human: what have we learned? JAMA. 2005; 293(19):2384–2390

[19] Galvin RS, Delbanco S, Milstein A, Belden G. Has the leapfrog group had an impact on the health care market? Health Aff (Millwood). 2005; 24(1):228–233

[20] Adler NE, Rehkopf DH. U.S. disparities in health: descriptions, causes, and mechanisms. Annu Rev Public Health. 2008; 29:235–252

[21] Koh HC, Tan G. Data mining applications in healthcare. J Healthc Inf Manag. 2005; 19(2):64–72

[22] Jette AM. 43rd Mary McMillan Lecture. Face into the storm. Phys Ther. 2012; 92(9):1221–1229

[23] Gawande A. Cowboys and Pit Crews. The New Yorker, May 26, 2011. Available at: http://www.newyorker.com/news/news-desk/cowboys-and-pit-crews. Accessed August 13, 2017

[24] American Physical Therapy Association. Vision Statement for the Physical Therapy Profession and Guiding Principles to Achieve the Vision. 2013. Available at: https://www.apta.org/Vision. Accessed August 14, 2017

[25] Hordichuk CJ, Robinson AJ, Sullivan TM. Conceptualising professionalism in occupational therapy through a Western lens. Aust Occup Ther J. 2015; 62 (3):150–159

[26] Swisher LL, Page CG. Professionalism in Physical Therapy: History, Practice and Development. St. Louis, MO: Elsevier Saunders; 2005

[27] Delany CM, Edwards I, Jensen GM, Skinner E. Closing the gap between ethics knowledge and practice through active engagement: an applied model of physical therapy ethics. Phys Ther. 2010; 90(7):1068–1078

[28] Edwards I, Delany CM, Townsend AF, Swisher LL. Moral agency as enacted justice: a clinical and ethical decision-making framework for responding to health inequities and social injustice. Phys Ther. 2011; 91(11):1653–1663

[29] American Physical Therapy Association. About Residency Programs. Available at: http://www.abptrfe.org/ResidencyPrograms/About/. Accessed August 14, 2017

[30] American Physical Therapy Association. Duke University Doctor of Physical Therapy Division Faculty Residency. Available at: http://www.abptrfe.org/APTA/ABPTRFE/ListingReport.aspx?id=0×01000000625e6e7b5f27f35b83e036ae269b68cff39905ba4cc3a0d5&type=Residency. Accessed August 14, 2017

[31] American Physical Therapy Association. About Fellowship Programs. Available at: http://www.abptrfe.org/FellowshipPrograms/Overview/. Accessed August 14, 2017

[32] Jones S, Bellah C, Godges JJ. A comparison of professional development and leadership activities between graduates and non-graduates of physical therapist clinical residency programs. J Phys Ther Educ. 2008; 22(3):85–88

[33] American Physical Therapy Association. Educational Leadership Institute (ELI) Fellowship. Available at: http://www.apta.org/eli/. Accessed August 14, 2017

[34] American Physical Therapy Association. What We Do. Available at: http://www.abptrfe.org/WhatWeDo/. Accessed August 14, 2017

[35] Kulig K. Residencies in physical therapy. Phys Ther. 2013; 94(1):151–161

[36] Furze JA, Tichenor CJ, Fisher BE, Jensen GM, Rapport MJ. Physical therapy residency and fellowship education: Reflections on the past, present, and future. Phys Ther. 2016; 96(7):949–960

[37] Rodeghero J, Wang YC, Flynn T, Cleland JA, Wainner RS, Whitman JM. The impact of physical therapy residency or fellowship education on clinical outcomes for patients with musculoskeletal conditions. J Orthop Sports Phys Ther. 2015; 45(2):86–96

[38] American Physical Therapy Association. Physical Therapy and Society Summit (PASS). Available at: http://www.apta.org/pass/. PASS Summit. Accessed August 14, 2017

[39] American Physical Therapy Association. Innovation Summit: Objectives. Available at: http://www.apta.org/InnovationSummit/Objectives/. Accessed August 14, 2017

[40] American Physical Therapy Association. Innovation 2.0. Available at: http://www.apta.org/Innovation2/. Accessed August 14, 2017

[41] American Physical Therapy Association. Membership and Benefits. Available at: http://www.apta.org/Membership/. Accessed August 14, 2017

[42] American Physical Therapy Association. Vision 2020. Available at: http://www.apta.org/Vision2020/. Accessed August 14, 2017

[43] American Physical Therapy Association. Direct Access in Practice. Available at: http://www.apta.org/DirectAccess/. Accessed August 14, 2017

[44] American Physical Therapy Association. Facilitating Access, Improving Care: Physical Therapists are Integral ACO Members. Innovation 2.0 Flynn. Available at: https://www.apta.org/Innovation2/FacilitatingAccessImprovingCare/. Accessed August 14, 2017

[45] Johnson MP, Abrams SL. Historical perspectives of autonomy within the medical profession: considerations for 21st century physical therapy practice. J Orthop Sports Phys Ther. 2005; 35(10):628–636

[46] Apker J, Propp KM, Zabava Ford WS, Hofmeister N. Collaboration, credibility, compassion, and coordination: professional nurse communication skill sets in health care team interactions. J Prof Nurs. 2006; 22(3):180–189

[47] Interprofessional Education Collaborative. Core Competencies for Interprofessional Collaborative Practice. Available at: https://nebula.wsimg.com/2f68a39520b03336b41038c370497473?AccessKeyId=DC06780E69ED19E2B3A5&disposition=0&alloworigin=1. Accessed August 14, 2017

[48] American Physical Therapy Association. Annual Checkup by a Physical Therapist. Available at: http://www.apta.org/AnnualCheckup/. Accessed August 14, 2017

[49] Centers for Disease Control and Prevention. Important Facts About Falls. Available at: https://www.cdc.gov/homeandrecreationalsafety/falls/adultfalls.html. Accessed August 14, 2017

[50] Ebersbach G, Ebersbach A, Edler D, et al. Comparing exercise in Parkinson's disease—the Berlin LSVT®BIG study. Mov Disord. 2010; 25(12):1902–1908

[51] Stevens JA, Corso PS, Finkelstein EA, Miller TR. The costs of fatal and non-fatal falls among older adults. Inj Prev. 2006; 12(5):290–295

[52] YouTube. Available at: https://www.youtube.com/watch?v=ihu517N7bVE. Accessed August 16, 2017

Glossary

Academic program: That aspect of the curriculum where students' learning occurs directly as a function of being immersed in the academic institution of higher education. The academic program is the didactic component of the curriculum that is managed and controlled by the physical therapy educational program and the college/university hierarchy. The academic program may occur in a traditional classroom setting or hybrid (combined traditional classroom and online).

Accountability: Active acceptance of responsibility for the many roles, obligations, opportunities, and actions of the physical therapist including self-regulation, advocacy, life-long learning and other behaviors that positively influence patient/client outcomes, the profession, and the health needs of society.

Acute Medical Rehabilitation: A hospital, or part of a hospital, that provides an intensive rehabilitation program to inpatients.

Administration: The skilled process of controlling, planning, directing, organizing, and managing human, technical, environmental, regulatory, and financial resources effectively and efficiently.

Administrative law: Administrative law is the body of law that governs the activities of administrative agencies of a government. Government agency action can include rulemaking, adjudication, or the enforcement of a specific regulatory agenda.

Advanced Beneficiary Notice: An Advanced Beneficiary Notice (ABN) is a written notice from Medicare (standard government form CMS-R-131), given to a patient prior to receiving certain items or services. The ABN provides formal notification from the provider that Medicare may deny payment for that specific procedure or treatment. The patient will be personally responsible for full payment if Medicare denies payment.

Advocacy: Advocacy is public support for or recommendation of a particular cause or policy. Advocacy is an important responsibility of physical therapists and physical therapist assistants.

Affective: Relating to the expression of emotion and feeling.

Affordable Care Act: The Affordable Care Act provides Americans with better health security by putting in place comprehensive health insurance reforms that expands coverage, holds health insurance accountable, lowers costs, guarantees more choices, and enhance the quality of life of Americans through improved health. The Affordable Care Act actually refers to two separate pieces of legislation—the Patient Protection and Affordable Care Act (P.L. 111-148) and the Health Care and Education Reconciliation Act of 2010 (P.L. 111-152)—that together expand Medicaid coverage to millions of low-income Americans and makes numerous improvements to both Medicaid and the Children's Health Insurance Program.

Altruism: The primary regard for or devotion to the interest of others. From the physical therapy perspective includes direct and indirect patient care, advocacy, community service, and volunteerism.

American Physical Therapy Association Clinical Site Information Form: The purpose of the APTA Clinical Site Information Form (CSIF) is for physical therapist and physical therapist assistant education programs to collect information from clinical education sites to facilitate clinical site selection and student placements, assess the learning experiences and practice opportunities available to students, and provide assistance with documentation relevant for accreditation.

American Physical Therapy Association: The American Physical Therapy Association is the official member organization of the profession of physical therapy in the United States.

Americans with Disabilities Act (ADA): The 1990 federal statute that prohibits discrimination against individuals with disability in employment and public accommodations.

Autonomous practitioner model: Refers to the ability to act according to one's knowledge and judgment, providing care within the full scope of practice as defined by existing professional, regulatory, and organizational rules.

Behaviorism: Behaviorism (also called behavioral psychology) refers to a psychological approach which emphasizes scientific and objective methods of investigation. The approach is only concerned with observable stimulus-response behaviors, and states all behaviors are learned through interaction with the environment.

Bundled payment: Bundled payment, also known as episode-based payment, episode payment, episode-of-care payment, case rate, evidence-based case rate, global bundled payment, global payment, package pricing, or packaged pricing, is defined as the reimbursement of health care providers (such as hospitals and physical therapists) on the basis of expected costs for clinically-defined episodes of care. It has been described as "a middle ground" between fee-for-service reimbursement and capitation, given that risk is shared between payer and provider.

Capitation: Capitation is a payment arrangement for health care service providers such as physicians or physical therapists. It pays providers a set amount for each enrolled person assigned to them, per period of time, whether or not that person seeks care (called the per-member-per-month fee). These providers generally are contracted with a type of health maintenance organization. The amount of remuneration is based on the average expected health care utilization of that patient, occasionally with greater payment for patients with significant medical history.

Caring: The consistent concern, empathy, and consideration for the needs and values of others.

Center Coordinator of Clinical Education (CCCE): Individual(s), employed by the clinical site, who administer, manage, and coordinate clinical instructor assignments and learning activities for students during their clinical education experiences. In addition, this person determines the readiness of persons to serve as clinical instructors for students, supervises clinical instructors in the delivery of clinical education experiences, communicates with the academic program (DCE) regarding student performance, and provides essential information about the clinical education program to physical therapy programs.

Claim: A request for payment that the patient submits to Medicare or other health insurance when the patient receives items and services that the patient believes are covered.

Clients: Individuals who are not necessarily sick or injured but can benefit from a physical therapist's consultation, professional expertise, or services. Clients may be individuals, businesses, school systems, families, caregivers, member of the public, and others who benefit from physical therapy services.

Clinical decision making: Clinical decision making is a balance of experience, awareness, knowledge and information gathering, using appropriate assessment tools, colleagues and evidence-based practice to guide making clinical decisions. Good, effective clinical decision making requires a combination of experience, knowledge of the research, and clinical skills.

Clinical education agreement: A legal contract that is negotiated between the entry-level academic institution and clinical education site that specifies each party's roles, responsibilities, and liabilities relating to student clinical education.

Clinical education consortium: A regional group that typically includes representatives (typically the DCE) from physical therapy and physical therapy assistant programs for the purpose of sharing resources, ideas, and efforts.

Clinical education experience: That aspect of the curriculum where the students' learning occurs directly as a function of being immersed within physical therapy practice. These dynamic and progressive experiences comprise all of the direct and indirect formal and practical "real life" learning experiences provided for students to apply classroom knowledge, skills, and behaviors in the clinical environment. These experiences can be of short or long duration (e.g., part-time and full-time experiences, internships that are most often full-time post-graduation experiences for a period of 1 year) and can vary by the manner in which the learning experiences are provided (e.g., rotations on different units that vary within the same setting, rotations between different practice settings within the same health care system). These experiences include comprehensive care of patients across the life span and related activities. (Synonym: Clinical learning experiences).

Clinical education program: Refers to programs, apart from the didactic curriculum, that provide professionals-in-training with practical and skills-oriented instruction under the supervision of a skilled practitioner.

Clinical education site: The physical therapy practice environment where clinical education occurs; that aspect of the clinical education experience that is managed and delivered exclusively within the physical therapy practice environment and encompasses the entire clinical facility.

Clinical expertise: Clinical expertise refers to the clinician's cumulated experience, education and clinical skills.

Clinical instructor (CI): An individual at the clinical education site, who directly instructs and supervises students during their clinical learning experiences. These individuals are responsible for carrying out clinical learning experiences and assessing students' performance in cognitive, psychomotor, and affective domains as related to entry-level clinical practice and academic and clinical performance expectations. (Synonyms: clinical teacher; clinical tutor; clinical supervisor).

Clinical Performance Instrument (CPI): American Physical Therapy Association-developed student evaluation instrument that is used to assess the clinical education performance of physical therapist and physical therapist assistant students. The Physical Therapist CPI consists of 24 performance criteria and the Physical Therapist Assistant CPI consists of 20 performance criteria.

Clinical practice guidelines: Guidelines that include recommendations, intended to optimize patient care, that are informed by a systematic review of evidence and an assessment of the benefits and harms of alternative care options.

Clinical reasoning: The process by which physical therapists collect cues, process information, come to an understanding of a patient problem or situation, plan and implement interventions, evaluate outcomes, and reflect on and learn from the process.

Clinical research question: A focused research question leads to a systematic planning of a research project such as an experimental design study or a systematic review.

Clinical site: The location, often away from the location of the didactic curriculum, where the clinical education curriculum is house.

Code of Ethics for the Physical Therapist: The Code of Ethics for the Physical Therapist (Code of Ethics) delineates the ethical obligations of all physical therapists as determined by the House of Delegates of the American Physical Therapy Association.

Coding: The process of assigning a code to something for the purposes of classification or identification. In healthcare this is the process of assigning a diagnostic code to the insurance bill.

Cognitive: Characterized by knowledge, awareness, reasoning, and judgment.

Coinsurance: An amount which the patient may be required to pay as a share of the cost for services after paying any deductibles. Coinsurance is usually a percentage (for example, 20%).

Commission in Accreditation of Physical Therapy Education: The Commission on Accreditation in Physical Therapy Education (CAPTE) is the only accreditation agency recognized by the United States Department of Education (USDE) and the Council for Higher Education Accreditation (CHEA) to accredit entry-level physical therapist and physical therapist assistant education programs.

Commission on Accreditation in Physical Therapy Education: The Commission on Accreditation in Physical Therapy Education (CAPTE) is an accrediting agency that is nationally recognized by the US Department of Education and the Council for Higher Education Accreditation. CAPTE grants specialized accreditation status to qualified entry-level education programs for physical therapists and physical therapist assistants.

Common law: Common law is the part of English law that is derived from custom and judicial precedent rather than statutes.

Communication: A verbal or nonverbal exchange between two or more individuals or groups that is: open and honest; accurate and complete; timely and ongoing; and occurs between physical therapists and physical therapist assistants, as well as between patients, family or caregivers, health care providers, and the health care delivery system.

Community service: Voluntary work intended to help a person or a cohort of persons performed within an altruistic framework.

Compassion: The desire to identify with or sense something of another's experience. Compassion is a precursor of caring.

Competencies: A set of standard criteria, determined by experts and defined by practice setting and scope, by which one is objectively evaluated.

Competent: Demonstrates skill and proficiency in a fluid and coordinated manner in rendering physical therapy care (physical therapist), or those aspects of physical therapy care (e.g., interventions) as directed and supervised by the physical therapist (physical therapist assistant).

Comprehension: The action or capability of understanding.

Constitutional law: Refers to rights carved out in the federal and state constitutions. The majority of this body of law has developed from state and federal Supreme Court rulings, which interpret their respective constitutions and ensure that the laws passed by the legislature do not violate constitutional limits.

Convergent versus divergent thinking styles: Convergent thinking is about learning facts, following instructions, and solving problems with one right answer. Divergent thinking is generating unique solutions and seeing various possibilities in response to questions and problems.

Copayment: An amount the patient may be required to pay as share of the cost for a medical service or supply, like a doctor's visit, hospital outpatient visit, or prescription drug. A copayment is usually a set amount, rather than a percentage. For example, the patient may pay $10 or $20 for a doctor's visit or prescription drug.

Critically appraised topic: A critically appraised topic (or CAT) is a short summary of evidence on a topic of interest, usually focused around a clinical question. A CAT is a shorter and less rigorous version of a systematic review.

Cultural and individual differences: The acknowledgment of and response to, age, gender, race, creed, national and ethnic origin, sexual orientation, marital status, health status, disability or limitations, socioeconomic status, and language.

Cultural competence: Cultural competence is a set of congruent behaviors, beliefs, attitudes and policies that come together in a system that enables effective work in cross-cultural situations. Competence implies having the capacity to function effectively as an individual and an organization within the context of the cultural beliefs, behaviors, and needs presented by consumers and their communities.

Cultural humility: Cultural humility is the ability to maintain an interpersonal stance that is other-oriented in relation to aspects of cultural identity that are most important to the person.

Culture: Refers to integrated patterns of human behavior that include the language, thoughts, communications, actions, customs, beliefs, values, and institutions of racial, ethnic, religious, or social groups.

Current Procedural Terminology: Current Procedural Terminology (CPT) is a medical code set that is used to report medical, surgical, and diagnostic procedures and services to entities such as health insurance companies and accreditation organizations.

Custodial Care: Non-skilled personal care, such as assistance with activities of daily living like bathing, dressing, eating, getting in or out of a bed or chair, moving around, and using the bathroom. It may also include the kind of health-related care that most people do themselves, like using eye drops. In most cases, medical insurances do not pay for custodial care.

Data collection: The process of gathering and measuring information on variables of interest, in an established systematic fashion that enables one to answer stated research questions, test hypotheses evaluate outcomes, and draw conclusions.

Database: A structured set of data, typically housed electronically, especially one that is accessible in various ways.

Deductible: The amount the patient must pay for health care or prescriptions before Original Medicare, the prescription drug plan, or your other insurance begins to pay.

Dental insurance: Dental insurance is an insurance coverage for individuals to protect against planned and unplanned dental costs. It insures against the expense of treatment and care of dental disease and accident to teeth. Often provided as a benefit of employment.

Department of Health and Human Services: The federal agency that oversees the Centers for Medicare and Medicaid Services, which administers programs for protecting the health of all Americans, including Medicare, the Marketplace, Medicaid, and the Children's Health Insurance Program (CHIP).

Diagnosis: Diagnosis is both a process and a label. The diagnostic process performed by the physical therapist includes integrating and evaluating data that are suggested by clinical scripts and obtained during the examination to describe the patient/client condition in terms that will guide the prognosis, the plan of care, and intervention strategies. Physical therapists and other healthcare personnel use diagnostic labels that identify the impact of a condition on function at the level of the system. Unique to physical therapists is the diagnostic labeling based upon the movement system.

Diagnostic labels: Traditionally, diagnostic labels focused on the pathology/pathophysiology to describe the diseased state of an individual. These labels typically identify disease or condition at the level of the cell, tissue, organ, or system (health condition). The most extensive listing of such diagnostic labels can be found in the *International Classification* of *Diseases*.

Diagnostic process: The diagnostic process includes collection and categorization of data, establishment of hypotheses, testing of each hypothesis by systematically ruling out alternatives, and confirmation or refutation of each hypothesis.

Differential diagnoses: A list of two or more conditions that share similar signs and symptoms.

Differential diagnosis: The process of differentiating between two or more conditions that share similar signs or symptoms.

Direct access: Direct access means the removal of the physician referral mandated by state law to access physical therapists' services for evaluation and treatment. Every state, the District of Columbia, and the US Virgin Islands allow for evaluation and some form of treatment without physician referral.

Director of Clinical Education (DCE): An individual who is responsible for managing and coordinating the clinical education program at the academic institution, including facilitating development of the clinical education sites and clinical educators. The DCE is also responsible for coordinating student placements, communicating with clinical educators about the academic program and student performance, and maintaining current information on clinical education sites. In some instances the DCE may be referred to as the Academic Coordinator for Clinical Education (ACCE).

Disability insurance: A program managed by the Social Security Administration that insures a worker in case of a mishap. Disability insurance offers income protection to individuals who become disabled for a long period of time, and as a result can no longer work during that time period.

Discharge summary: The summary note, often copied to the referring physician, written at the termination of an episode of care.

Doctor of Physical Therapy degree: Doctor of Physical Therapy (DPT) degree is a post-baccalaureate degree that takes 2-3+ years to complete. As of 2017, all accredited and developing physical therapist programs are DPT programs.

Doctor of Physical Therapy: A Doctor of Physical Therapy (DPT) is a graduate of an accredited Doctor of Physical Therapy program and is considered a clinical doctor who is educated in the science of physical therapy.

Domains of learning: The domains of learning can be categorized as cognitive domain (knowledge), psychomotor domain (skills) and affective domain (attitudes). This categorization is best explained by the Taxonomy of Learning Domains formulated by a group of researchers led by Benjamin Bloom in 1956.

Durable medical equipment: Certain medical equipment, such as a walker, wheelchair, or hospital bed, that is ordered by a healthcare practitioner for use by the patient.

Eight-minute rule: The eight-minute rule governs the process by which rehabilitation therapists determine how many units of treatment should be billed to Medicare for the outpatient therapy services they provide on a particular date of service. A therapist must provide direct, one-on-one therapy for at least eight minutes to receive reimbursement for a time-based treatment code.

Electronic health record: The electronic health record (EHR) is a digital version of the patient's comprehensive medical history. Information can be created and managed by authorized providers in a digital format capable of being shared with other providers across more than one health care organization. EHRs are built to share information with other health care providers and organizations—such as laboratories, specialists, medical imaging facilities, pharmacies, emergency facilities, and school and workplace clinics—so they contain information from all clinicians involved in a patient's care.

Electronic medical record: The electronic medical record (EMR) is a digital version of the medical record documenting activity from one practitioner or, when used by many health care practitioners, from one episode of care.

Empathy: The ability to understand and share the feelings of others.

Employment law: Employment law is a broad area encompassing all areas of the employer/employee relationship except the negotiation process covered by labor law and collective bargaining.

Entry-level program: The program which prepares a physical therapist or physical therapist assistant for the profession of physical therapist or physical therapist assistant. Once successfully completed and all requirements met, the student may sit for the national board examination.

Equal Pay Act: The Equal Pay Act of 1963 is a United States labor law amending the Fair Labor Standards Act, aimed at abolishing wage disparity based on sex. It was signed into law on June 10, 1963, by John F. Kennedy.

Ethical and legal behaviors: Those behaviors that result from a deliberate decision-making process that adheres to an established set of standards for conduct that are derived from values that have been mutually agreed on and adopted for that group.

Evaluation: A dynamic process in which the physical therapist makes clinical judgments based on data gathered during the examination.

Evidence-based practice: Evidence-based practice is the integration of clinical expertise with the best available external clinical evidence from systematic research into the decision-making process for patient care.

Examination: A comprehensive and specific testing process performed by a physical therapist that leads to diagnostic classification or, as appropriate, to a referral to another practitioner. The examination has three components: the patient/client history, the systems reviews, and tests and measures. Specific tests and measures are used to add items to the differential diagnosis list, remove items from the differential diagnosis list, or to confirm a differential diagnosis.

Excellence: Excellence is physical therapy practice that consistently uses current knowledge, evidence, and theory while understanding personal limits, integrates judgment and the patient/client perspective, partners with other experts when needed, embraces advancement, challenges mediocrity, and works toward the development of new knowledge.

Exempt or non-exempt employee: According to the Fair Labor Standards Act (FLSA), which governs most jobs, employees are either "exempt" (hourly) or "nonexempt" (salary). Nonexempt employees are typically paid by the hour and are entitled to overtime pay it they work more than 40 hours per week. Exempt employees, on the other hand, do not get overtime pay.

Family and Medical Leave Act: The Family and Medical Leave Act of 1993 (FMLA) is a United States labor law requiring covered employers to provide employees with job-protected and unpaid leave for qualified medical and family reasons.

Federation of State Boards of Physical Therapy: The mission of the Federation of State Boards of Physical Therapy (FSBPTE) is to protect the public by providing service and leadership that promote safe and competent physical therapy practice. The FSBPTE has six focus areas: examinations, membership, states' rights and responsibilities and professional standards, education, leadership, and organization and financial stability.

Fellowship: A community of interest, activity, feeling, or experience.

First professional position: The first paid position following graduation from the entry-level professional program and successfully completing the Physical Therapy Board Examination.

Flipped classroom: An instructional strategy and a type of blended learning that reverses the traditional learning environment by delivering instructional content, often online, outside of the classroom. Activities, including those that may have traditionally been considered homework, are moved into the classroom.

Good Samaritan law: Good Samaritan laws generally provide basic legal protection for those who assist a person who is injured or in danger. In essence, these laws protect the "Good Samaritan" from liability if unintended consequences result from their assistance.

Health benefits: The health care items or services covered under a health insurance plan. Covered benefits and excluded services are defined in the health insurance plan's coverage documents.

Health care provider: A person or organization that is licensed to give health care. Doctors, physical therapists, physical therapist assistants, nurses, and hospitals are examples of health care providers.

Health insurance marketplace: A service that helps people shop for and enroll in affordable health insurance. The federal government operates the marketplace, available at HealthCare.gov, for most states. Some states run their own marketplaces.

Health Insurance Portability and Accountability Act (HIPAA): The "Standard for Privacy of Individually Identifiable Health

Information" (also called the "Privacy Rule") of HIPAA assures health information is properly protected while allowing the flow of health information needed to provide and promote high quality health care and to protect the public's health and well-being.

Health insurance: Health insurance is a type of insurance coverage that pays for medical and surgical expenses incurred by the insured. Health insurance can reimburse the insured for expenses incurred from illness or injury, or pay the care provider directly.

Health Maintenance Organization Act: The Health Maintenance Organization (HMO) Act of 1973, informally known as the federal HMO Act, is a federal law that provides for a trial federal program to promote and encourage the development of HMOs. The federal HMO Act amended the Public Health Service Act, which Congress passed in 1944.The Act facilitated the development of a class of insurance known as Health Maintenance Organizations.

Health maintenance organization: A type of health insurance plan that usually limits coverage to care from doctors who work for or contract with the health maintenance organization (HMO). HMOs generally will not cover out-of-network care except in an emergency. An HMO may require the subscriber to live or work in its service area to be eligible for coverage. HMOs often provide integrated care and focus on prevention and wellness.

Home health care: Health care services and supplies a doctor decides is necessary to receive in the home under a plan of care established by the doctor. Medicare only covers home health care on a limited basis as ordered by the doctor.

Homebound: From a healthcare viewpoint homebound indicates that the patient hasn't the functional ability to leave the home save for an emergent situation or medical appointment. Classified as "homebound" permits the patient to access additional healthcare benefits such as physical therapy in the home.

Hospice: A special way of caring for people who are terminally ill. Hospice care involves a team-oriented approach that addresses the medical, physical, social, emotional, and spiritual needs of the patient. Hospice also provides support to the patient's family or caregiver.

Immigration Reform and Control Act: The Immigration Reform and Control Act was passed and signed into law on November 6, 1986. The purpose of this legislation was to amend, revise, and reform/re-assess the status of unauthorized immigrants set forth in the Immigration and Nationality Act.

Informed consent: Informed consent is permission granted in the knowledge of the possible consequences, typically that which is given by a patient to a healthcare practitioner for treatment with full knowledge of the possible risks and benefits.

Inpatient prospective payment system: Hospitals that have contracted with Medicare to provide acute inpatient care and accept a predetermined rate as determined by the admitting diagnosis as payment in full.

In-service: Professional content presentation, typically performed by an expert, to facilitate continuous improvement in clinical, administrative, or behavioral performance.

Integrated clinical experience: The integrated clinical experience (ICE) is a series of courses during the didactic portion of the curriculum in which students work with clients in a healthcare arena. The ICE is separate from clinical education. ICEs are typically part-time and provide early exposure to authentic clients in a healthcare arena. Students, under the supervision of a licensed therapist, are asked to perform clinical examination techniques and interventions parallel to the didactic curriculum.

Integrity: Steadfast adherence to high ethical principles or professional standards.

International Classification of Diseases: The International Classification of Diseases (ICD) is the international standard diagnostic tool for epidemiology, health management, and clinical purposes. Its full official name is International Statistical Classification of Diseases and Related Health Problems. Maintained by the World Health Organization, the ICD is designed as a healthcare classification system, providing a common language for classifying diseases.

Interprofessional education: Interprofessional education (IPE) is an important pedagogical approach for preparing health professions students to provide patient care in a collaborative team environment. The appealing premise of IPE is that once health care professionals begin to work together in a collaborative manner, patient care will improve.

Intervention: The purposeful and skilled interaction of the physical therapist with the patient/client and, when appropriate, with other individuals involved in care (i.e., physical therapist assistant), using various methods and techniques to produce change.

Interview: An interview is a formal meeting in which one or more persons question, consult, or evaluate another person.

Journal club: A method of continuing education in which persons with a common clinical background formally review current literature.

Leadership: Leadership is having a vision and sharing it with others, having the ability to motivate, being a server, possessing empathy, having good managerial and organizational skills, being able to communicate effectively, taking risks and fostering an environment of continuous improvement, and being thorough.

Learning theories: Learning theories are conceptual frameworks describing how knowledge is absorbed, processed, and retained during the learning process. Cognitive, emotional, and environmental influences, as well as prior experience, all play a part in how understanding is acquired, influenced, or changed and knowledge and skills retained.

Legibility: The quality of being sufficiently clear to permit reading.

Letter of medical necessity: A letter to the insurance provider requesting payment of a medical service or item. The letter describes the medical necessity, cost, alternatives, and time frames associated with the service or item. Letters of medical necessity, especially when related to durable medical equipment, adaptive equipment, or assistive equipment, are often written by the attending physical therapist.

Liability: Liability insurance is an insurance policy that protects an individual or business from the risk that they may be sued and held legally liable for something such as malpractice, injury or negligence. Intentional damage and contractual liabilities are typically not covered by these policies.

Licensure: Licensure is the granting or regulation of licenses, as for professionals.

Life insurance: A type of insurance that pays out a sum of money either on the death of the insured person or after a set period.

Long-term care: A continuum of fee-for-service living arrangements ranging from independent living to assisted living to nursing home care that may include variety of non-medical services provided to people who are unable to independently perform basic activities of daily living, like dressing or bathing.

Long-term care insurance: A type of insurance which covers the fee-for-service expenses associated with long-term care.

Malpractice insurance: Medical professional liability insurance, sometimes known as medical malpractice insurance, is one type of professional liability insurance which protects physicians and other licensed health care professionals (e.g., physical therapists and physical therapist assistants) from liability associated with wrongful practices resulting in bodily injury, medical expenses and property damage, as well as the cost of defending lawsuits related to such claims. A medical professional liability insurance policy covers bodily injury or property damage as well as liability for personal injury such as mental anguish.

Managed care: Managed care is a healthcare system in which patients agree to visit only certain doctors and hospitals, and in which the cost of treatment is monitored by a managing company. The general philosophy of managed care is the loss of flexibility in choosing providers in return for lower costs.

Medicaid: Medicaid in the United States is a social health care program for families and individuals with limited financial resources. Medicaid is a government-sponsored insurance program for persons of all ages whose income and resources are insufficient to pay for health care.

Medically necessary care: Health care services or supplies needed to diagnose or treat an illness, injury, condition, disease, or its symptoms and that meet accepted standards of medicine.

Medicare Advantage Plan: A synonym for Medicare C.

Medicare Fee Schedule: A fee schedule is a complete listing of fees used by Medicare to pay doctors or other providers/suppliers. This comprehensive listing of fee maximums is used to reimburse a physician and/or other providers on a fee-for-service basis. CMS develops fee schedules for physical therapists, physicians, ambulance services, clinical laboratory services, and durable medical equipment, prosthetics, orthotics, and supplies. Many other insurance carriers utilize a form of the Medicare fee schedule to reimburse providers.

Medicare Part A: Also known as hospital insurance. Part A covers inpatient hospital stays, care in a skilled nursing facility, care in an acute medical rehabilitation facility, hospice care, and some home health care.

Medicare Part B: Also known as outpatient insurance. Part B covers certain doctors' services, outpatient care (including physical therapy), medical supplies, and some preventive services.

Medicare Part C: Upon entering the coverage age for Medicare, patients may choose the traditional plan (Medicare Part A and Part B) or Medicare Part C. Medicare Part C is known as Medicare Advantage Plan. Medicare Part C is a type of Medicare health plan offered by a private company that contracts with Medicare to provide the patient with all Part A and Part B benefits. Medicare Advantage Plans include health maintenance organizations, preferred provider organizations, private fee-for-service plans, special needs plans, and Medicare Medical Savings Account Plans. Most Medicare Advantage Plans offer prescription drug coverage.

Medicare Part D: Also known as prescription drug coverage. Part D adds prescription drug coverage to traditional Medicare, some Medicare Cost Plans, some Medicare Private-Fee-for-Service Plans, and Medicare Medical Savings Account Plans. These plans are offered by insurance companies and other private companies approved by Medicare.

Medicare Summary Notice: A notice the patient receives after the doctor, other health care provider, or supplier files a claim for Part A or Part B services in Original Medicare. It explains what the doctor, other health care provider, or supplier billed for, the Medicare-approved amount, how much Medicare paid, and what the patient must pay.

Medicare: Medicare is a single-payer, national social insurance program, administered by the U.S. federal government since 1966, currently using about 30–50 private insurance companies across the United States under contract for administration. Medicare is funded by a payroll tax, premiums and surtaxes from beneficiaries, and general revenue. It provides health insurance for Americans aged 65 and older who have worked and paid into the system through the payroll tax. It also provides health insurance to younger people with some disabilities status as determined by the Social Security Administration, as well as younger people with end stage renal disease and amyotrophic lateral sclerosis. Benefits are typically defined under the subsets of Medicare Parts A, B, C, and D.

Medigap insurance: Medigap is the common term used for Medicare Supplement Insurance. Medical Supplemental Insurance is sold by private insurance companies to fill "gaps" in Original Medicare coverage.

Mentorship: Mentorship is the guidance provided by a mentor—especially an experienced person—in a company or educational institution. Mentorship may also be provided by former teachers, previous colleagues, and trusted friends. Mentorship can be formal or informal.

Mission statement: A formal summary of the aims and values of a department, company, organization, or individual.

Modifiers: Along with the Current Procedural Terminology code, a service or procedure can be further described by using 2-digit modifiers. The Modifier Reference Guide lists Level I (CPT-4), Level II (non-CPT-4 alpha numeric), and Level III (local) modifiers. Level I and II modifier definitions are contained in the Healthcare Common Procedure Coding System (HCPCS).

National health insurance: National health insurance (NHI) —sometimes called statutory health insurance (SHI)—is legally enforced health insurance that insures a national population against the costs of health care. It may be administered by the public sector, the private sector, or a combination of both. Funding mechanisms vary with the particular program and country.

Nihilism: Nihilism is the rejection of all religious and moral principles, often in the belief that life is meaningless.

One on one versus group therapy: The Current Procedural Terminology lists specific codes for physical therapists to utilize when treating patients one on one and in a group. Medicare publishes comprehensive guides to assist the therapist in determining if the therapy provided is one on one or in a group.

Order: A physician (and, depending on the jurisdiction, a dentist, nurse practitioner, physician assistant, or physician assistant) provides an order for service. The order typically contains a diagnosis and recommendations for intervention. In some jurisdictions, qualified physical therapists do not require an order prior to evaluating and treating specific outpatient conditions.

Organizational culture: Organizational culture is a system of shared assumptions, values, and beliefs, which governs how people behave in organizations. These shared values have a strong influence on the people in the organization and dictate how they dress, act, and perform their jobs.

Organizational structure: Organizational structure is a system that consists of explicit and implicit institutional rules and policies designed to outline how various work roles and responsibilities are delegated, controlled and coordinated. Organizational structure also determines how information flows from level to level within the company.

Orientation: Orientation is the process of inculturation to an organization. Orientation typically includes a review of policies and procedures, learning about the history of the organization, a review of the job description, a tour of the physical plant, introductions to key employees, and the completion of specific job-specific compliances. The orientation "period" is classically 90 days.

Patient values: Patient values are the beliefs, expectations, needs, and pre-existing expectations that the patient brings to a specific episode of care. Incorporating the patient values into the care plan includes listening to, informing and involving patients in their care. The patient values are an instrumental part of patient-centered care.

Patient/client management model: An element of physical therapist patient care that leads to optimal outcomes through examination, evaluation, diagnosis, prognosis, and intervention. Includes the development of the patient-therapist collaborative alliance, discovery through mutual inquiry, co-setting of goals, and agreement on the intervention plan.

Patient-centered care: Patient-centered care is the provision of care that is respectful of, and responsive to, individual patient preferences, needs and values, and ensuring that patient values are included in all clinical decision making.

Patients: Individuals who are the recipients of physical therapy direct intervention.

Patient-therapist collaborative alliance: As part of the patient/client management model, the collaborative alliance describes the partnership with patient to facilitate a trusting relationship, mutually inquiry, mutual goal setting, and agreement of intervention.

Performance improvement: Performance improvement (PI) (also known as continuous quality improvement) originated from the theory of Edward Deming. PI is the belief that all organizational processes require period formal periodic review and only through improving policies can an organization improve the quality of product delivered.

Per-member-per-month fee: Per-member-per-month fee is the reimbursement model for many capitation agreements under the health maintenance organization umbrella. The provider of services is reimbursed a specific dollar amount per month for reach patient assigned to a particular primary care physician whether or not the patient receives skilled services.

Philosophy: Broad context and theoretical framework provided for a program purpose, organization, structure, goals, and objectives. Typically an elaboration of the mission statement.

Physical therapist assistant: A person who is a graduate of an accredited physical therapist assistant program and who assists the physical therapist in the provision of physical therapy. The physical therapist assistant may perform physical therapy procedures and related tasks that have been selected and delegated by the supervising physical therapist.

Physical therapist professional entry education: First level of education that prepares student to enter the practice of physical therapy.

Physical therapist: Physical therapists (PTs) are highly educated graduates of an accredited physical therapy program, licensed health care professionals who can help patients reduce pain and improve or restore mobility—in many cases without expensive surgery and often reducing the need for long-term use of prescription medications and their side effects.

Physical Therapy Clinical Performance Instrument: An assessment tool, developed by the American Physical Therapy Association, that is used to assess the clinical education performance of entry-level doctor of physical therapy students.

Physical therapy personnel: This includes all persons who are associated with the provision of physical therapy services, including physical therapists, physical therapist assistants who work under the direction and supervision of a physical therapist, and other support personnel such as aides, clerks, billers, and coders.

Physical therapy: Therapy for the preservation, enhancement, or restoration of movement and physical function impaired or threatened by disease, injury, or disability that utilizes therapeutic exercise, physical modalities, assistive and adaptive devices and technology, and patient education and training.

Piaget's Theory of Cognitive Development: Jean Piaget's theory of cognitive development suggests that children move through four different stages of mental development. His theory focuses not only on understanding how children acquire knowledge, but also on understanding the nature of intelligence. He believed that children took at active role in the learning process, acting much like little scientists as they perform experiments, make observations, and learn about the world. As kids interact with the world around them, they continually add new knowledge, build upon existing knowledge, and adapt previously held ideas to accommodate new information. Piaget proposed four stages of cognitive development: the sensorimotor, preoperational, concrete operational, and formal operational period.

PICO: PICO (alternately known as PICOT) is a mnemonic used to describe the four elements of a good clinical question. It stands for: **P**—Patient/Problem; **I**—Intervention; **C**—Comparison; **O**—Outcome.

Plan of care: Statements that specify the anticipated goals and the expected outcomes, predicted level of optimal improvement, specific interventions to be used, and proposed duration and frequency of the interventions that are required to reach the goals and outcomes. The plan of care includes the anticipated discharge plans and time-period for reassessment.

Political action committee: Often referred to as a "PAC." A PAC is an organization that raises money privately to influence elections or legislation, especially at the federal level.

Post-graduate education: With regard to a physical therapist with the entry-level doctor of physical therapy degree this includes residencies and fellowships.

Pregnancy Discrimination Act: The Pregnancy Discrimination Act (PDA) of 1978 is a United States federal statute. It amended Title VII of the Civil Rights Act of 1964 to "prohibit sex discrimination on the basis of pregnancy." The Act covers discrimination "on the basis of pregnancy, childbirth, or related medical conditions."

Pre-tax benefits: Pretax payroll deductions are qualified deductions that lower your employees' taxable wages. You subtract their contributions from their gross wages before figuring their tax withholding. Some pretax deductions reduce taxable wages for income tax; others reduce taxable wages for Social Security and Medicare taxes.

Preventive services: Health care to prevent illness or detect illness at an early stage, when treatment is likely to work best (for example, preventive services include Pap tests, flu shots, and screening mammograms).

Primary care physician: The doctor seen first for most health problems. He or she ensures the patient receives the needed care. Many insurances require the primary care doctor to approve a referral to a specialist.

Private insurance: Private health insurance often offered through employers or other organizations is typically defined as non-government-sponsored health insurance.

Pro bono physical therapy: Physical therapy services provided free of charge—often to underserved or uninsured individuals or cohorts.

Professional behavior: Professional behavior is the conduct, aims, or qualities that characterize or mark a profession or a professional person.

Professional Behaviors Assessment Tool: The intent of the Professional Behaviors Assessment Tool is to identify and describe the spectrum of professional behaviors necessary for success in the practice of physical therapy. The tool is intended to represent and be applied to student growth and development in the classroom and the clinic. It also contains behavioral criteria for the practicing clinician. Each professional behavior is defined and then broken down into developmental levels with each level containing behavioral criteria that describe behaviors that represent possession of the professional behavior they represent. Each developmental level builds on the previous level such that the tool represents growth over time in physical therapy education and practice.

Professional duty: Professional duty is the personal commitment to meeting one's ethical, moral, and legal obligations to provide effective physical therapy services to individual patients/clients, to serve the profession, and to positively influence the health of society.

Professional Identity: Professional identity is defined as one's professional self-concept based on attributes, beliefs, values, motives, and experiences.

Professional: A person who is educated to the level of possessing a unique body of knowledge, adheres to ethical conduct, requires licensure to practice, participates in the monitoring of one's peers, and is accepted and recognized by the public as being a professional.

Professionalism: Professionalism is the competence or skill expected of a professional.

Prognosis: The determination by the physical therapist of the predicted optimal level of improvement in function and the estimated amount of time needed to reach that level.

Psychomotor: Refers to motor activity that is preceded by or related to mental activity.

Public dissemination: Public dissemination means to broadcast a message to the public without direct feedback from the audience.

Reconstruction aide: Reconstruction aides were the precursor to physical therapists. Reconstructions were "on-the-job trained" and typically had backgrounds in exercise or massage.

Reevaluation: The process of incorporating the results of selected tests and measures into a review of the diagnosis, prognosis, and plan of care.

Reexamination: The process of performing selected tests and measures after the initial examination to evaluate progress and to modify or redirect interventions.

Referral: A written order from the primary care doctor to see a specialist or get certain medical services. In many Health Maintenance Organizations (HMOs), a referral must be generated prior to receiving medical care from anyone except the primary care doctor.

Reflection: The purpose of reflection is to facilitate learning from a particular practical experience. Reflection will help make connections between what is taught in theory and what needs to be done in clinical practice.

Reflection-in-action: A conscious effort to think about an activity or incident in real time to facilitate consideration of what is positive, negative or challenging about the activity or incident and, if appropriate, plan how it might be enhanced, improved or done differently in the future.

Reflection-on-action: Reflection on action is the retrospective contemplation of practice in order to uncover the knowledge used in a particular situation, by analyzing and interpreting the information recalled. The reflective practitioner may speculate how the situation might have been handled differently and what other knowledge would have been helpful.

Reliability: Reliability in statistics and psychometrics is the overall consistency of a measure. A measure is said to have a high reliability if it produces similar results under consistent conditions. For example, measurements of people's height are often extremely reliable.

Research agenda: The research agenda is a fluid document outlining one's planned research and publishing plans. Typically presented as a conceptual framework, the research agenda documents the starting and potential end point of the research line and highlights which areas have been completed or remain pending.

Research design: The research design refers to the overall strategy which integrates the different components of the study in a coherent and logical way, thereby ensuring an effective address of the research problem; it constitutes the blueprint for the collection, measurement, and analysis of data.

Residency: Residency programs are post-professional programs intended to train physical therapists in a specialty area.

Respite Care: Temporary care provided in a nursing home, hospice inpatient facility, or hospital so that a family member or friend who is the patient's caregiver can rest or take some time off. Typically not covered by insurance.

Retirement: Retirement is the point where a person stops employment completely. A person may semi-retire by reducing work hours. Many people choose to retire when they are eligible for private or public pension benefits, although some are forced to retire when physical conditions no longer allow the person to work

Salary: Salary is the monetary remuneration for work performed.

Scope of practice: Describes the procedures, actions, and processes that a healthcare practitioner is permitted to undertake in keeping with the terms of the professional license. Defined primarily by the state practice act but strongly influenced by administrative policy.

Screening: Determining, through specific tests and measures, the need for further examination or consultation by a physical therapist or for referral to another health professional.

Search engine: A web search engine is a software system that is designed to search for information on the World Wide Web. Search engines are often used by researchers to identify and investigate pertinent published literature.

Self-actualization: Self-actualization is the realization or fulfillment of one's talents and potentialities.

Servant leadership: The servant-leader focuses primarily on the growth and well-being of people and the communities to which they belong. While traditional leadership generally involves the accumulation and exercise of power by one at the "top of the pyramid," servant leadership is different. The servant-leader shares power, puts the needs of others first and helps people develop and perform as highly as possible.

Service learning: Service learning is a teaching and learning strategy that integrates meaningful community service with instruction and reflection to enrich the learning experience, teach civic responsibility, and strengthen communities.

Service-based supervised (or untimed) CPT codes: Specific codes to perm services such as conducting and evaluation or applying hot/cold packs. Time is not important; only one code can be billed regardless of the time to perform the evaluation or assessment.

Sexual harassment: Sexual harassment typically occurring in a workplace, or other professional or social situation, involves the making of unwanted sexual advances or obscene remarks.

Single payer system: Single-payer healthcare is a healthcare system financed by taxes that covers the costs of essential healthcare for all residents, with costs covered by a single public system.

Skilled nursing facility: A healthcare facility along the healthcare continuum, with the staff and equipment to give skilled nursing care and, in most cases, skilled rehabilitative services and other related health services to patients with a skilled need.

Social responsibility: The promotion of a mutual trust between the physical therapist as a part of the profession and the larger public. This trust necessitates a response to societal needs for health and wellness.

Spiritual competence: As a subset of multicultural competencies, spiritual and religious competencies are defined as a set of attitudes, knowledge, and skills in the domains of spirituality and religion that every psychologist should have to effectively and ethically practice psychology, regardless of whether or not they conduct spiritually.

Stark and Anti-Kickback: The Federal Anti-Kickback Statute and Stark Law are often confused. The Anti-Kickback Statute is a criminal law that prohibits the knowing and willful payment of remuneration to induce or reward patient referrals or the generation of business involving any item or service payable by federal health programs. The Stark Law prohibits physicians

form referring patient to receive designated health services payable by Medicare or Medicaid form entities with which he physician or an immediate family member has a financial interest.

Statistics: The practice or science of collecting and analyzing numerical data in large quantities, especially for the purpose of inferring proportions in a whole from those in a representative sample.

Statutory law: The term used to define written laws, usually enacted by a legislative body. Statutory laws vary from regulatory or administrative laws that are passed by executive agencies, and common law, or the law created by prior court decisions.

Student physical therapist assistant: A student matriculated in an accredited entry-level physical therapist assistant program.

Student physical therapist: A student matriculated in an accredited entry-level physical therapy program.

Student placement forms: A questionnaire distributed by physical therapy education programs to clinical education sites requesting the number and type of available placements for students to complete clinical education experiences.

Supervision: A process where two or more people actively participate in a joint effort to establish, maintain, and elevate a level of performance; it is structured according to the supervisee's qualifications, position, level of preparation, depth of experience, and the environment in which the supervisee functions.

Tax bracket: Tax bracket is the range of incomes taxed at a given rate.

Teaching: Teaching is the occupation, work, or profession of being an educator.

Team behaviors: The sum total of each team member's personal background, skills, and personal traits or behaviors. As individuals get to gradually accept each other in a team, understanding individual behavior is an essential step in the initial stage of team development.

Team roles: Formal roles are the external, defined positions that are associated with given responsibilities and are usually allocated according to the position or ability of each person. Individuals in a team will also tend to adopt informal roles that depend more on their character than on any specific knowledge or position.

The Hypothesis Oriented Algorithm for Clinicians: The Hypothesis Oriented Algorithm for Clinicians (HOAC) is primarily a linear model that uses a systematic approach to generating, testing, and reformulating hypotheses about the diagnosis and the patient/client response to intervention.

Therapy Cap: Medicare Part B helps pay for medically necessary outpatient physical and occupational therapy, and speech-language pathology services. There are limits on these services when obtained from most outpatient providers. These limits are called "therapy caps" or "therapy cap limits."

Time-based (constant attendance) CPT codes: Specific codes which allow for variable billing in 15-minute increments when a practitioner provides a patient with one-on-one services, such as manual therapy or gait training.

Title VII of the Civil Rights Act: Title VII of the Civil Rights Act of 1964 is a federal law that prohibits employers from discriminating against employees on the basis of sex, race, color, national origin, and religion. It generally applies to employers with 15 or more employees, including federal, state, and local governments.

Treatment: The intervention; the therapeutic service received by the patient. Also: The sum of all interventions provided by the physical therapist to a patient/client during an episode of care.

Universal classroom design: The goal of universal design (UD) is to use a variety of teaching methods to remove any barriers to learning and give all students equal opportunities to succeed. UD doesn't specifically target kids with learning and attention issues; it is about building in flexibility that can be adjusted for *every* student's strengths and needs.

Validity: The degree to which accumulated evidence and theory support specific interpretation of test scores entailed by proposed use of a test. The degree to which a test measures what it is intended to measure; a test is valid for a particular purpose for a particular group.

Vision 2020: Vision 2020 served as the vision statement fo the phsyical therapy profession from its adoption by the 2000 House of Delegates until the 2013 House of Delages adopted the curent vision statement.

Vision statement: A road map for a department, company, organization, or individual. Indicates both what the company wants to become and aids in guiding transformational initiatives by setting a defined direction for the company's growth

Worker's compensation health insurance: Workers' compensation is a form of insurance providing wage replacement and medical benefits to employees injured in the course of employment in exchange for mandatory relinquishment of the employee's right to sue his or her employer for the tort of negligence.

Index